Also by Brenda Watson, CNC

HEART of PERFECT HEALTH

The Startling Truths About Heart Disease
And The Power You Hold To Stop It

BRENDA WATSON, CNC

with Leonard Smith, MD and Jamey Jones, BSc

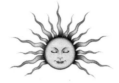

RENEW LIFE PRESS and INFORMATION SERVICES
198 Alt. 19 South
Palm Harbor, FL 34683
1-800-830-4778

Art Direction, Design and Photography
© 2012, michael black, BLACK SUN ®
www.michaelblack.com

Medical Illustrations
© 2012, Adam Questell, A KYU Design
www.akyudesign.com

Printed in China

ISBN 978-0-9802163-7-0

Library of Congress Control Number 202909180

A Note to the Reader

For my dad, Henry Furr.

CONTENTS

HEART of PERFECT HEALTH

The Startling Truths About Heart Disease
And The Power You Hold To Stop It

BRENDA WATSON, CNC

with Leonard Smith, MD and Jamey Jones, BSc

ACKNOWLEDGMENTS

What an amazing team I have! It is continually gratifying to see the way we produce unique and educational books time after time. I am blessed with the creative people in my life. To bring another book of this magnitude to fruition is amazing to me.

First and foremost I have to thank Jamey Jones. She is an amazing force in her ability to not only take my vision but take difficult concepts and bring them to life. She has really stepped up to the plate with *Heart of Perfect Health*. We have somewhat departed from conventional thought in connecting cardiovascular disease with the gut, but the science is there. Jamey used all of it to make this book the cutting-edge piece it is. Thank you, Jamey, because without you this would not be possible. You are a young brilliant talent who will continue to grow and inspire.

Thank you, Leonard Smith, MD, my friend, teacher, and mentor. To have Dr. Smith's contribution to this book is an honor for me. I have always known how brilliant he is, but he really brought the knowledge of integrative medicine and personal experience as a surgeon to the subject of cardiovascular disease. Dr. Smith worked as a vascular surgeon and has spent the last 30 years in functional medicine. The gift of knowledge he brings to this book cannot be measured. It has truly been rewarding to work with him all these years. He not only is my co-author; he also makes sure everything is accurate and scientifically sound.

I interviewed six doctors, including Dr. Smith, in *Heart of Perfect Health*. Their contributions have brought light to a subject that is only beginning to be illuminated in both conventional medicine and integrative medicine.

William Davis, MD, has contributed one of the most profound works on diet and health in his book Wheat Belly. I am so proud to have his interview in my book. Dr. Davis has revealed to the world the problems we face as a result of the processing and hybridization of wheat and other grains. Heart disease, as well as other diseases, is the direct result of what and how we eat. The issue of wheat in the diet has long been a concern for me. Dr. Davis not only does his research; he also proves it with the health of his patients. I applaud you, Dr. Davis, and thank you so much.

Dwight Lundell, MD, is a cardiac surgeon who has focused on educating people about the underlying cause of heart disease—inflammation. Thank you so much for your insight on cardiovascular disease. Your input gives another voice of experience that heart disease can be prevented when we look to the root causes.

R. Ernest Cohn, MD, NMD, DC, was interviewed about chelation therapy and nutritional therapies for heart disease and other chronic conditions. I was very happy to have chelation therapy explained so that people know they have options. Dr. Cohn, you provided an excellent explanation about alternative methods of healing. Thank you for contributing this information.

Thomas Levy, MD, JD, has taught me so much about vitamin C deficiency as an underlying cause of not only cardiovascular disease but many other chronic diseases as well. He is a pioneer in his ability to see outside the box. Please accept my sincere thanks for your contribution.

Rick Sponaugle, MD, my friend and teacher, thank you for your efforts in continually helping your patients with inflammation, chronic health problems, and detoxification. You are an inspiration, and I feel grateful to have your input in this book. Your description of how gut connections affect us in many ways is much needed.

A very special thanks to Jerry Adams, who has worked diligently beside me and my team to make sure we can deliver this book to everyone. I cannot say enough about the importance of remaining focused in order to accomplish the production of a book like this one. Jerry does this very well, and I want him to know he is appreciated for his efforts.

This book would not even be here without the vision and creative talent of Michael Black. This is my third book with Michael, and I think it is the most important one. I gave Michael creative control over this book, and he has taken it to another level for me. I strive to produce books that teach people with visuals. Michael has made it possible for me to bring to the world a simple yet elegant presentation of cardiovascular disease and its associated conditions. Not only that, but he also is a master cook and photographer. He brings the recipes and photos to life with his creative spirit.

We have had a remarkable team in the creation of *Heart of Perfect Health*. Adam Questell has done an outstanding job in the creation of all the medical illustrations. Adam takes our guidance and creates the most amazing pictures. This is close to my heart, as visuals are important in my teaching.

Big thanks to our editor Leda Scheintaub and proofreader Liana Krissoff. You two are incredible in your efficiency and attention to detail.

Also a special thanks to my team at ReNew Life and Advanced Naturals. I feel the love and support you give me as we all strive to educate and help people achieve better health. You all support this effort by your actions that keep us moving ahead. I really appreciate each and every one of you.

Another invaluable person involved in this book is Brenda Valen. Brenda has been my executive assistant for many years now. I could not function without her support. She keeps me on track and is always there for me. I cannot say how much this means to me.

I was able to tell the health stories about my sister, Sandee, my husband, Stan, and my father in this book. My gratitude to them runs deep, as they have shared in this health journey with me in many ways throughout my life.

As always, my husband, Stan, has given me constant love and support toward any effort I undertake. Thank you for truly understanding my heart.

Brenda Watson

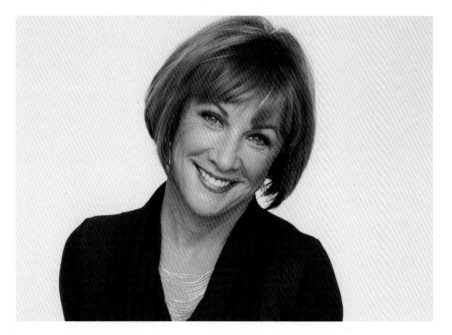

PREFACE

Heart disease is the number one killer of men and women in this country. Take a moment to think about this. How has it already affected someone in your family? I know it has, because one in three people have some form of cardiovascular disease.

In my own family heart attack and stroke have taken the lives of not only my father but many other members of my family. That was my inspiration for writing this book. I want people to understand that they have the power to change their health if only they educate themselves and take initiative. By making the right choices optimal health can be achieved. It doesn't have to be difficult; simple lifestyle changes can make all the difference.

I have been a Natural Health Care Practitioner for over 20 years. My area of focus is the digestive system, so writing a book on cardiovascular health was not something I ever saw myself doing. But my understanding of the relationship of the gut to all chronic disease, in addition to the personal challenges my family has faced with heart attack and stroke, provided the impetus for bringing this information to people who desperately need it in today's world.

This book delves into the science supporting the fact that heart disease is not only preventable but is in many cases reversible. All that is missing is the knowledge to help make it happen. *Heart of Perfect Health* is my contribution to help people understand that it is within their power to take control of their health anytime they choose. This book empowers you to be your own health advocate.

Heart of Perfect Health will not only explain the underlying causes of cardiovascular disease; it also will give you the tools you need to get started on a healthy program that can reduce your risk of heart attack or stroke. You will also find new cutting-edge approaches to health that will help you with any chronic health condition.

To accomplish any task, a toolbox containing a variety of tools is needed. This is certainly true with cardiovascular disease. You will find that the markers of heart disease are easy to monitor yourself. But what are those disease markers? This book will show you some you know, and some you probably do not.

Most people know that high cholesterol is a marker for cardiovascular disease. The link between high cholesterol and heart disease is well-entrenched in our psyche. You may be surprised to discover that the total overall cholesterol number is not as important as digging deeper into the HDL/LDL ratio, and learning the condition in which these types of cholesterol are found. This information is still new for many people, and even many doctors. In *Heart of Perfect Health*, you will get in-depth information about new types of testing that may well save your life by giving you a more accurate view of your heart disease risk.

You will also understand the importance of personally monitoring blood pressure. Did you know that high blood pressure often goes undetected? It's called the silent killer for a reason; you may not know you have it. In this book we highlight new information on some of the underlying causes of high blood pressure you haven't considered.

I think one of the most startling facts this book will reveal is how sugar affects cardiovascular disease possibly more than any single factor. A diet high in sugar—including the sugar found in carbohydrates—triggers a cascade in the body that affects cholesterol, blood pressure, obesity, blood sugar levels, and more. Sugar initiates a vicious cycle that affects most heart disease markers.

Heart of Perfect Health covers the most commonly known markers for cardiovascular disease, and will also reveal underlying causes that even many doctors do not consider. What about environmental toxins? The onslaught of chemicals in our food, air, and water is contributing to heart attack and stroke and literally killing us. We certainly are not getting this information from our mainstream medical establishments.

Finally, and closest to my heart, you will learn what role the gut plays in the development of heart disease. I would not be writing this if the gut was not an important source of the problem. In *Heart of Perfect Health* you will found out how our Gut Protection System (what I call the body's GPS), which is the internal modulator of our health, is at the center of it all. You will learn how all chronic health conditions have an origin in the gut, and how optimal digestive health is the foundation upon which total-body health, including heart health, is built.

You will see the testimonials of people who have used the programs in this book to turn their health around. After watching so many of my family members die of cardiovascular disease, it was exciting for me to see my husband and sister regain their health. To know that I helped them become healthy is a gift in life I cherish.

Heart of Perfect Health also gives interviews with cutting-edge doctors who have helped change the way we look at cardiovascular disease and the negative impact the food industry has had on our health. The outdated and poorly supported idea that a low-fat, high-carbohydrate diet is a heart-healthy diet has been perpetuated for decades, but it is just plain wrong, and these doctors help give credible scientific evidence to prove it.

Finally, *Heart of Perfect Health* gives us the diet, lifestyle, and supplement choices to help us avoid the fate of heart disease. In the "Love Your Heart" section of this book, you will be given a simple eating plan, delicious recipes, and the HOPE Formula—High Fiber, Omega-3s, Probiotics, and Enzymes—to help you build your health from the base up. Taking control of your health in this way, by addressing diet and building digestive health can change your life.

The number of people who are obese and dying of cardiovascular disease continues to grow at an alarming rate in this country and throughout the world. This is not just a health crisis but an economic crisis that affects everyone. Together we can help stop this debilitating pandemic. By each one of us making healthy choices, together we can help change the world.

By following the program in *Heart of Perfect Health* you are taking the first steps toward a better and more vibrant life. You are making a conscious choice to take control of your health. I applaud that choice. And I'm right there with you.

Your partner in health,

Brenda Watson

TRUTHS ABOUT HEART DISEASE

"The various features and aspects of human life, such as longevity, good health, success, happiness, and so forth, which we consider desirable, are all dependent on kindness and a good heart."

—Dalai Lama XIV

Chapter 1

Heart Disease Is Killing Us

The Stats: What Are We Facing Here?

The stats tell it all: The number one cause of death in the United States is heart disease. That's right, more than any other disease—even cancer (a close second)—heart disease is the most likely to kill you. Add the heart disease death rate to that of stroke, a complication of heart disease, and you'll find you are about 30 percent more likely to drop from heart disease or its complications than from any other cause.

FACT:

One in three American adults has one or more types of cardiovascular disease.

Despite this frightening death sentence, heart disease doesn't seem to be scaring us. It is estimated that one in three American adults has one or more types of cardiovascular disease (CVD).[1] That's more than 82 million adults, or one third of the U.S. population. No wonder we're dying of heart disease. The United States is currently facing a "diabesity" epidemic, or a substantial increase in the prevalence of diabetes and obesity. Diabetes and obesity are both risk factors for heart disease.

According to the American Heart Association, every 34 seconds someone in the United States dies of a heart attack. By the time you finish reading this paragraph, another person will have lost their life. Sadly, many people do not even know they have heart disease until they experience a heart attack. Each year about 785,000 Americans have their first heart attack, and another 470,000 experience their second or subsequent heart attack.[2] I don't know about you, but I want to do everything I can to take my name off that list.

Heart disease is not only a problem in the United States. According to the World Health Organization, cardiovascular disease is also the leading cause of death worldwide, representing about 30 percent of all global deaths. It is the leading cause of death in every region of the world except Sub-Saharan Africa, where infectious diseases still kill more people than any other cause.[3]

At the beginning of the twentieth century, CVD accounted for 10 percent of all deaths worldwide. At the beginning of the twenty-first century, it accounts for nearly half of all deaths in developed countries, and about 25 percent in developing countries.[4,5]

Let's take a look at heart disease deaths across the nation. What do we see?

It's obvious from the first map that much of the eastern and largely the southeastern United States is in some trouble. Compare that map to the second map, of obesity in the United States,[6] and you'll notice a similarity.

Again, the southeastern United States is in some trouble: Rates of obesity are highest in the Southeast. If you look at the obesity map over time, however, you will see the entire country getting fatter year by year. It just so happens the Southeast is in the lead. Take a look at the third map to see obesity rates in 1996.

And ten years before that?

The Fattening of America

As a whole, this country is becoming fat, or as science calls it, obese. Obesity is defined as body mass index (BMI) over 30. BMI is calculated by dividing a person's weight (mass) in kilograms by the square of the person's height in meters. BMI is a widely accepted measure of obesity. The trend of increasing obesity is important when considering cardiovascular disease, as obesity is an independent risk factor for the development of CVD.[7] This means that if you

Death Rates

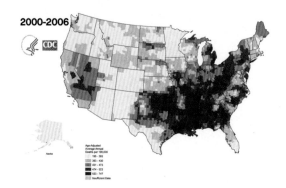

Obesity Rates

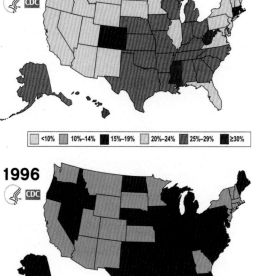

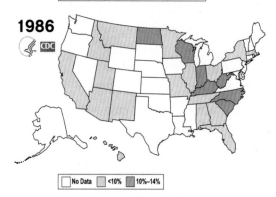

Almost half a million women die each year from heart disease.

are obese but have no other risk factor for cardiovascular disease—such as high LDL cholesterol, high blood pressure, or diabetes—you are still at risk of developing heart disease. As America fattens, do we wonder why so many people die of heart disease?

Heart Disease in Women

Heart disease has long been thought of as a man's disease, but this idea is mistaken. Heart disease or stroke will kill one out of every two women. Compare this to breast cancer, which kills one out of every 25 women, and you can see the extent of the problem. It gets worse—42 percent of women who have a heart attack die within one year, compared to only 24 percent of men.[8] A total of almost half a million women die each year from heart disease.[9] While the reason for this discrepancy is not completely understood, women tend to develop heart disease at an older age—about ten years later than men—and usually have coexisting chronic health conditions that may contribute to the poorer outcomes in women.

Another likely explanation for the higher heart disease death rate in women over men is the fact that symptoms of a heart attack in women differ from those in men. Men tend to experience the classic heart attack symptoms of chest pain and chest pressure, whereas women often experience subtle symptoms

that mimic less-critical health conditions, like gastrointestinal distress, anxiety, or stress.[10]

In one study of more than 500 female cardiac patients who had suffered a heart attack within the last four to six months, almost all the women suffered symptoms as early as one month before the attack. The most frequent of those early symptoms were unusual fatigue, sleep disturbance, and shortness of breath. Other reported symptoms included indigestion and anxiety.[11] In contrast to men, during the heart attack itself symptoms of shortness of breath, weakness, fatigue, cold sweats, and dizziness were experienced. Less than half of the women experienced any chest pain, pressure, or chest tightness, as are common in men.

Symptoms of Heart Attack in Women

- Anxiety
- Arm pain
- Back pain
- Chest pain
- Cold sweats
- Dizziness
- Indigestion
- Jaw pain
- Nausea
- Shortness of breath
- Sleep disturbance
- Unusual fatigue
- Weakness

Adding to these symptoms, another survey of 52 women found that pain of the jaw, arm, back, or chest, shortness of breath, fatigue, nausea, and sweating were all reported as acute symptoms by women who had experienced heart attack.[12] In women who experience symptoms or signs of heart disease, the majority have either no narrowing of the arteries, or less than 50 percent narrowing.[13] Narrowing of the arteries, or stenosis, is another characteristic common in men. What's more, about 64 percent of women who die suddenly from heart disease display no previous symptoms at all.[14] That's a scary statistic.

The story continues. Young women have twice the risk of dying after coronary bypass surgery, and experience twice the incidence of heart failure as men.[15] Prevalence of cardiovascular disease is actually lower in women than men, and women develop signs of cardiovascular disease about ten years later than men, yet women are still dying from the disease more than men. Further, death rates from heart disease are dropping overall, yet they drop slower in women than in men. In women younger than 55, however, death rates are actually increasing.[16] Though women tend to develop heart disease later in life than men, those women who do develop CVD under the age of 50 are more likely than men to die after a heart attack or coronary artery bypass graft (CABG) surgery.[17]

It is thought that hormones present in women prior to menopause may exert a protective cardiovascular effect,[18] providing an explanation for the later development of CVD in women.

As women reach the menopausal years, cardiovascular risk factors increase. It is thought that aging and hormonal changes contribute to the increase in cardiovascular disease. For years women were given menopausal hormone therapy, which was thought to decrease cardiovascular disease.

Why Are There So Many Names for Heart Disease?

Between cardiovascular disease, heart disease, coronary heart disease, coronary artery disease, peripheral artery disease, atherosclerosis, heart attack, stroke, cardiac arrest, heart failure, heart arrhythmia (that's not all—I think I made my point), there are enough heart conditions to confuse anyone. Why are there so many, and what do we need to know about these conditions? Let's break it down.

The term *heart disease* is used to describe a range of diseases that affect the heart. Heart disease includes coronary artery disease (also known as coronary heart disease), heart rhythm conditions (arrhythmias), heart infections, and heart defects present at birth (congenital heart defects). The terms *heart disease* and *cardiovascular disease* are often used interchangeably. *Cardiovascular disease* refers to a class of diseases associated with damage to the arteries—those of the heart and of other areas of the body. For example, peripheral artery disease involves the same processes as coronary artery disease, only in the peripheral arteries, and not in arteries of the heart.

The Women's Health Initiative, a large study initiative funded by the National Institutes of Health to address the most common causes of death, disability, and impaired quality of life in postmenopausal women, included a clinical trial on postmenopausal hormone therapy involving more than 25,000 women. This trial was stopped after **investigators found that the associated health risks of the combination hormone therapy—including increased risks of cardiovascular disease and breast cancer—outweighed the benefits.**[19] See chapter 10 for more information on hormones and heart health.

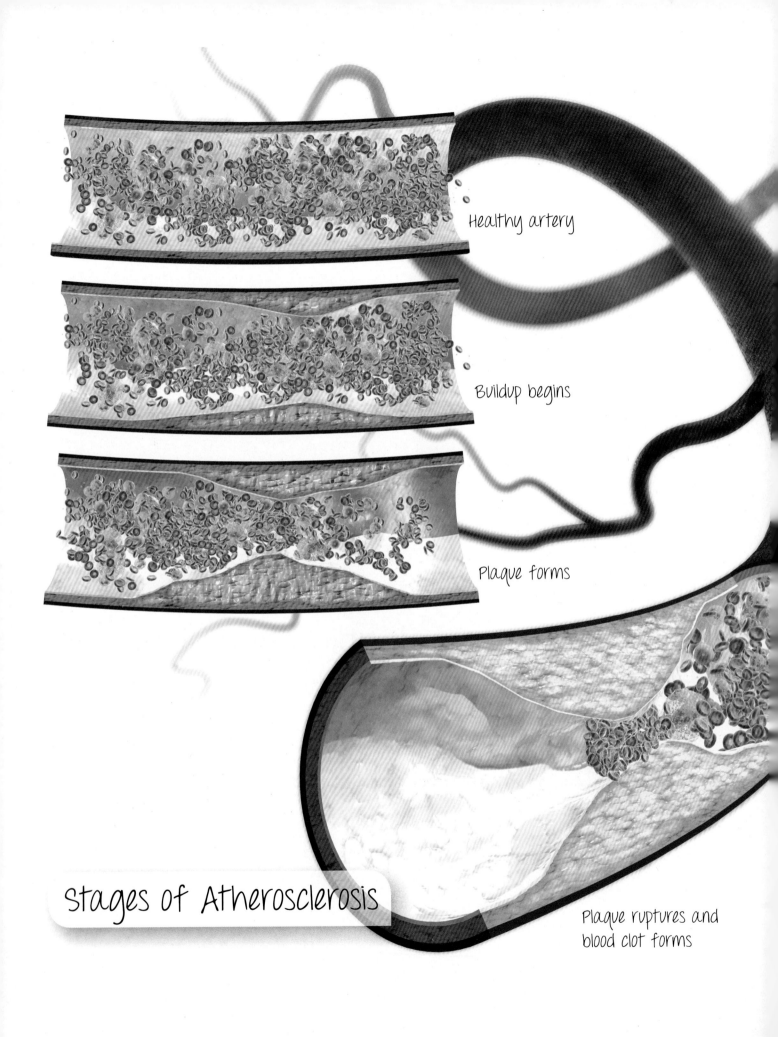

Healthy artery

Buildup begins

Plaque forms

Plaque ruptures and
blood clot forms

Stages of Atherosclerosis

Atherosclerosis: An Underlying Feature of Cardiovascular Disease

Atherosclerosis, also known as hardening of the arteries, deserves particular attention, as it is the main underlying feature of coronary artery disease, peripheral artery disease, and cerebrovascular disease—all representing the majority of cardiovascular disease. Simply put, atherosclerosis is the buildup of plaque in the arteries. Atherosclerotic plaque in the arteries is like having rusty pipes.

As plaque builds up in the arteries, the internal diameter of the artery decreases, eventually blocking blood flow through the artery and making it less flexible. When the arteries are narrowed as they are in heart disease, blood flow to the heart is restricted. Angina, or chest pains, may be experienced as a result of the restricted blood flow, and can progress to heart attack, which results from blocked blood and oxygen supply to the heart.

Over time, coronary heart disease may weaken the heart so that it can no longer pump enough blood to the rest of the body, a chronic condition known as heart failure. Congestive heart failure involves the buildup of fluid in areas of the body such as the lungs, liver, gastrointestinal tract, or arms and legs, due to the inability of the heart to pump blood throughout the body.

Another complication of heart disease, as a result of atherosclerosis, is stroke. Blood clots often form at the site of atherosclerosis. If a blood clot forms in an artery leading to the brain, and the artery is narrow enough, it may block blood flow to the brain. When blood flow to the brain is cut off, the brain cannot get the blood and oxygen it requires. In other cases a blood clot will break off from an artery and travel up the artery until it lodges in a narrower section. This results in the same blockage of blood and oxygen to the brain. Without blood and oxygen, brain cells die, which can cause permanent damage.

What Happens During Atherosclerosis?

Though there are many different types of heart disease, those associated with atherosclerosis are the most common and the most reversible. That's right—atherosclerosis is reversible.[20] Not only is it preventable, it's reversible. Before we talk about that, though, let's take a closer look at what happens during atherosclerosis.

It was once thought that the plaque buildup associated with atherosclerosis was caused by the accumulation of cholesterol in arteries. Though this idea has since been refuted, many people are still under the impression that cholesterol is the main factor in heart disease. It's true that cholesterol does build up in plaque, and it's true that oxidized LDL cholesterol (more on that in the next chapter) plays a role, but more important than cholesterol is the presence of an overall inflammatory process gone awry.

Inflammation is the body's normal response to wounds or infections. Ordinarily the inflammatory process is resolved in due time as the body returns to homeostasis, or balance. If inflammation does not completely resolve, which we will later learn can happen for a number of reasons, chronic low-grade inflammation ensues. Inflammation plays an ongoing role in all stages of atherosclerosis—from initiation, through progression, to the end complications of blood clot formation and/or plaque rupture.[21]

Atherosclerosis begins with dysfunction of the artery lining, also known as endothelial dysfunction. Endothelial dysfunction is covered in more detail in chapter 9. Suffice to say, it involves inflammation: The artery lining becomes inflamed and attracts white blood cells and oxidized fat proteins (such as oxidized LDL cholesterol, which is discussed in the next chapter), all of which take up residence in the arterial wall. Once there, the white blood cells begin to consume the oxidized fat proteins (as a way of destroying them), and the white blood cells are then considered foam cells. That's right, these foam cells actually eat up rancid fat, getting bigger and bigger.

The stuff inside these foam cells looks like pus, not something I want building up in my arteries—how about you? This process triggers further inflammatory response, which leads to the accumulation of fat and cholesterol in addition to minerals like calcium and free radicals. The calcium content accumulated during this process contributes to the calcification of the plaque, giving it the characteristic hardening, from which the name hardening of the arteries comes. The accumulation of all these substances just under the lining of the arteries is known as atherosclerotic plaque.

Now, let's find out how all this happens. Instead of starting with the final problem (heart disease) as modern traditional medicine tends to do, let's back up and take a look at what's at the heart of the problem.

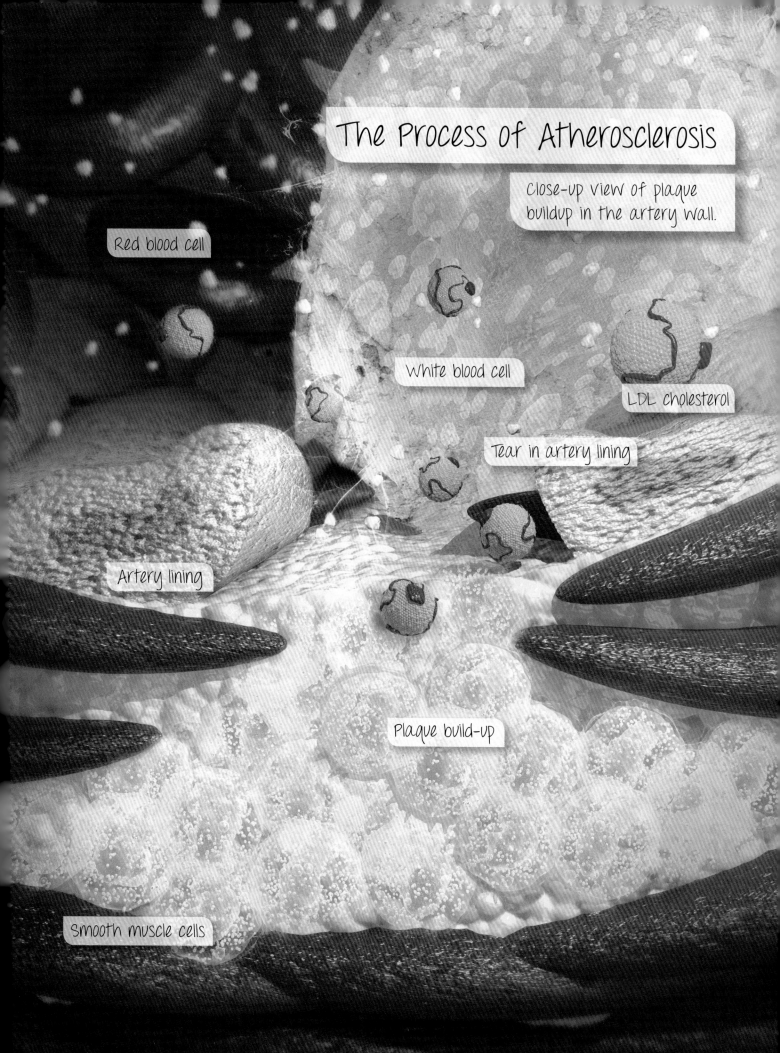

The Process of Atherosclerosis

Close-up view of plaque buildup in the artery wall.

Red blood cell

White blood cell

LDL cholesterol

Tear in artery lining

Artery lining

Plaque build-up

Smooth muscle cells

"Health is the thing that makes you feel that now is the best time of the year."

—Franklin P. Adams

Chapter 2
Cholesterol Is Not All Bad

When most people think of cholesterol, they think of it as a bad thing—something to get rid of; something that causes heart disease. But did you know that cholesterol is essential to life and is present in every cell in the human body? Although most people think of cholesterol as harmful, it is a crucial factor in many different functions of the body:

- Cholesterol is present in the cell membrane, or the protective lining around each cell, strengthening the cell wall and aiding the exchange of nutrients and wastes across the cell membrane.[1]

- Cholesterol is a major component of myelin in the central nervous system.[2] Myelin insulates nerve cells and is essential to the proper functioning of the nervous system. Cholesterol also acts as an antioxidant in the brain, protecting against oxidative damage associated with aging.[3]

- Cholesterol is a steroid precursor, vital to the production of adrenal steroids such as cortisol (the stress hormone) and reproductive hormones such as testosterone and estrogens.[4]

- Cholesterol is needed for the production of vitamin D from UVB sun exposure.[5]

- Cholesterol is a precursor for the production of bile acids, which help break down fats for digestion.

In order to understand why cholesterol doesn't entirely deserve the bad reputation it has acquired, we need to take a closer look at what cholesterol is and what it does.

LDL Cholesterol Particle

Close-up view of an LDL
cholesterol particle.

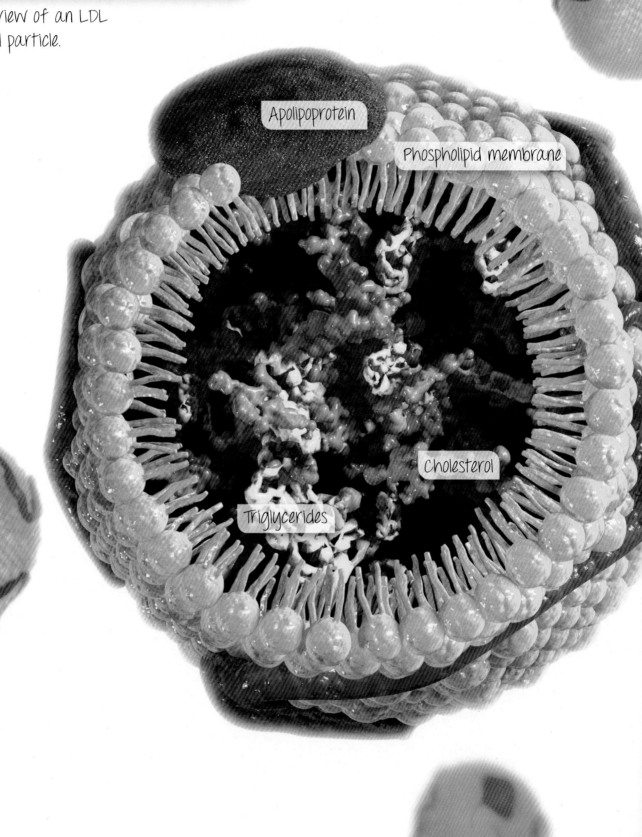

Apolipoprotein

Phospholipid membrane

Cholesterol

Triglycerides

Cholesterol—Let's Break It Down

There are two main forms in which cholesterol is found in the bloodstream: Low-density lipoprotein (LDL), i.e., cholesterol in the low-density fraction of blood, and high-density lipoprotein (HDL), i.e., cholesterol in the high-density fraction of blood.

LDL cholesterol is often labeled "bad" cholesterol and HDL labeled "good." This is a misnomer, however. Cholesterol is carried around in the body by molecules called lipoproteins. The cholesterol itself has nothing to do with being "good" or "bad" but, rather, the lipoprotein carrier of the cholesterol (LDL and HDL), as well as the state in which these carriers are found (e.g., particle size, density, oxidation, etc.—more on this later), determine whether the cholesterol is "good" or "bad."

Cholesterol needs a carrier because it is a fatlike substance and needs to travel through the bloodstream, which is a watery substance (remember: oil and water don't mix). Think of lipoproteins as vehicles—the LDL is a dump truck, carrying cholesterol from the liver to different areas of the body (arteries, for example), and HDL is a pickup truck, picking up cholesterol from different areas of the body and bringing it back to the liver for removal.

In conventional thought, maintaining healthy levels of these two types of lipoproteins is important, as high levels of LDL and low levels of HDL are risk factors for heart disease. Think about it—if you have too much LDL, which carries cholesterol from the liver to the arteries, and not enough HDL, which helps remove cholesterol from the arteries, cholesterol builds up in artery walls, which triggers atherosclerosis. This is only part of the story, however. As you will see, focusing only on HDL and LDL cholesterol can also serve to mislead you and your doctor. This is because the state in which the cholesterol particles are found plays the most important role in cardiovascular risk, not just the amount of cholesterol in the two fractions of blood. More on that later.

The term describing high blood levels of cholesterol is hypercholesterolemia, also called high cholesterol. It refers to high levels of total cholesterol, made up of both LDL and HDL cholesterol. The following highlights the standard measured blood cholesterol levels and how they are viewed by conventional doctors.

Total Cholesterol

< 200 mg/dL	Normal
200–239 mg/dL	Borderline high
> 240 mg/dL	High

LDL Cholesterol

< 100 mg/dL	Optimal
100–129 mg/dL	Near optimal
130–159 mg/dL	Borderline high
160–189 mg/dL	High
> 190 mg/dL	Very high

HDL Cholesterol

> 60	High/optimal
< 40 in men	Low
< 50 in women	Low

Some experts recommend lowering LDL cholesterol to below 70 mg/dL,[6] but this recommendation misses the mark. It is more important to consider the condition in which LDL cholesterol is found, rather than simply the total amount of cholesterol carried by the LDL particle. Most people are surprised to learn that LDL cholesterol is rarely actually measured—it's calculated based on measured total cholesterol, HDL, and triglyceride levels,[7] so it's more an estimation than an actual measured level. And it is an estimation that is prone to frequent, sometimes dramatic, inaccuracies.

Triglycerides are a type of fat found in the blood and in fat cells. They are the basic storage unit for fat in the body. When you eat, your body converts calories it doesn't use right away into triglycerides, which are stored in fat cells. Triglyceride levels are usually measured along with cholesterol levels. The following highlights measured blood triglyceride levels and how they are viewed by most doctors:

Triglyceride levels

< 150 mg/dL	Normal
150–199 mg/dL	Borderline high
200–499 mg/dL	High
> 500 mg/dL	Very high

Though levels less than 150 mg/dL are considered normal, the American Heart Association recommends a level of 100 mg/dL or lower as being optimal.[8] Like elevated cholesterol, elevated triglycerides are an independent risk factor for cardiovascular disease, meaning that if you have high triglycerides, and no other risk factors, you are still at increased risk.

Most physicians rely on the standard cholesterol panel of tests including total, HDL, and LDL cholesterol, and triglyceride levels. These tests only tell part of the story, however. High levels of total and/or LDL cholesterol may indicate a problem, but more testing is needed to assess the condition of the LDL particles, which more accurately determines heart attack risk.

The Bigger, the Better

When it comes to cholesterol levels, there is more to it than simply the amounts of total cholesterol and cholesterol in the LDL and HDL fractions of blood. Among the most important issues to consider is the size of LDL particles. The size of LDL particle is related to its atherogenicity, or its ability to trigger atherosclerosis, the process underlying heart disease and heart attacks. Standard blood cholesterol levels do not consider the size of the LDL particle. These tests only take into consideration the amount of cholesterol in the low-density (LDL) fraction, the high-density fraction (HDL), and total (total cholesterol).

Small, dense LDL particles are more destructive, their compact size allowing them to easily burrow into the artery wall. Once formed, small, dense LDL particles persist in the bloodstream several days longer than large LDL particles, are more tightly adherent to the artery wall, and are

TIP:

Omega-3 fish oils help to decrease harmful small, dense LDL cholesterol and increase less harmful large, buoyant LDL cholesterol.

more likely to trigger inflammatory responses, effects that all lead to atherosclerosis. A pattern of excessive small LDL particles is sometimes called "pattern B" to distinguish it from a normal pattern of mostly large LDL particles called "pattern A." The presence of high numbers of small, dense LDL particles is strongly associated with cardiovascular disease, and is nearly always found in people with metabolic syndrome and diabetes,[9] both conditions associated with heightened risk for heart disease.

People with pattern B are more likely to also have low HDL levels, elevated triglyceride levels, and tend to have high blood sugar levels, prediabetes and type 2 diabetes.[10] People with pattern B who have normal LDL cholesterol levels are still at increased risk of developing atherosclerosis, despite the seemingly normal values. In fact, it is possible for two people with the same LDL cholesterol levels to have completely different LDL patterns. This partly explains why more than 50 percent of people who have a heart attack also have normal cholesterol levels.

The tests used to detect particle size are not part of the standard blood lipid profile. Several laboratories nationwide perform these lipoprotein tests. Among the available lipoprotein assessments are LipoScience's NMR (nuclear magnetic resonance) profile, which uses an MRI device to determine the size of the LDL particles; Atherotech's VAP lipoprotein test; HDL Labs, which also uses an NMR approach; and Berkeley HeartLab, which uses an electrophoretic method.

All of these techniques yield additional insights into lipoprotein composition and number, including the most important LDL particle size. People with normal LDL cholesterol levels and heart disease, or a family history of heart disease, would most certainly benefit from these tests. People who are overweight, or have abnormally high blood glucose, prediabetes, or diabetes, are also often surprised at how different lipoprotein testing values are compared to standard lipid values.

The most effective way to reduce the proportion of small LDL particles is through diet, exercise, and maintaining a healthy weight. Omega-3 fatty acids from fish oil—EPA (eicosapentaenoic acid) and DHA (docosahexaenoic acid)—substantially reduce the number of small LDL particles.[11] Fish oils are particularly heart healthy, as discussed later in the Love Your Heart section. Interestingly, the statin drugs used to lower LDL cholesterol levels do not specifically decrease small, dense LDL cholesterol but, rather, reduce total LDL, regardless of size.[12]

Diet is the most effective strategy to reduce the expression of small LDL particles. Because consuming carbohydrates in any form triggers the formation of small, dense LDL particles, reducing consumption of carbohydrates yields reductions in small, dense LDL particles. High-carbohydrate intake increases levels of triglycerides, and triglycerides are required for the process that leads to formation of small, dense LDL particles. Therefore, the higher the triglyceride level, the greater the number of small LDL particles.[13]

Small, Dense LDL Particles

Close-up view of small, dense LDL particles, which more easily penetrate and damage the artery lining, leading to atherosclerosis..

Red blood cell

LDL cholesterol

Endothelial cell (artery lining)

MYTH:
Cholesterol is bad.

Ironically, reducing the fat in the diet and following a low-fat, high-carbohydrate diet can decrease total LDL levels, but shifts LDL particles from large to small, dense LDL particles. It may therefore appear that LDL cholesterol is lower, but in reality the underlying pattern switches to a more harmful form of increased numbers of small, dense LDL particles.

Oxidized LDL

The oxidation of LDL cholesterol particles is a crucial step in the process of atherosclerosis. Oxidation occurs when LDL particles react with free radicals, highly reactive molecules produced during many biological processes, such as metabolism, immune response, and detoxification. The oxidation of fat molecules in the LDL particles results in the creation of reactive oxidized LDL particles, which trigger inflammation, a main feature of atherosclerosis. The oxidized LDL more easily damages the lining of the artery, slipping underneath the artery lining (the endothelium), where it triggers the accumulation of inflammation-producing white blood cells known as macrophages. These inflammatory cells accumulate along with more cholesterol and fats, forming the atherosclerotic plaque that is characteristic of heart disease.

Think of an oxidized LDL particle as a normal LDL particle that got hit by a free radical: like an innocent guy who got punched in the face, then turned into a bully who picks a fight with anyone he encounters. When he comes across a bigger bully—the macrophage—he's met his match. The macrophage consumes the oxidized LDL particle.

LDL cholesterol

Oxidized LDL

Close-up view of LDL particles reacting with free radicals. LDL becomes oxidized and more harmful to arteries.

Free radical

oxidation

FACT:

Cholesterol is found in every cell in your body. It's not the cholesterol we should be worried about, but instead we should worry about the state in which it is found.

This process repeats over and over again, recruiting additional macrophages into the fray, changing what started off as a fight into a full-fledged war—oxidized LDLs and macrophages scuffling in our arteries. All this fighting causes more inflammation and attracts yet more oxidized LDL and macrophages to join the fight. The result is a buildup of atherosclerotic plaque inside the artery wall. This war in the coronary arteries is what kills more Americans than any other disease.

Oxidized LDL particles are strongly correlated with cardiovascular disease. In fact, elevated levels of oxidized LDL have been considered a stronger predictor of heart disease risk than even standard lipid measures and other traditional risk factors such as smoking status and obesity.[14] To help avoid oxidation of LDL particles, antioxidants are helpful. A diet high in vegetables and fruits is generally high in antioxidants, including flavonoid-rich foods like blueberries and other berries, and deeply colored vegetables such as peppers, green tea, and cocoa. Oxidized LDL can form as a result of smoking, consuming trans fats, fructose, deep-fried foods, and processed cured meats, having high blood sugar, and taking in too much omega-6 fatty acid (found in many commercial vegetable oils such as corn oil and soybean oil).

Dietary Cholesterol—Not as Bad as You Think

Many people think that eating a diet high in cholesterol—for example, a diet high in egg yolks—raises cholesterol levels. You may have been told to not eat eggs every morning as a way of controlling cholesterol levels. This notion is mistaken.

Cholesterol is obtained two ways: The body produces cholesterol (much of it in the liver), and cholesterol is absorbed from the small intestine, either from food or from bile salts passing through the intestine from the gallbladder. To balance out the production and absorption of cholesterol, the body is constantly using cholesterol to produce hormones and to maintain the integrity of cell membranes.

The body also gets rid of some cholesterol through the production of bile salts in the liver. Bile salts, made of cholesterol and other steroid acids bound to sodium, are sent from the liver to the gallbladder, where they are held until needed for digestion of fat. When you eat a fatty meal, bile is secreted into the small intestine from the gallbladder, and lipase is secreted into the small intestine by the pancreas,

MYTH:
Dietary cholesterol increases cholesterol levels.

both to help break down fat. In this way, some cholesterol is excreted from the body with intestinal waste, and some of this cholesterol is reabsorbed into the bloodstream so that it can be reused.

Cholesterol Recycling

Cholesterol forms bile salts in the liver.

Bile salts are secreted into the small intestine when a fatty meal is eaten to help break down fats.

Some cholesterol in bile salts is reabsorbed from the small intestine into the body, reentering the bloodstream for reuse.

Some cholesterol is excreted with feces. This amount increases with dietary fiber.

Although some cholesterol is absorbed from food, dietary cholesterol has little impact on blood cholesterol levels.[15] This is because the body's process of cholesterol recycling is regulated in such a way that when there is an increase in cholesterol from the diet, the body will make less. Conversely, if there is not enough cholesterol taken in from food, the body will make more cholesterol to compensate. Because of this cholesterol recycling process, dietary cholesterol intake contributes less to blood cholesterol levels than we are led to believe.

The body produces about 800 milligrams, on average, of cholesterol daily. Most people consume between 0 and

FACT:

Cholesterol levels have little to do with dietary cholesterol intake. Cholesterol is recycled in the body. When the body absorbs more cholesterol from high-cholesterol foods, the liver will produce less. When you don't eat enough cholesterol, the liver will produce more. Most people can eat an egg a day without worrying about raising cholesterol levels.

400 milligrams (200 milligrams average) of cholesterol daily. For each 100 milligrams of dietary cholesterol consumed over 400 milligrams, there is a slight increase of 2.17 mg/dL total cholesterol, 0.31 mg/dL increase in HDL, and 0.77 mg/dL increase in LDL cholesterol.[16] One study in people with moderately high cholesterol levels demonstrated that eating seven eggs per week resulted in only minor changes in total and LDL cholesterol.[17] Further, a Harvard study of 38,000 men and 80,000 women demonstrated that eating up to one egg per day was not associated with increased cardiovascular risk.[18]

Role of Inflammation

As mentioned at the beginning of this chapter, cholesterol is an important component of many different functions in the body. When cholesterol is paired with the process of inflammation is when it becomes a problem. This begins with the oxidation of LDL cholesterol. Remember the bully (the oxidant) who started a fight (with LDL cholesterol) that ended in war (atherosclerosis)? Think of inflammation as the gunfire of that war. Inflammation plays an important role throughout the entire process of atherosclerosis—in fact, atherosclerosis is known as an inflammatory disease.[19] Not only does inflammation occur along with the accumulation of fats in the arteries, but it is related to most of the risk factors for heart disease as well. See chapter 6 for more information on the role of inflammation in heart disease.

The role of inflammation in the body is primarily to protect against harm. Unfortunately, the inflammatory process itself can result in harm. In a healthy state, inflammation will resolve before too much damage is done. Far too often, however, chronic, low-grade inflammation—sometimes called silent inflammation because you cannot feel it—continues for long periods of time. It is this chronic, low-grade inflammation that is found in most chronic diseases, including heart disease.

Gut Connection to Cholesterol

Where does inflammation come from? There are actually many different sources of inflammation, but one very important (and often overlooked) source is the gut. That's right—there is a direct connection between the gut and the heart. There is an intricate array of capillaries connected to the gut, carrying nutrients and anything absorbed from the gut throughout the body. Further, the lymphatic system also connects the gut to the bloodstream. What gets through the gut lining will

There is a direct connection between the gut and the heart.

have an effect on the circulatory system. When inflammation is present in the gut, which may result from a variety of factors (covered in depth in chapter 7), there will be inflammation throughout the body. Cool the inflammation in the gut, and you will help to cool the inflammation throughout the body.

One example of this gut connection is found with low-grade inflammation induced by endotoxemia. Endotoxemia is the presence of bacterial toxins (endotoxins) in the bloodstream. Endotoxins enter the bloodstream through the digestive system, usually as a result of a change in gut microbial balance and/or damage to the intestinal lining, causing increased permeability, or "leaky gut."[20] A study in ten healthy adults found that a very low dose of endotoxin promoted a low-grade inflammatory response, and a reduction in the ability of HDL particles to remove cholesterol from artery walls.[21] This study shows that it wouldn't take much of a gut imbalance or leaky gut to promote inflammation and affect the function of good cholesterol.

Interestingly, an increase in the friendly gut bacteria known as bifidobacteria was found to be protective against the increase in endotoxins after eating.[22] Probiotics, or friendly gut bacteria, are known to have an anti-inflammatory effect in the gut. This may explain the protective effect seen with bifidobacteria.

Another interesting gut connection to cholesterol also involves gut bacteria. The gut is populated with 100 trillion bacteria. These bacteria consist of beneficial, neutral, and potentially harmful species. In healthy people, these bacteria strike a balance with higher amounts of beneficial and neutral bacteria and low amounts of potentially harmful bacteria. When this balance is disrupted, which can occur for many reasons (covered in more detail in chapter 7), poor health results—of the gut, and of other areas of the body. It has been shown that certain beneficial gut bacteria, also known as probiotics, are able to reduce cholesterol levels. Studies using probiotic bacteria in fermented food products and in capsules have found a cholesterol-lowering effect.

TIP:

The gut connection to cholesterol involves the absorption and reabsorption of cholesterol in the gut. Gut imbalances, digestive conditions, and poor diet can all affect cholesterol levels.

There are a few possible ways in which probiotics may affect cholesterol levels.[23]

- The gut bacteria may assimilate cholesterol, using it as a nutrient.

- Enzymes produced by the bacteria may break down bile salts (which contain cholesterol).

- Cholesterol may bind to bacterial cells walls and be excreted with waste.

- Bacteria may promote the inhibition of cholesterol production in the liver (digested gut contents travel from the gut directly to the liver via the portal vein).

Because cholesterol is recycled and reabsorbed from the small intestines, the gut plays a major role in cholesterol metabolism. What passes through the gut also plays a role. Dietary fiber, found in vegetables, fruits, legumes, and whole grains, has an effect on cholesterol. There are two main types of dietary fiber—soluble and insoluble. Soluble fiber is the type most beneficial for cholesterol. It acts as a sponge, absorbing the cholesterol and moving it out of the body.

Different types of soluble fiber have been found to effectively lower blood levels of LDL cholesterol. For each gram of soluble fiber in the diet, it is estimated that cholesterol levels will decrease by 1.08 to 1.12 mg/dL.[24] I recommend getting 35 grams of dietary fiber daily. If you can't get that much from diet alone, add a fiber supplement. See the Love Your Heart section for more information on the benefits of fiber.

Soluble Fiber Absorbs Cholesterol in the Gut

Inside the digestive tract, soluble fiber absorbs cholesterol from food. The fiber dissolves into digestive contents, carrying cholesterol out of the body.

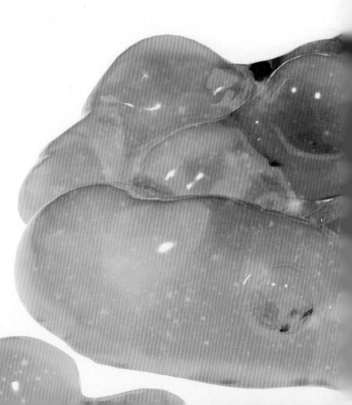

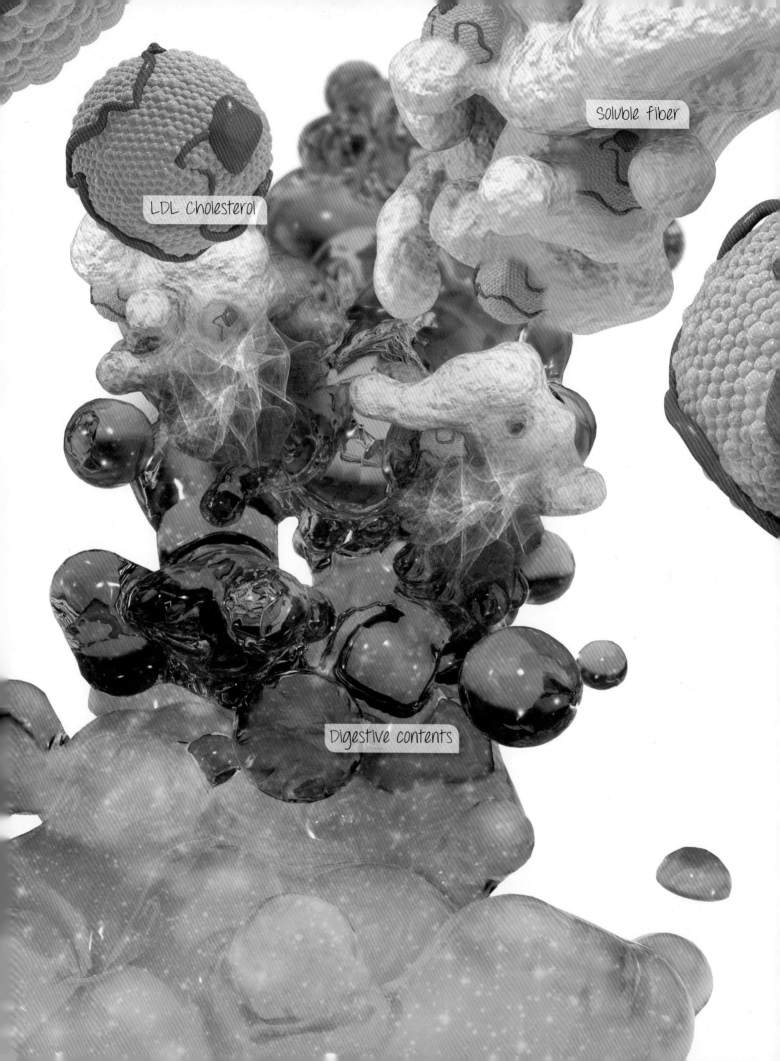

Controversy surrounds the use
of statin drugs. Statin drugs are
one of the most prescribed
medications in the United States.

Remember, however, there is more to the story than simply lowering cholesterol. Knowing the condition in which LDL particles are found will help you to more completely address the underlying causes of heart disease. Probiotics and fiber go a long way to helping improve other heart disease risk factors, as you will learn in later chapters.

The Role of Sugar and Carbohydrates

Low-fat diets have been widely recommended for reduction of heart disease risk because saturated fat increases LDL cholesterol. The problem with these recommendations is that a low-fat diet often becomes a high-carbohydrate diet, known to reduce HDL cholesterol, raise triglycerides,[25] and increase levels of small,

dense LDL cholesterol[26]—all factors that increase heart disease risk.

When low-fat diet recommendations were first made back in the 1970s, to maintain good taste the food industry began to replace fat with carbohydrates, often in the form of sugar, in processed foods. Thus began the implementation of the low-fat, high-carbohydrate diet craze. The result, as is discussed in more detail in chapters 4 and 5, is an unprecedented increase in obesity, diabetes, and heart disease—the opposite effect to that intended. Indeed, maintaining a moderate fat intake while reducing carbohydrates has been found to be more effective in preventing heart disease than reducing overall fat intake.[27] Unfortunately, this is not the Standard American Diet (SAD). I want to help change that.

There is a widely held misconception that a low-fat diet is heart healthy. The problem is that when dietary fat is reduced, it must be replaced by another macronutrient—either carbohydrates or protein. In most cases carbohydrate intake increases. This is where everything goes wrong. As we will see throughout this book, a high-sugar, high-carbohydrate diet contributes to the metabolic imbalances that lead to cardiovascular disease.

Standard Treatment

The standard treatment for dyslipidemia, or high total and LDL cholesterol, high triglycerides, and low HDL cholesterol, should begin with lifestyle changes. These include a healthy diet, regular exercise, weight loss if overweight, and no smoking. For people with high triglycerides, omega-3 fish oils are recommended by the American Heart Association as standard treatment.

Unfortunately, prescription medications—statin drugs for lowering LDL cholesterol and fibrates for lowering triglycerides and raising HDL—are often pushed more than lifestyle changes. Of all prescribed drugs in 2010, Americans spent the most money on Lipitor, a statin drug.[28] The generic statin simvastatin (Zocor) was the second-most prescribed drug that same year.

Pharmaceutical companies have been very successful at selling the idea that LDL cholesterol causes heart disease, but in reality, it doesn't. High levels of LDL may be a marker for heart disease, but it's more important to look at the types of LDL cholesterol. Modified LDL—whether oxidized LDL or small, dense LDL—is more powerfully associated with heart disease than large, light and fluffy LDL. Standard blood tests, upon which statin prescription is based, don't detect these different LDL types. Further, inflammation plays an important role in the development of heart disease.

So why have statins been found to reduce heart disease risk if simply lowering LDL cholesterol doesn't address the whole problem? Very interestingly, although statins do lower LDL cholesterol, it has also been found that they have anti-inflammatory effects.[29] It is likely the anti-inflammatory effect underlies at least some of the benefits of statin drugs. This begs the question: Could the inflammation be quelled by other non-pharmaceutical means? It certainly can. More about this in chapter 6.

TIP:

The widely recommended, so-called healthy low-fat diet turns out to be a high-sugar, high-carbohydrate diet—not heart-healthy at all.

Why My Husband's Cholesterol Changed My Life: Stan's Story

For many years, cholesterol has been a measure of good health, especially heart health. Never did I think I would be writing about it, since my focus has always been on gut health. But over the last ten years I have discovered that all health—whether of the heart, joints, brain, or any other system of the body—has a direct connection to the digestive system. This unfolding discovery, in addition to the fact that high cholesterol levels in my husband, Stan, threatened his life, gave me the passion to take his experience and share it with others so they may benefit from what he's learned after years of frustration trying to manage this condition.

About ten years ago, while being assessed for insurance coverage, we found Stan's total cholesterol level to be outrageously high—over 800 mg/dL! Needless to say, we were in shock. At the time, we were growing our company and under a lot of stress. We immediately went to a doctor. Even before the appointment, we decided he should start right away with diet changes and extra supplements to see if that would help. Stan was overweight at the time, and his biggest challenge was sugar consumption.

Just over two weeks later we arrived at the doctor's office with a second lab report of Stan's latest blood work. After about two weeks, he had been able to get his cholesterol down from 800 to 582 mg/dL, with only diet changes and additional supplementation. The doctor was still in shock from his high cholesterol levels, however, and wanted to put him on statins right away. Stan was less than excited about that.

The doctor was also very blunt about his need to change his diet and lose weight. Stan asked the doctor to give him a month to implement diet changes and continue supplementation with omega-3 fish oil and fiber. Most doctors would probably not agree to this, since Stan's cholesterol levels were so high, but our doctor was a proponent of healthy eating and knew about the heart benefits of omega-3s.

So off we went, with Stan determined to get his cholesterol down without resorting to statin drugs. He knew about the detrimental effects statins can have and wanted to avoid them if possible. Before his next appointment, he lost about ten pounds and had augmented his omega-3 fish oil and fiber supplementation. The next cholesterol panel came back from the lab with his total cholesterol at 216 mg/dL. Wow! And his LDL to HDL ratio fell into a good range. The doctor was pleased, and Stan left the office determined to maintain a healthy cholesterol level.

If I could press a repeat button now, it would describe Stan's story over the past ten years. He gets his cholesterol down, but then begins to slip back to his old eating habits, and up it goes again. Repeat story. I think Stan is like millions of Americans. Their cholesterol levels might not get as high as his, but they struggle with consistently keeping their levels down. They struggle with diet and lifestyle changes. They struggle with weight. They struggle with stress. So we get stuck in our usual patterns and have a hard time getting out. We get lost in the events of our lives, and forget about our health for a while. The state of our health teeters between good and bad, over and over again.

Finally Stan hit bottom with a little help from me. It was late 2009; around Halloween, to be exact (a fitting time of year, with all that Halloween candy). I had some traveling to do, and before I left, I cleaned out all sugary foods from the house. I left in the hopes of finding a sugar-free house upon return. No such luck. Ice cream, chocolate syrup, and candy greeted my arrival. At this time Stan's weight was also up, and his cholesterol skyrocketed.

As he dug into his second bowl of ice cream, I lost it. We needed a heart-to-heart talk. I told him he had to get serious and change his lifestyle so that we could be sure to have a life together after working so hard all these years. He said to me, "I tried diet and lifestyle changes. That doesn't work for me." I told him I didn't want to become his coach because I didn't want to become a nag, but something had to be done.

Life has a funny way of working out sometimes. When you put something out there—a thought, a need, a desire—the answer will show up for you. The next day I was at the bank. The banker, who has been a friend for many years, said hello. But I didn't recognize him at first. "Scott?" I said. I couldn't believe how different he looked. He told me he had lost 30 pounds, and I asked how. He told me about a program he had followed to lose the weight. I told Stan about it right away, and off we went.

Stan started a healthy eating program. The program is what we are presenting in the Love Your Heart section of this book. The program was so simple he could do it himself with no help from me. Over two months he lost 15 pounds, and brought his total cholesterol down to 179 mg/dL. He continued to lose a total of 40 pounds, and maintains a healthy weight to this day. His cholesterol has also remained in the healthy range.

There is more to Stan's story, as you will see in chapter 5. We have begun a wonderful journey that has not only changed his life, but our life and our relationship. I'm excited to share it with you. ∎

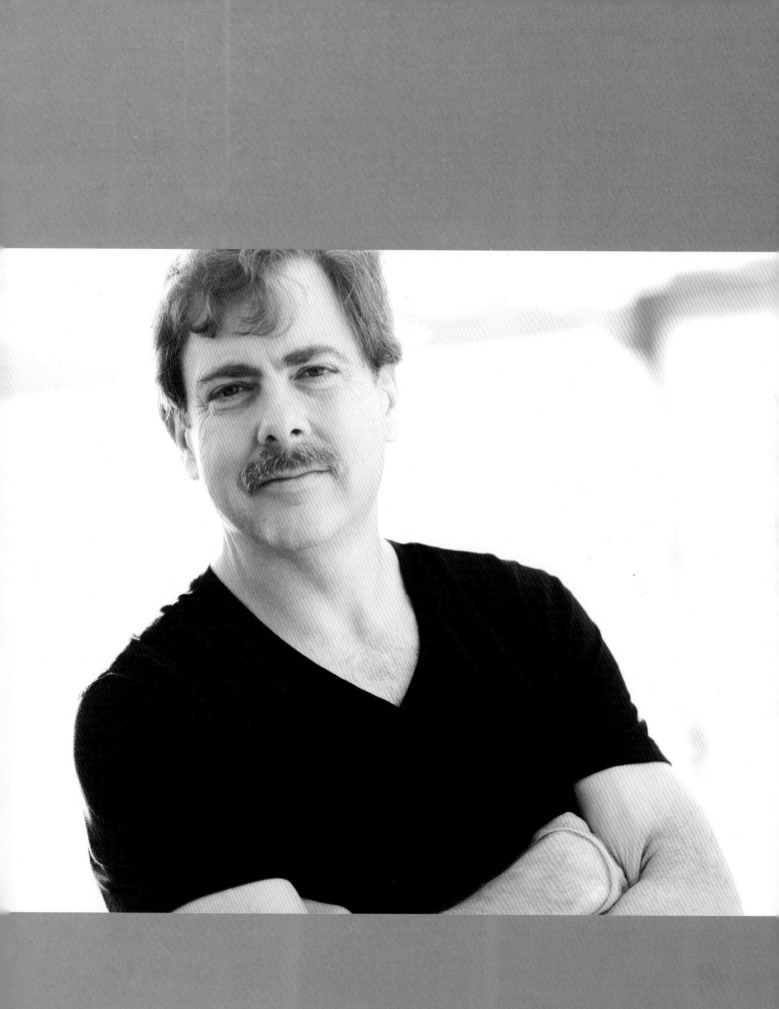

Gut Bacteria Affect Statin Drug Success. Gut bacteria play a role in cholesterol metabolism primarily because the site of reabsorption of cholesterol is the gut lining, the home of gut bacteria. An interesting study has found that the composition of bacteria in the gut affects whether statins work effectively or not.[30] Not everyone responds to statin drugs with lower cholesterol levels to the same degree.

Gut bacteria and their role in modifying bile acids may be the reason. The study found that, in **people who responded best to statin drugs, bile acids played a role with an enhanced LDL cholesterol–reducing response in the presence of specific gut bacteria such as lactobacillus.** Other researchers have recognized the potential role of probiotics in cholesterol metabolism,[31] calling for more research into the role of gut bacteria and response to statins.

Controversy surrounds the use of statin drugs. Public outcry sounded when the American Academy of Pediatrics revised recommendations for the treatment of high cholesterol in children, recommending that children as young as eight years old with high cholesterol take statin drugs.[32] There are limited data showing that statins are safe in children of this age, and long-term studies are lacking. Due to the rapid growth and development that occurs at this young age, the safety of this recommendation is questioned.

As we've seen in this chapter, the standard view of cholesterol does not tell the whole story. Whether you have high cholesterol or low cholesterol, plenty of "good" cholesterol or low levels of "bad" cholesterol, you may be at risk for heart disease. You might need to take a closer look at what kind of LDL cholesterol you have, and what other risk factors you have. The next chapters will discuss more risk factors you might not know you have.

Tips to Improve Your Blood Lipid Levels

See the Love Your Heart section for more information about how to develop a heart-healthy lifestyle.

- Eat a diet low in grain-based, refined, and starchy carbohydrates and sugars, and high in vegetables, healthy fats, and lean proteins, nuts and seeds.
- Avoid processed foods, refined sugars, grain-based carbs, and starchy foods (especially pasta, breads, and cereals made from wheat; potatoes; white rice; packaged snack foods, etc.).
- Exercise regularly.
- If overweight, lose weight.
- Be sure to get 35 grams of fiber daily. Add a fiber supplement if necessary.
- Supplement your diet with omega-3 fish oils.
- Optimize your vitamin D level.
- Eat a variety of vegetables for antioxidant nutrients.
- Balance your gut with probiotics.

"When you have your health, you have everything. When you do not have your health, nothing else matters at all."

—Augusten Burroughs

Chapter 3

High Blood Pressure— Take It Seriously

Many people underestimate the harm caused by high blood pressure, also known as hypertension. If a high blood pressure reading is taken during a routine checkup, it might be dismissed by the patient as the result of a recent stressful event, or from nervousness due to the checkup itself.

Some people think that if they were to have high blood pressure they would feel it. This is not at all true, however. About one in three U.S. adults has high blood pressure.[1] Another 25 percent have prehypertension, or blood pressure numbers in the high-normal range.[2] Together, those two groups make up well over half of U.S. adults, yet more than 22 percent of people with high blood pressure don't know they have it. For these reasons and more, high blood pressure is known as the "silent killer," silently increasing the risk of heart disease and stroke.

Blood Pressure—Let's Break It Down

As the heart pumps blood through the arteries, the blood pushes against the artery walls, creating pressure—blood pressure. There are two types of blood pressure: systolic and diastolic pressure. Systolic pressure refers to the pressure exerted when the heart pumps, and diastolic pressure refers to the pressure exerted against the artery as the heart relaxes between pumps. This is why blood pressure levels read as two numbers, systolic over diastolic (like 120/80). Systolic pressure is

MYTH:

If you had high blood pressure, you would know it.

FACT:

High blood pressure is known as the "silent killer" because more than 22 percent of people with high blood pressure don't know they have it.

higher than diastolic because when the heart pumps, it pushes blood through the arteries, which increases pressure against the arteries. When it rests, blood slows and the pressure is lessened.

Blood pressure is measured with a blood pressure cuff, also known as a sphygmomanometer. Blood pressure is generally measured during regular checkups. A phenomenon, known as white-coat hypertension, which occurs in 25 percent of people, causes blood pressure to rise during a doctor's visit, usually as a result of nervousness. If high blood pressure is measured during a doctor's visit, you will likely be advised to monitor your blood pressure throughout the day with a blood pressure cuff to be sure you do not have chronically elevated blood pressure, which requires treatment. The following highlights standard measured blood pressure levels.

Blood Pressure

Systolic	Diastolic	
< 120	< 80	Normal
120–139	80–89	Prehypertension
140–159	90–99	Stage 1 hypertension
> 160	> 100	Stage 2 hypertension

We see from these standard guidelines that blood pressure of 140/90 is considered the threshold for high blood pressure. In 2006 researchers found that people with blood pressure ranging from 120/80 to 139/89 were at increased risk of developing cardiovascular disease when compared to people in the normal range.[3] This helped establish the prehypertension range, creating the need for people to maintain an even lower blood pressure.

Blood Pressure

Close-up view of pressure exerted by blood on the artery walls.

The Life Extension Foundation recommends an even lower optimal blood pressure level of 115/75, based on studies that found each 20/10 increment over 115/75 doubles the risk of heart attack, heart failure, stroke, or kidney disease in individuals 40 to 70 years old.[4] Even in people with normal blood pressure at age 55, 90 percent will go on to develop high blood pressure at some point.[5] That is an astounding statistic. Are you paying attention yet? Blood pressure is not something to be ignored.

Even in people with normal blood pressure at age 55, fully 90 percent will go on to develop high blood pressure.

When blood pressure is raised, the heart must work harder to pump blood throughout the body. Over time, an overworked heart muscle will thicken as it tries to pump blood. A thickened heart may result in less blood pumped throughout the body, known as reduced cardiac output, which may eventually lead to heart failure, or the inability of the heart to pump enough blood throughout the body.

High blood pressure also damages the arteries. Increased blood pressure contributes to thickening of the artery walls and creates microscopic tears, which can trigger or worsen atherosclerosis and lead to heart disease, heart attack, stroke, and even death.

There are two main types of hypertension: primary and secondary. Primary hypertension refers to high blood pressure for which a specific cause is not identified. Most people with high blood pressure have primary hypertension. Secondary hypertension refers to high blood pressure triggered by an underlying cause. Many medical conditions can cause secondary hypertension, including diabetes, kidney disease, and endocrine disorders (such as thyroid dysfunction). Certain medications, such as corticosteroids, nonsteroidal anti-inflammatory drugs (NSAIDs), certain cold medicines, and oral contraceptives, can also trigger high blood pressure.

There are three main processes contributing to increased blood pressure in the arteries:

1) Fluid retention, which increases blood volume

2) Increased blood flow

3) Artery stiffness

Perhaps it's not the sodium that is the major contributor to cardiovascular risk, but the overall poor quality of the diet instead.

Fluid retention is largely controlled by the kidneys, which regulate the balance of water and salt. If the kidneys lose their efficiency at excreting sodium, or salt, or if excess dietary sodium is consumed, blood volume will increase, and thus blood pressure will increase. Low potassium intake can also contribute to salt retention, as potassium balances the effects of sodium. This explains why it may be important to watch salt intake when dealing with hypertension. The cardiovascular benefits of reducing dietary salt intake have been questioned, however.[6,7] Perhaps it's not the sodium that is the major contributor to cardiovascular risk, but the overall poor quality of the diet instead.

Increased blood flow increases blood pressure. As a simple example, systolic blood pressure—the pressure exerted when the heart pumps—is higher than diastolic because blood flow increases as the heart pumps. Other factors leading to increased blood flow will increase blood pressure. Both exercise and stress have this effect. Temporary increases, as seen with exercise and stressful events, in small doses generally are not harmful to the arteries. Chronic stress, however, can cause sustained increases in blood pressure.

TIP:

Chronic stress can raise blood pressure. If your life is stressful, find ways to relieve the stress. Rest more, find a calming activity you enjoy, and ask for help when you need it.

Artery stiffness also contributes to blood pressure. As we age the arteries lose some of their natural flexibility, becoming stiffer. This is one reason why so many older adults have high blood pressure. Artery stiffness is also triggered by certain detrimental processes in the body, as we will learn. Stiff arteries increase resistance in the artery wall, which increases blood pressure.

Oxidant/Antioxidant Balance

One main contributor to blood pressure levels is the oxidant and antioxidant balance in the body. As we learned in chapter 2 with oxidative LDL, oxidation is a damaging process. Remember the LDL particle that got punched in the face? Think of the punch itself as oxidation, and the one punching as the oxidant. Enter the peacekeeper—the antioxidant. The antioxidant essentially extends a helping hand to the harmful oxidant, turning the potential fight into a friendly handshake. Antioxidants basically keep the peace. They travel around the body, and when they encounter a bully, they make the situation peaceful. They do this by neutralizing free radicals, the oxidants.

Dark Chocolate Saves the Day! In one study involving 44 patients with untreated stage 1 hypertension or prehypertension, eating 6.3 grams of dark chocolate per day lowered blood pressure by 2.9/1.9 mm Hg over 18 weeks.[8] This is a relatively small decrease, but considering it's a relatively small piece of chocolate, and no other changes were made, the results are notable. I say, why not? Have your chocolate. Find a high-quality dark chocolate—milk chocolate won't work—and be sure it's low in sugar.

The oxidant/antioxidant balance is important when it comes to high blood pressure because oxidation reduces the production of an important vasodilator, nitric oxide,[9] which contributes to high blood pressure. Think of a vasodilator as something that relaxes the arteries. Stiff arteries, as we have learned, increase blood pressure due to their inflexibility.

A diet high in colorful fruits and vegetables, as well as certain antioxidant supplements, can be protective against the oxidation that leads to high blood pressure. Coenzyme Q10, vitamin C, vitamin E with mixed tocopherols and tocotrienols, and garlic are all heart-healthy antioxidants.

> # A diet high in colorful fruits and vegetables, as well as certain antioxidant supplements, can be protective against the oxidation that leads to high blood pressure.

Relaxed arteries, as are found when there is enough nitric oxide produced by the cells lining the blood vessels, help to reduce blood pressure.

Oxidation also triggers an inflammatory process. Remember from chapter 2 that inflammation is like the gunfire of war—it harms everything in its path. Not only does oxidation itself decrease amounts of nitric oxide, but so does the ensuing inflammation.[10] Under these conditions, the relaxing nitric oxide doesn't have a chance. Arteries become stiff and blood pressure increases.

Role of Inflammation

The role of inflammation in the development of many chronic diseases is now well established.[11] Atherosclerosis itself is known as an inflammatory disease because inflammation plays a primary role throughout the entire process. In this book, you are beginning to understand the importance of tracing back to the root causes of heart disease, rather than simply treating symptoms (usually in the form of pharmaceutical drugs), as traditional medicine tends to do. We will find that most times when we trace back to the initial factors leading to heart disease, inflammation is involved. This is also the case with high blood pressure.

Chronic, low-grade inflammation has been associated with high blood pressure, and is now known to precede its development. Since inflammation has been found to come before

TIP:

Chronic, low-grade inflammation—called silent inflammation because you might not even know you have it—is a major feature of, and underlying risk factor for, heart disease.

high blood pretssure, this suggests it may be a cause of high blood pressure. Researchers use one particular inflammation marker, C-reactive protein (CRP), as a way to detect underlying inflammation in the body. CRP is produced when the body is inflamed. During acute infections, CRP levels in the blood are greatly increased. Under chronic, low-grade inflammatory conditions—silent inflammation that cannot be felt—CRP levels are detected at lower amounts, yet still higher than normal.[12] CRP levels are one of the best markers of silent inflammation. See chapter 6 for more information.

Two large studies have found elevated CRP levels to precede the development of hypertension. In the Women's Health Study, involving more than 20,000 women, the women with normal blood pressure and higher levels of CRP over the course of almost eight years were more likely to later develop high blood pressure than those women with normal CRP levels, even if they had no other conventional cardiovascular risk factors.[13]

Another study in men took these findings even further. Almost 400 middle-aged men with normal blood pressure were followed for 11 years. Over that time 33 percent developed high blood pressure. Men with hs-CRP levels (high-sensitivity CRP, a very sensitive test that detects CRP in the blood) equal to or greater than 3.0 mg/L were more likely to develop high blood pressure than those with levels below 1.0 mg/L.[14] This was true even after researchers ruled out features of the metabolic syndrome and lifestyle factors, meaning the results were not due to other factors that might put the men at greater risk of developing high blood pressure. Even if the men were totally healthy, if they had underlying chronic, low-grade inflammation, they were still more likely to develop high blood pressure.

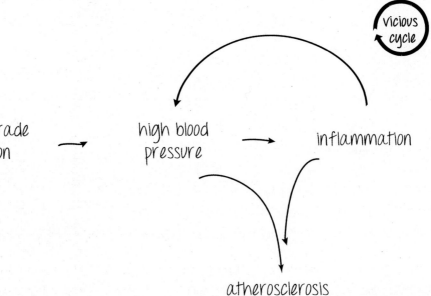

Gut inflammation has systemic effects, and contributes to heart disease.

One main way in which inflammation contributes to high blood pressure is by increasing artery stiffness. As mentioned previously, artery stiffness is a main feature of high blood pressure. When arteries are stiff, pressure increases inside the blood vessel. Increased inflammation, as measured by hs-CRP blood levels, in addition to other inflammatory chemicals, has been related to measures of artery stiffness.[15]

Not only does inflammation precede high blood pressure, but it is also a result of high blood pressure.[16] The increase in pressure exerted on the artery wall triggers an inflammatory process known as endothelial dysfunction (endothelium is a fancy word for the lining of the artery). Endothelial dysfunction is basically the first step in atherosclerosis, the development of plaque in the arteries. Endothelial dysfunction indicates something has gone wrong in the artery wall. Chapter 9 highlights the important role of endothelial dysfunction as the initiator of heart disease.

Inflammation comes both before and after high blood pressure, highlighting its important role in the development of heart disease, which itself is known as an inflammatory disease. The questions to ask, then, are: Where is this inflammation coming from, and how can it be quelled?

Although it has been established that chronic, low-grade inflammation is an underlying feature of high blood pressure, heart disease, and, indeed, most chronic diseases, it is not entirely understood where this inflammation is coming from. Inflammation response involves an intricate array of immune cells and chemicals, and may be present in most any area of the body. It is well known that foreign invaders like pathogens, allergens, and toxins trigger acute inflammatory responses. Could they also trigger chronic, low-grade inflammation? Let's look to the gut to find out.

Gut Connection to High Blood Pressure

Gut dysfunction often involves inflammation. Take irritable bowel syndrome (IBS), one common bowel disorder, as an example. IBS can be triggered by a disturbance in the balance of intestinal bacteria known as dysbiosis. This imbalance may be the result of an infection, dietary changes, or from certain medications such as antibiotics. The result is chronic, low-grade inflammation.[17] Indeed, people with IBS have higher levels of hs-CRP than healthy people,[18] indicating the systemic effects of gut inflammation. As we have learned, an elevated CRP level can lead to high blood pressure, and is an independent risk factor for heart disease.

How Sugar and Carbs Affect Blood Pressue

In another study, a low-carbohydrate diet led to similar weight loss as a low-fat diet with the added fat-absorbing drug Orlistat, but the low-carbohydrate diet was more effective at lowering blood pressure.[20] To understand how a high-carbohydrate diet might contribute to high blood pressure, an animal study found that it decreased nitric oxide and worsened the antioxidant/oxidant balance.[21] In one study looking at the short-term effects of various sugars on blood pressure, both glucose and sucrose (table sugar, which itself is made of fructose and glucose) were found to raise systolic blood pressure in healthy young men.[22] These are just a few examples of the harmful effects of a diet high in refined carbohydrates and sugars, the Standard American Diet (SAD).

Air pollution from large cities is usually transported hundreds of miles.

Toxins and Blood Pressure

Most people know air pollution is harmful. Some people even know that air pollution is bad for your heart. But many people who do not live in major cities don't tend to worry much about air pollution. What they don't realize is that air pollution from large cities is usually transported hundreds of miles. This means air pollution can be found just about everywhere, even in rural, seemingly pristine areas.[23] One major component of air pollution is particulate matter, which is made up of an array of chemicals, gases, and metals. Exposure to particulate matter at high concentrations is able to raise blood pressure within hours to days.[24] Even at levels commonly encountered, airborne pollutants can increase blood pressure.[25]

Air pollution brings about oxidative stress, primarily by impairing the protective function of nitric oxide—remember the chemical responsible for relaxing the blood vessels. Because air pollution cannot always be avoided, supporting the body's detoxification functions is important, especially by increasing the amount of antioxidants consumed. Colorful fruits and vegetables and certain vitamins and antioxidant supplements will help counteract oxidative stress.

Heavy metals should also be considered in the discussion of high blood pressure. Heavy metal exposure can be measured in the hair because metals are stored in the body long term, and hair represents a measure of long-term exposure to heavy metals. Levels of nickel, cadmium, copper, chromium, and lead have all been found to be higher in hair samples of men with high blood pressure compared to men with normal blood pressure.[26] Arsenic exposure has also been found to be related to high blood pressure in a dose-dependent fashion—meaning the higher the arsenic level, the higher the blood pressure.[27]

Another study, based on data from more than 10,000 participants of the National Health and Nutrition Examination Survey (NHANES), found that cadmium levels in blood were associated

TIP:

Because air pollution and certain toxins cannot always be avoided, supporting the body's detoxification functions is important. Increase the amount of antioxidants you consume with a diet high in colorful fruits and vegetables, and antioxidant supplements if needed.

with increased blood pressure.[28] Interestingly, this association was not as strong in smokers as it was in nonsmokers, even though smoking is a major source of cadmium exposure. This suggests that the cadmium is coming from another source. Air pollution, industrial exposure, and certain foods are other means of exposure to cadmium.

Mercury is another important heavy metal to consider here. Mercury is the most dangerous of all the heavy metals.[29] In the body, mercury impairs the function of the mitochondria, the energy producers of cells. This creates oxidative stress and reduces antioxidant defenses, which we have seen can lead to high blood pressure.

Lead exposure also plays a role here. In women aged 40 to 59 years, blood lead levels well below the U.S. occupational exposure limit guidelines (40 micrograms/dL) were associated with risks of high blood pressure.[30] The relationship was strongest in postmenopausal women, thought to be due to the decreased

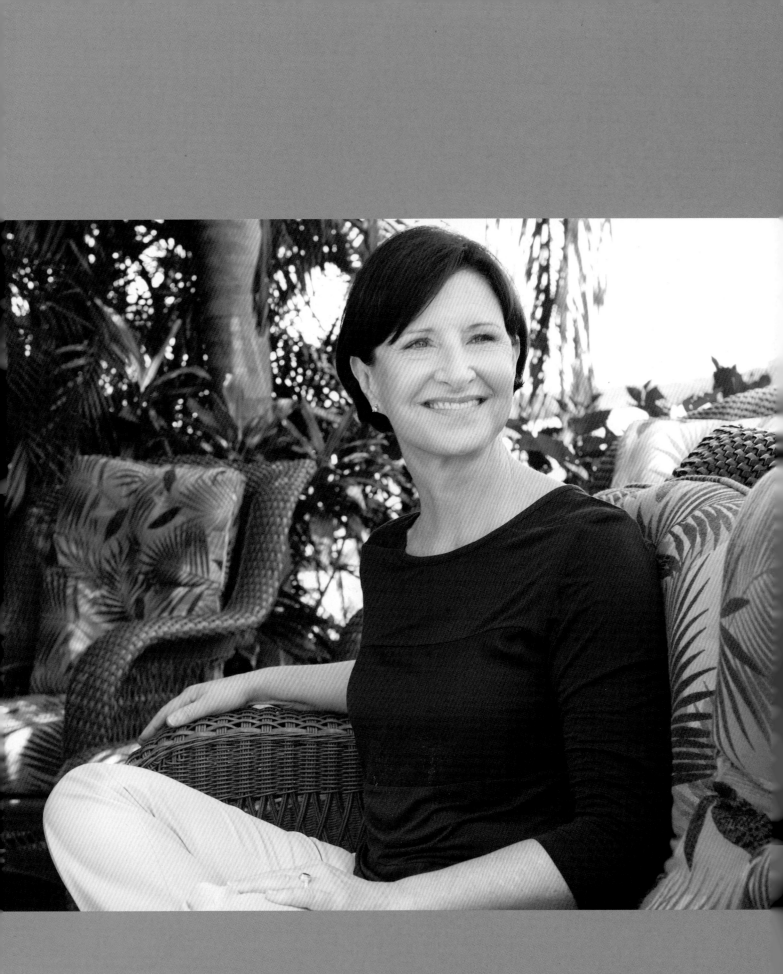

How Blood Pressure Creeps Up on You with Age: Sandee's Story

My sister Sandee has always worked really hard to stay healthy. Sandee is in her fifties and, like many of us baby boomers, she wants to stay off medications as she gets older. Sandee has seen the ramifications of being overmedicated by observing our father, who died earlier than he should have. Due to decades of bad habits, and a lack of knowledge from an early age about how to help himself naturally, two things, in combination, happened. First, he thought doctors were going to save him from his bad habits. Second, he spent years taking medications, never addressing diet or lifestyle. Sandee took all this to heart, as did I.

Sandee works as an advisor for a dietary supplement company, and hears daily from people who are fed up with taking so many medications. These people are looking for alternative solutions. Over the years, she has observed that people are starting to realize that the idea of a "miracle pill" is a joke. To Sandee, it is disheartening to listen to hundreds of people who have followed the advice of their doctors, only to discover the direction they were given not only didn't solve their heart problems, but in many ways made the problems worse.

So, when I say Sandee had a wake-up call with her own health, you can see how important it was for her to solve it without medication, as she has so much experience helping other people with the same problems.

When she discovered her high blood pressure, she was shocked. She said, "When the doctor took my blood pressure, it was 171/100. She told me I had to go on blood-pressure-lowering medication. I felt so depressed. My first thought was: No. I will not end up dependent on medication when I know I have the ability to solve this."

Sandee did leave the doctor's office with a prescription, but also with a very determined mind-set to be off of the medication within three to six months. She knew the key to her success would be to lose weight and, especially because of her family history, eliminate sugar from her diet. She knew she had the tools to make this work.

I will never forget her words to me: "This blood pressure thing is a creeper. You don't feel it, so you don't know anything is wrong." This is why monitoring blood pressure is so important for us all.

Was Sandee successful in her quest to get off the medication? See page 105 to find out. ∎

levels of estrogen found in women after menopause. Estrogen is thought to help protect against high blood pressure.[31] The association of lead levels with high blood pressure also exists in men.

One way in which toxins may increase blood pressure is by decreasing amounts of the body's most potent antioxidant, glutathione.[32,33] Glutathione is the body's main antioxidant, helping to neutralize oxidation and bind with toxins so they can be removed from the body. If the body is overburdened with toxins, the antioxidant protection of glutathione is depleted.

Standard Treatment

Standard treatment for high blood pressure should begin with lifestyle changes. Unfortunately, either due to the doctor's choice to simply prescribe a drug, or due to the patient's inability to change his or her lifestyle, these recommendations are not often followed. A healthy diet high in fruits, vegetables, and low-fat dairy, and low in salt, in addition to exercising, maintaining a healthy weight, quitting smoking, and managing stress will all help to control high blood pressure. This is where you should begin.

When medications are prescribed, diuretics, or water pills, are often prescribed first. Other medications may replace or be added to the diuretic. These include angiotensin-converting enzyme (ACE) inhibitors, angiotensin II receptor blockers, beta blockers, calcium channel blockers, or renin inhibitors.

Common blood pressure medication side effects include:[34]

- Constipation
- Dehydration
- Dizziness, light-headedness, or fainting
- Drowsiness
- Dry mouth
- Frequent urination at night
- Headaches
- Increased sensitivity to cold
- Increased sensitivity to sunlight
- Potassium loss
- Tender, swollen, or bleeding gums
- Upset stomach

In most cases, lifestyle changes are your best bet to get high blood pressure under control without having to rely on medications for what might be the rest of your life. As we are beginning to see, with high blood pressure, and indeed with any of the risk factors for heart disease, there are interconnected processes that cannot be ignored. To simply treat each sign or symptom with its corresponding drug misses the larger picture that is the harmonious integration of different systems of the body in bringing about homeostasis—or healthy balance. Learning what the body needs, and doesn't need, to bring about this state is the way to reduce your risk of heart disease.

Tips for Helping Reduce High Blood Pressure

See the Love Your Heart section for a complete program to support heart health.

- Eat a diet high in colorful foods—mostly from vegetables and fruits—for plenty of antioxidants.

- Lower your sugar and carbohydrate intake, and the consumption of processed foods.

- Lower your sodium intake and consider a potassium supplement if you are not taking a multivitamin and mineral formula with plenty of potassium.

- If you're overweight or obese, lose weight.

- Add antioxidant supplements if needed. Coenzyme Q10, vitamin C, and vitamin E (with mixed tocopherols and tocotrienols) are helpful.

- Reduce the stress in your life. Find a relaxing activity you enjoy, and do it regularly.

- Monitor your blood pressure regularly.

- If you are not supplementing with omega-3 fish oil, consider adding this heart-healthy nutrient.

- Eat a piece of dark chocolate (low in sugar) every day.

"Every human being is the author of his own health or disease."

—Siddhartha Gautama

Chapter 4

High Blood Sugar– Know Your Risk

When most people think of high blood sugar, also known as high blood glucose, they think of diabetes, a condition in which high blood sugar is a main feature. Diabetes affects more than 25 million people in the United States. What's more, prediabetes, a milder form of high blood sugar that precedes diabetes, affects 79 million people.[1] That means more than 100 million people have diabetes or prediabetes. Unfortunately, many of these people don't even know it.

> ## More than 100 million people have diabetes or prediabetes, and many of these people don't even know it.

What do diabetes and blood sugar have to do with heart disease, you may ask? Well, an elevated blood sugar level is a risk factor for the development of heart disease in people with and without diabetes.[2] So even if you are healthy and have no other risk factors for heart disease (such as high cholesterol or high blood pressure), if your blood sugar is high, you are at higher risk of developing heart disease.

Unfortunately, when most people think of heart disease, blood sugar is not the first thing to come to mind, and it might not come to mind at all. I want to help change that. High blood sugar is one risk factor for heart disease that needs to be taken more seriously.

High Blood Sugar—Let's Break It Down

To understand how blood sugar rises, we have to understand how it is controlled. The main controller of blood glucose is insulin. Insulin is a hormone secreted by the islet cells of the pancreas, helping to move glucose from the blood into cells for use as energy. Glucose is a form of sugar that has been broken down by the complete digestion of carbohydrates. It is considered the body's main source of energy, utilized by nearly every cell. Blood glucose levels rise because there is either not enough insulin to move glucose into the cells, or because the insulin that is present does not work effectively, a condition known as insulin resistance. The following highlights standard measured blood glucose and insulin levels.[3,4]

Fasting Plasma Glucose Test

Plasma Glucose	Diagnosis
> 99 mg/dL	Normal
100–125 mg/dL	Prediabetes
> 126	Diabetes*

Oral Glucose Tolerance Test

2-hour Plasma Glucose	Diagnosis
> 139	Normal
140–199	Prediabetes
> 200	Diabetes*

HbA1c Test

Hemoglobin A1c	
4.5–5.6%	Normal
5.7–6.4%	Prediabetes
> 6.5%	Diabetes*

*These tests are confirmed by repeating the test on a different day.

Fasting or 2-hour Insulin Test

Insulin	
6–35 IU/mL	Normal*

*Levels vary depending on the test and the lab.

Myth:

Only diabetics need to worry about blood sugar.

The fasting plasma glucose test is the most common blood sugar test, taken first thing in the morning before eating. Adding the other tests will provide more information than the fasting blood glucose test alone. The hemoglobin A1c test (HbA1c) is a measure of average blood sugar levels over the previous several months, whereas the other blood glucose tests measure blood glucose in the moment. We see that, similar to the addition of a prehypertension category in the evaluation of high blood pressure, the addition of a prediabetes category has been made to the evaluation of blood sugar levels. Interestingly, in 2003 the fasting plasma glucose range for prediabetes lowered from 110–125 mg/dL to 100–125 mg/dL,[5] and in 1997 the range for diabetes lowered from 140 or more, to 126 or more.[6]

The Life Extension Foundation recommends an even lower normal blood glucose range of 75–85 mg/dL, based on a 22-year study in healthy, non-diabetic men that found that those with blood glucose levels above 85 mg/dL are at a 40 percent increased risk of heart attack.[7] Further, Life Extension recommends an insulin level of 5 IU/mL or less, as levels over this may trigger the development of insulin resistance.[8]

Fact:

Many people with diabetes and prediabetes do not even know they have it. Further, accepted "normal" levels of blood sugar continue to be lowered as researchers discover the dangers of even mildly elevated blood sugar.

Insulin Resistance—Where It All Begins

Blood glucose is generally measured more often than insulin, so the focus tends to remain on blood sugar, and not insulin. But since insulin regulates blood sugar levels, it's important to look at what has gone wrong with insulin in order to understand why blood sugar rises. Insulin resistance is what happens when cells do not respond to the action of insulin. Basically, insulin acts as a key to the cell—insert the insulin key, and the cell will open its doors to glucose, taking it in from the bloodstream, which lowers blood glucose levels. Think of insulin resistance as a broken keyhole. With insulin resistance, the insulin key no longer fits into its keyhole, so the doors of the cells do not open, and glucose cannot get into the cells from the bloodstream. Thus, blood glucose levels rise.

Cells need glucose to make energy. When they do not get it, and blood glucose levels rise, a message is sent to the pancreas to produce more insulin, which raises blood insulin levels to help shuffle glucose into cells, normalizing blood glucose levels. Increased insulin levels and insulin resistance can occur even with normal blood glucose levels. This raised insulin level can lead to more insulin resistance and, eventually, decreased insulin secretion from the pancreas due to overworked pancreatic islet cells, all creating a vicious cycle that raises blood glucose levels over time.[9]

About one-third of the most insulin resistant people among healthy individuals is at increased risk of developing cardiovascular disease.[10] Insulin resistance is the main feature of a condition known as the metabolic syndrome. Metabolic syndrome is a common condition, and is, itself, associated with increased risk in men and women for both cardiovascular disease and type 2 diabetes.[11] Insulin resistance also plays a role in the development of Alzheimer's disease.[12] In fact, Alzheimer's disease is also known as type 3 diabetes. It is thought that chronic increased levels of insulin in the blood (which is what leads to insulin resistance) result in a decrease in insulin crossing the blood brain barrier, which affects glucose metabolism in the brain. Glucose is the main energy source of brain

Bloodstream

Insulin

Glucose

Insulin receptor

Cell membrane

Insulin Resistance

Close-up view of insulin resistance. The insulin receptor on the right is able to receive insulin and open the channel for glucose to enter the cell, lowering blood glucose levels, a process known as insulin sensitivity. The insulin receptor on the left is unable to receive insulin, the channel remains closed to glucose, and blood glucose levels remain high, a process known as insulin resistance.

cells.[13] This disruption of glucose balance in the brain may affect many areas of brain function, including cognitive function. This highlights the far-reaching effects of high blood sugar and insulin.

we would be without a strong defense. But when inflammation persists, when it does not properly resolve, when it lays low, yet active, we have cause for worry. And we have a trigger for heart disease.

We have learned that insulin resistance is an early trigger of heart disease. And since we're in the habit of looking for the root cause of what has gone wrong in this increasingly complicated picture of heart disease, why not ask: What causes insulin resistance? As with both conditions previously covered in this book—high cholesterol and high blood sugar—inflammation is also at the root cause of insulin resistance.[14]

When inflammation persists, when it does not properly resolve, when it lays low, yet active, we have cause for worry. And we have a trigger for heart disease.

Role of Inflammation

Chronic, low-grade inflammation triggers the development of insulin resistance. Without getting too complicated, the process of inflammation involves an array of hormonelike molecules (cytokines and chemokines), transcription factors (DNA-binding proteins that affect gene expression), enzymes, and proteins, all playing an intricate role in the development of insulin resistance.[15] Inflammation is a necessary process in the body, helping to defend us against invading pathogens, toxins, and unwanted invaders. If we had no inflammation,

Chronic, low-grade inflammation, also known as silent inflammation because it cannot be felt, is measured in the blood by the presence of high-sensitivity C-reactive protein (hsCRP). As with high cholesterol and high blood pressure, raised hsCRP levels have been found to be related to insulin resistance.

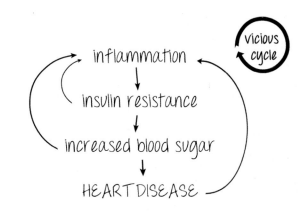

Not only does inflammation trigger insulin resistance and then increased blood sugar, but insulin resistance and increased blood sugar both trigger inflammation.[16,17] This creates a vicious cycle that perpetuates the inflammation. It's easy to see how chronic, low-grade inflammation is maintained.

Rather than treating the eventual signs, symptoms, or diseases, as modern medicine tends to do, we take a look at the larger picture...

If inflammation comes before insulin resistance, we must ask the question: What causes the inflammation? This is how we connect the dots. Rather than treating the eventual signs, symptoms, or diseases, as modern medicine tends to do, we take a look at the larger picture, trace back the steps leading to heart disease, so that we can try to remove the fuels of the fire before it flares up and into a full-blown forest fire of heart disease.

AGEs are Aging You

Hyperglycemia, or high blood sugar, contributes to the production of molecules in the body called AGEs (advanced glycation end products). AGEs are aptly named molecules produced naturally by the body, accumulating with age. They contribute to certain age-related chronic diseases such as diabetes, heart disease, and Alzheimer's disease, as well as to the aging process itself.[18] As a contributor to heart disease, AGEs are able to modify the LDL cholesterol particle so that it can be more easily oxidized.[19] As we have learned, oxidation of LDL cholesterol is a main factor contributing to the development of atherosclerosis. AGEs therefore play an important role in the development of heart disease.

In addition to being produced inside the body, AGEs may also be obtained from outside sources. Tobacco smoke is a primary contributor of AGEs. Certain foods, especially those cooked at high heat and in the absence of water, are high in AGEs. Foods high in processed carbohydrates and sugar increase AGEs because they increase blood sugar. It is impossible to eliminate the production or consumption of all AGEs, but reducing them may help reduce the inflammation and damage they inflict in the body. To reduce the amount of AGEs in the body, maintain healthy blood sugar levels and reduce your consumption of foods cooked at high heat.

Fat—an Organ Itself

Previously, fat was thought to merely be the storage house of excess energy. While energy

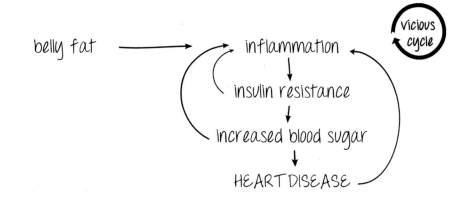

storage is certainly a function of body fat, it has recently been recognized that body fat functions as an endocrine organ that plays a major role in metabolism.[20] Body fat, or adipose tissue, produces a multitude of hormonelike chemicals collectively known as adipokines, some of which are inflammatory, and some anti-inflammatory. Adipokines have many functions, including regulation of satiety (feeling of fullness), carbohydrate and fat metabolism, and insulin sensitivity. Insulin sensitivity is the opposite of insulin resistance, involving the sensitivity of a cell to the function of insulin. People with more insulin sensitivity have better regulation of blood sugar,

because the key of insulin fits into the keyhole of the cell, opening the door so that glucose can enter, thus lowering blood glucose levels. Insulin resistance is a lack of insulin sensitivity, and body fat plays a major role in regulating this process.

The most concerning fat is belly fat—the fat surrounding the organs inside the abdomen. Belly fat is also known as visceral fat, or visceral adipose tissue (VAT). Not only do you have FAT, but now you have VAT. And VAT is one thing you don't want to have. VAT is the most metabolically active fat in the body, and contributes to the chronic inflammation underlying heart

...and trace back the steps leading to heart disease, so that we can try to remove the fuels of the fire before it flares up and into a full-blown forest fire of heart disease.

Toxins and undigested food particles

Harmful bacteria

Probiotics

disease.[21] If you tend to accumulate fat in your midsection, you're at increased risk for heart disease. See chapter 5 for more information about VAT, why it may be killing you, and what you can do about it.

The chronic, low-grade inflammation we have been talking about throughout this book originates, in large part, from the gut.

Before you let out a sigh of relief because you are slim and without belly fat, you may still have silent inflammation. Although belly fat is a primary source of inflammation, it is not the only source. It is true that the heavier an individual is, the more likely they are to be insulin resistant, but even slender people can still have insulin resistance. Likewise, not all overweight individuals will have insulin resistance. This means there are more sources of inflammation. One important source of inflammation is the gut.

Leaky gut

Capillary

Lymphatic capillary

Lymphatic vessel

Intestinal lining

The Gut Connection

Close-up view of the intestinal lining. When the gut is out of balance (dysbiosis) pathogenic bacteria can gain the upper hand and destroy the intestinal lining (leaky gut). Bacterial toxins then enter the bloodstream and can trigger metabolic imbalances such as inflammation and insulin resistance that contribute to heart disease.

Gut Connection to High Blood Sugar

An obvious gut connection to high blood sugar involves food, since the gut lining acts as the interface between the food that passes through the body and systemic circulation. Certainly what we eat affects our blood sugar. I'll cover this in the next section.

First, I want to talk about the gut as an important source of inflammation. The chronic, low-grade inflammation we have been talking about throughout this book originates, in large part, from the gut. A condition known as metabolic endotoxemia is largely responsible for this gut connection. Metabolic endotoxemia creates inflammation, leading to metabolic imbalances such as insulin resistance and high blood sugar—both initiating factors in the development of heart disease.

Metabolic endotoxemia involves an increase in the bacterial toxin lipopolysaccharide (LPS), also known as an endotoxin, in the bloodstream. Endotoxins are those toxins produced inside the body, compared to exotoxins, which come from our environment. *Endotoxemia* means "endotoxin in the bloodstream." *Metabolic* refers to the metabolic dysfunction that ensues. LPS is a cell wall component of certain intestinal bacteria, shed when the bacteria die in the intestines. (Bacteria have a short lifespan and are always reproducing in the intestines.) LPS enters the bloodstream when intestinal permeability is increased. Increased intestinal permeability is also known as leaky gut, or leaky gut syndrome, and is triggered by many different factors. (Here we go again, looking back to the root cause. Sometimes it takes a while to trace back to it, but it will always give you the answers you are looking for.) Read chapter 7 for more information on leaky gut and what causes it.

Metabolic endotoxemia triggers inflammation, leading to weight gain and diabetes.[22] The question remains, of course: What causes metabolic endotoxemia? Well, we already know LPS comes from the cell walls of Gram-negative bacteria, and we know that it can enter the bloodstream through a leaky gut. Blood levels of LPS are also increased when you eat a high-fat meal.[23] Very interestingly, changes in the gut bacteria, collectively known as the gut microbiota, control metabolic endotoxemia, inflammation, and associated disorders.[24] Yes, you read that correctly. The bacteria residing in your gut have been found to control the endotoxemia-induced inflammation that may result from eating a high-fat diet.

What's more, consuming probiotics (beneficial bacteria) or prebiotics (fibers that feed the gut's own beneficial bacteria) has been found in animal models to reduce the increase of metabolic endotoxemia by increasing the beneficial gut bacteria bifidobacteria, and by improving the function of the gut barrier.[25] To quote the conclusion of one study, "It would be useful to develop specific strategies for modifying gut microbiota in favor of bifidobacteria to prevent the deleterious effect of metabolic diseases."[26] Indeed, bifidobacteria have been found to improve gut barrier function and reduce LPS

TIP:

Increasing levels of bifidobacteria in the gut may help to prevent the harmful effects of insulin resistance and high blood sugar. The beneficial gut bacteria bifidobacteria help to protect the lining of the intesine by reducing leaky gut and protecting against metabolic endotoxemia, all helping to guard against the metabolic imbalances that lead to heart disease.

levels in the blood. And prebiotics have been found to reduce blood sugar levels in people with diabetes.[27]

Dietary fiber is another consideration related to the gut-heart connection. Dietary fiber helps to slow the absorption of carbohydrates, which helps regulate blood glucose levels, helping to avoid the development of insulin resistance, a known contributor to high blood pressure. It has been found that increasing the amount of dietary fiber in Western diets can help prevent the development of high blood pressure.[28] Most Americans only consume between 10 to 15 grams of fiber each day, less than half the 35 grams they should be getting.

How Sugar and Carbs Affect Blood Sugar

The main source of blood glucose is dietary carbohydrates, which come in the form of complex carbs such as whole grains, legumes, and vegetables, and simple carbs such as fruits, sugars, and sweeteners. The rise of blood glucose levels after eating depends on the source of the carbohydrate, its method of preparation, and the composition of the total meal.[29] Contrary to popular belief, the classification of a carbohydrate as simple or complex does not necessarily determine its effects on blood glucose levels.[30] Rapidly absorbed carbohydrates, which increase blood sugar and insulin levels, may be simple or complex carbs in certain cases. Taking into

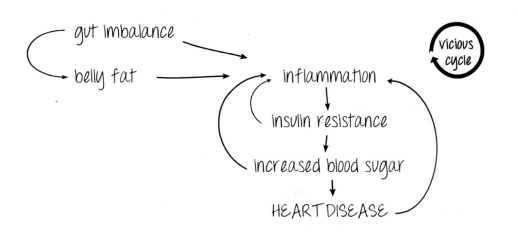

High Blood Sugar—the Devastating Health Condition My Father Faced

When most people think of high blood sugar, diabetes comes to mind. But what most people don't consider is prediabetes—a milder form of diabetes, which, along with diabetes, affects 40 percent of people over age 20. Many of these people have high blood sugar and don't even know it. This is why it is so important that I help build awareness of the devastating consequences of high blood sugar, and about how diet, weight, and lifestyle solutions for high blood sugar are crucial.

I have lost many family members, on both my mother's and father's sides, to conditions related to high blood sugar. When I was a child my grandfather and uncles even had limbs removed as a result of diabetes, and I remember thinking that it was a disease that could not be controlled. My family talked about it as if it was just fate, a way of life. They would say, "Your grandfather has diabetes and his leg will not heal." I thought it was just something that happened when you got old. It was scary. It's probably one of the reasons natural solutions appealed to me later in life. Knowing what I know now, it amazes me that people would end up amputating arms or legs from a condition that could have been prevented or even reversed!

The most important influence on my viewpoint of high blood sugar is the fact that diabetes was one of the most critical factors leading to my father's heart disease, and eventually his death. What happened to my father? Simply put, too much sugar for too long.

Until about the age of 55, my father was an alcoholic. When he quit drinking, he immediately substituted mass amounts of sugar, in the form of ice cream and other desserts, for the alcohol. By the time he turned 63, when he retired, he had gained 30 pounds and had full-blown type 2 diabetes. He was on medication, and he thought that since he took a pill to keep his blood sugar in check, he could continue to eat whatever he wanted.

Yet another doctor-promoted idea, my father thought he could consume artificial sugars (NutraSweet) without any problems. Since the doctor told him it was OK (my dad, like so many people, thought that doctors know everything), he consumed massive amounts of NutraSweet. I'll explain later why I think this was another factor contributing to his death.

After retiring, he also became more sedentary, which didn't help. About 10 years after being diagnosed with diabetes, Dad suffered a stroke. With his cardiologist (yet another doctor added to the mix), he decided to have triple bypass surgery, during which they removed the great saphenous vein in his leg to use for the artery bypass. Remember, he had diabetes, so healing his leg turned into the biggest nightmare of all. This is when it really escalated, with more doctors, and more medications.

After all this, my sisters and I hoped that the doctors and good ole dietitians would give him a healthy diet program to follow. What a joke that was! Their idea of a good diet for heart disease and diabetes was not just laughable, it was pathetic and sad.

A year later my Dad was on 17 medications and suffering more that ever. With all the medications, we had to consult with someone to determine what interactions existed between the medications. We had to figure out how to sort through the contraindications, since none of the doctors talked to each other. What a mess! It became very important for someone in the family to help keep track of all this because it was overwhelming for my dad, who placed doctors on a pedestal, never questioning their recommendations. Heaven forbid—just take the pills and hope for the best. That was his mentality.

The bottom line is he still had diabetes that could have been controlled with the proper diet and lifestyle changes. Interestingly, at this time I had entered the natural/integrative health arena. I observed all this thinking that there had to be a better way to help him. Finally, I realized that if he was going to hear my message, it had to come from—guess who?—a doctor—an integrative, holistic-minded doctor. What better messenger than that? Find out what happened next on page 122. ■

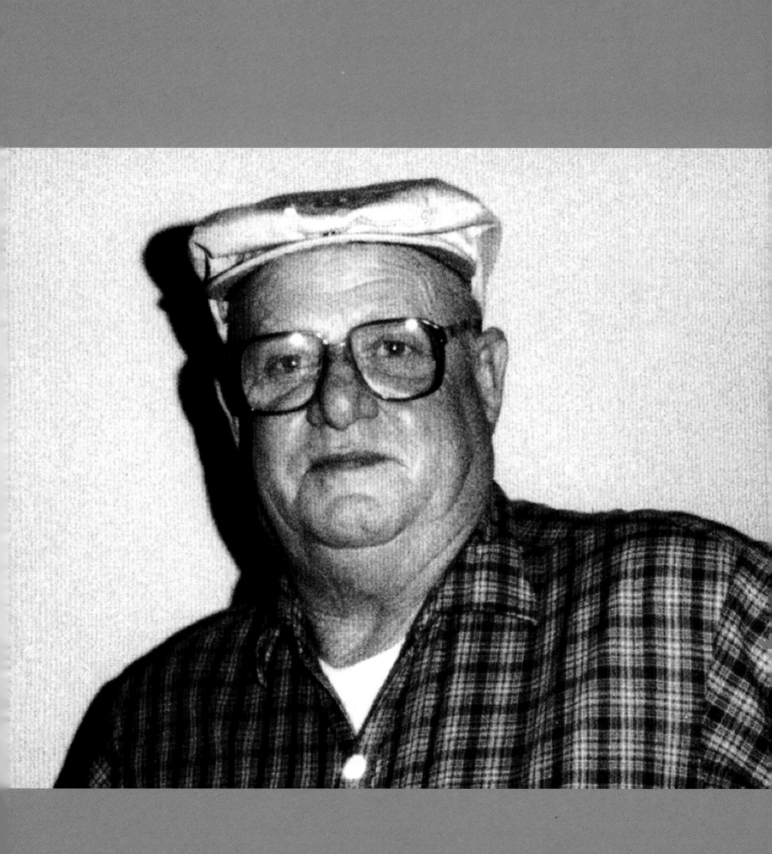

consideration the entire meal is also necessary, as dietary fat slows the absorption of glucose and dietary proteins increase the release of insulin, both helping to lower the rise of blood glucose levels after eating.[31]

Carbohydrates are broken down into sugars primarily by the digestive enzyme amylase, secreted in the mouth and the small intestine. The sugars are further broken down, if needed, into the simplest form of sugar, glucose, by disaccharidase enzymes on the lining of the small intestine. Glucose is small enough to pass through the intestinal lining into the bloodstream. This is the source of blood glucose.

Both the type and amount of dietary carbohydrate is important when considering the effects of carbohydrates on blood glucose levels.[32] Because different types of carbohydrates affect blood sugar differently, the glycemic index was created. The glycemic index is a measure of the change in blood glucose two hours after eating a carbohydrate-containing food. This value is then compared to an equivalent amount of glucose or white bread, creating a scale from 1 to 100.

A low–glycemic index diet certainly has a better effect on blood sugar levels than the Standard American Diet (SAD), but low-glycemic diets are usually still very high in carbohydrates.[33] When a low-glycemic index diet is compared to a low-carbohydrate diet in people with type 2 diabetes, blood sugar control and HDL-cholesterol levels are more greatly improved, and medication reduction or elimination is better, on the low-carbohydrate diet.[34]

When a low-carbohydrate diet was compared to the standard low-fat, high-carbohydrate diet in obese adults, after one year follow-up both groups had lost similar amounts of weight, but the diabetics in the low-carb group had more favorable effects on triglyceride levels, HDL cholesterol levels, and blood sugar control compared to the diabetics in the low-fat, high-carbohydrate diet.[35] We see from these examples (and there are many more) that following a low-carbohydrate diet has beneficial effects in people with high blood sugar.

Dietary fiber is a type of carbohydrate that is not degraded like other common forms of carbohydrate, and so it does not contribute to raised glucose levels. In fact, dietary fiber intake, particularly soluble fiber, helps to lower blood glucose and insulin levels in healthy people and in people with diabetes.[36] Further, high dietary fiber intake has been shown to help prevent the development of diabetes.[37]

Dietary fiber helps to slow the absorption of glucose, which serves to regulate blood glucose levels. Unfortunately, while experts recommend at least 35 grams of fiber daily, the Standard American Diet only averages about 10 to 15 grams of fiber per day. There is clearly a lack of dietary fiber in the diets of most people. I believe this lack of fiber is a primary reason so many people develop cardiovascular disease.

Refined and processed carbohydrates, certain vegetable starches (like potatoes), and sugars

TIP:

Dietary fiber helps slow the absorption of sugar from food, promoting healthy blood sugar levels. High dietary fiber intake helps prevent the development of both diabetes and heart disease. I recommend at least 35 grams of fiber daily.

raise blood glucose levels the most. (Notice these are all low-fiber foods.) Refined whole grain products—such as whole wheat breads, crackers, and muffins—can also raise blood sugar considerably, despite the "whole grains." The problem is that these foods are still processed, which makes them easier to break down into sugars in the digestive tract. In fact, as pointed out by William Davis, MD, two slices of whole grain bread can raise blood sugar more than two tablespoons of sugar can.[38] (See the complete interview with Dr. Davis at the end of this chapter.) Most people think they are eating healthy by choosing whole grain processed breads, crackers, and muffins, but this couldn't be further from the truth.

Standard Treatment

For most people with high blood sugar, lifestyle changes like diet and exercise are usually recommended first. When diabetes is confirmed, medications are often prescribed without giving proper attention to diet and exercise. There are several classes of medications for type 2 diabetes, each of which works to lower blood sugar. These classes include: meglitinides, sulfonylureas, dipeptidyl peptidase-4 inhibitors, biguanides, thiazolidinediones, and alpha-glucosidase inhibitors. Some of these medications come with significant side effects, which is one reason why a focus on prevention, or reversal, of diabetes is needed. If these medications are not successful at lowering blood sugar levels, insulin production by the pancreas may be greatly reduced, and insulin administration may be necessary.

Glucose Meters

In the United States alone, about 7 million people have undiagnosed diabetes. Fully 79 million more people have prediabetes. Many people have chronically elevated blood sugar and do not even realize it. Luckily, by taking control of your health, changing your diet, and exercising regularly, it is possible to completely reverse or prevent the development of diabetes.

Because so many cases of high blood sugar go unnoticed, it is imperative that you determine your blood sugar level. A glucose meter is an easy at-home finger-prick test that uses one drop of blood to assess blood glucose levels. Usually it is only recommended as a way to monitor blood sugar levels throughout the day in people already diagnosed with diabetes, but a glucose meter can be a powerful tool to help you get even mild blood sugar elevations under control, before it's too late.

Testing blood sugar with a glucose meter first thing in the morning, and again one to two hours after eating (and even again at about 5 P.M. to detect blood glucose levels after lunch is completely absorbed) provides a glimpse of how certain foods affect your blood sugar.[39] The glucose meter can serve as a tool to help you refine your diet according to how your glucose rises after certain foods. Glucose meters can be purchased over the counter or online, and are relatively inexpensive. Don't wait until you are already diagnosed with diabetes to monitor your blood glucose.

Use a glucose meter to monitor your blood sugar levels and to determine which foods raise your blood sugar. If you determine you have elevated blood glucose levels in the diabetes or prediabetes range after using the glucose meter, be sure to visit your doctor to have your blood sugar tested through a local lab to confirm these results. The glucose meter cannot be used to diagnose diabetes, but rather to monitor blood glucose levels throughout the day.

Tips For Helping Reduce High Blood Sugar
See the Love Your Heart section for a complete program to support heart health.

- Eat a diet low in grain-based, refined, and starchy carbohydrates and sugars, and high in vegetables, healthy fats, and lean proteins, nuts, and seeds.
- Increase your fiber intake.
- Exercise regularly.
- If you are overweight or obese, lose weight.
- Supplement with omega-3 fish oil and vitamin D3.
- Balance your gut with probiotics.
- Monitor your blood sugar with a glucose meter.

interview

Dr. William Davis

Brenda sits down with cardiologist and author of *Wheat Belly: Lose the Weight and Find Your Path back to Health*

BW: Dr. Davis, first I want to thank you for taking the time to do this interview. As a cardiologist, you bring an especially interesting perspective to this book. Tell me, how has your practice changed over time?

WD: Fifteen years ago I was doing what I was trained to do: lots of angioplasty, stents, atherectomies, and all that fancy stuff that helps restore blood flow. I couldn't help but realize how pointless it was to put in three stents, do an atherectomy, laser, or whatever, and the patient still comes back in six months for more procedures. Back then, no one ever asked why this was happening in the first place.

Then statin drugs came on the scene, changing the equation a bit. Doctors thought that statins would be an answer, and they were a small answer, perhaps, but the disease still persisted.

Then my own mother died of heart disease, which really made me turn the corner and ask some very serious questions. I realized that heart disease would continue unless the underlying causes were addressed.

I got involved with CT heart scanning, which is a way to "score" atherosclerotic plaque by measuring coronary calcium as an indirect means of quantifying coronary atherosclerosis. I couldn't help but start to think, "If John Smith's heart scan score is 500 (which is very high), can we stop it?" You see, if you do nothing, atherosclerotic plaque will grow at a horrifying rate of 30 percent per year. Being able to track plaque with the heart scan turned me from a doctor who tried to stop the acute event to a doctor trying to track the disease and put a stop to it, maybe even reverse it.

BW: Do you think people are missing the boat by only looking at cholesterol levels?

WD: The world is focused on cholesterol and lipids. I call that the "kindergarten version of heart disease causation." Semi-arbitrarily, cholesterol was chosen as the thing to measure to indirectly gauge the behavior of lipoproteins, the particles in the bloodstream that carry cholesterol.

You and I now have access to direct testing for lipoproteins. When you test lipoproteins and track plaque, you start to learn lessons that are entirely different from those gained by cholesterol testing. You'll learn, for instance, that carbohydrates are the incredible underlying cause for the number one cause for heart disease—the most common abnormality, which is small LDL particles. You start to realize this whole notion of reducing cholesterol is a silly notion, that if somebody reduces cholesterol in the diet, the true measures of heart disease—lipoproteins—are not reduced.

This changed my course in diet away from minding fats and cholesterol toward minding carbohydrates. So I had people remove wheat from their diets. Three months later they would come back 20 or 30 pounds lighter with no more acid reflux. Their blood sugar dropped—

both fasting and HbA1c. Small LDL dropped dramatically. And that's when we started to see much more powerful, profound control over coronary plaque growth.

BW: Your message is in line with my own: Wheat is not the healthy grain it's made out to be. What is a wheat belly?

WD: A wheat belly is the accumulation of deep visceral fat around the abdominal organs, such as the liver, intestinal tract, and kidneys, expressed on the surface as the protuberant fat that hangs over the beltline. Some call it "love handles" or a "muffin top," but I call it a "wheat belly."

I call it a wheat belly because wheat is the most extravagant trigger of visceral fat accumulation. It is the result of consuming a food, modern wheat, that increases blood sugar and, thereby, insulin to very high levels, higher than table sugar, higher than many candy bars. All you need to do is to consult a table of glycemic index and see that two slices of whole wheat bread increase blood sugar higher than sucrose, higher than a Snickers bar. Repetitive high blood sugar and insulin triggers a cascade of events that leads to insulin resistance, a common condition in which the body no longer responds to insulin. This leads to accumulation of visceral fat.

To make matters worse, modern wheat is a source of the gliadin protein that is degraded in the gastrointestinal tract to opiate-like compounds that trigger appetite. Wheat consumers eat, on average, 400 more calories per day, mostly wheat and other carbohydrates, while people who avoid wheat consume, on average, 400 calories less per day—without imposing any restriction on calories. Four hundred calories per day times 365 days per year can yield as much as 41.7 pounds per year. That's a lot of weight, and much of it gets deposited around the waistline, the wheat belly.

Conventional advice, such as that in the Dietary Guidelines for Americans that you may recognize as the USDA Food Pyramid or the new Food Plate, recommends that grains, refined and whole, serve as the biggest portion of your diet, the largest segment of the pyramid and plate. This is the advice, I believe, that has led to a nation experiencing the largest epidemic of weight gain and diabetes ever witnessed in human history.

BW: Most people have no idea that eating two slices of whole wheat bread can raise blood sugar more than 2 tablespoons of sugar can. You state that even the glycemic index of a Mars candy bar is less than that of whole wheat bread! People eat wheat bread thinking it's healthy. I see it all the time. It's a difficult viewpoint to get across, but you do it well in your book. How is it that 2 slices of whole wheat bread can raise blood sugar more than 2 tablespoons of sugar itself?

WD: Most of the carbohydrate in wheat is a form called amylopectin A. Unlike other forms of amylopectin, such as those found in beans and rice, the amylopectin A branching structure is highly and rapidly digestible by the enzyme amylase in the mouth and stomach, more than other forms of amylopectin, increasing blood sugar faster and higher than nearly all other foods.

Experiencing repetitive blood sugar highs is not good for you. Repetitive blood sugars highs are accompanied by high insulin levels; this is the process that leads to insulin resistance and visceral fat accumulation, the signature wheat belly. But there's more to it. While your primary care doctor often dismisses after-meal blood sugars as high as 190 mg/dl as harmless, they are far from it. High blood glucose provokes the process of glycation, or glucose-modification of the proteins of the body. If we glycate the proteins in the lenses of our eyes, we get cataracts. If we glycate the cartilage cells in cartilage, the cartilage becomes brittle, degrades, and leads to arthritis. If we glycate the cells lining our arteries, we get stiff arteries, hypertension, and atherosclerosis (heart attacks and stroke). In other words, glycation is a fundamental unhealthy process that underlies multiple health conditions, as well as aging. People with diabetes, who experience high blood sugars on a daily basis, age faster, die younger (eight years on average), and experience the phenomena of aging earlier in life, all from this process of glycation.

Any food consumed repeatedly that increases blood sugar to high levels will add to this irreversible process of glycation. Eating more "healthy whole grains" is one such repetitive process, since most people do so several times per day, seven days a week. Glycate the various proteins of your body and a host of health conditions develop, as well as accelerated aging.

Modern wheat no more resembles the wheat of Moses than a chimpanzee resembles a human—in fact, a chimpanzee is closer to a human than modern wheat is to ancient wheat.

"Modern wheat is not the product of genetic modification; it is the product of genetic manipulations that are far worse: cruder, less precise, and sometimes downright bizarre."

BW: You've done a lot of research into the origins of wheat, and the hybridizations that have occurred since wheat was first cultivated. How is the wheat we eat today different from the wheat of even 100 years ago?

WD: This is an absolutely crucial point: The wheat you are sold today as bread, rolls, bagels, and ciabattas is nothing like the wheat of our mothers' age, very different from the wheat of the early twentieth century, and nothing like the wheat of the Bible.

The wheat of the Bible, for instance, is emmer wheat, a wild-growing, 4½-foot-tall, 28-chromosome plant. Modern wheat is a 2-foot tall, short, stocky plant with an unusually large seed head, and 42 chromosomes.

People are concerned about the process of genetic modification or genetic engineering. Modern wheat is not the product of genetic modification; it is the product of genetic manipulations that are far worse: cruder, less precise, and sometimes downright bizarre. Modern wheat is the product of extensive hybridizations—i.e., crossing two strains repeatedly to winnow out certain genetic qualities such as reduced height and tolerance to drought, crossing with non-wheat grasses to introduce unique genes, and techniques like chemical, gamma ray, and high-dose x-ray irradiation of wheat seeds and embryos to induce mutations, a process called chemical or radiation mutagenesis. Clearfield wheat, for instance, now grown on nearly 1 million acres in the Pacific Northwest and marketed by the

BASF Corporation (the world's largest chemical manufacturer), was created in the genetics laboratory by exposing wheat seeds and embryos to the mutation-inducing industrial toxin sodium azide, poisonous to humans and known to explode when mishandled (like pouring down a sink). Incidentally, in the marketing for Clearfield wheat, BASF claims that Clearfield wheat is not the product of genetic modification, but the product of "traditional breeding methods." In fact, much of the wheat industry has been hiding behind

code of modern industrial wheat underlie the quadrupling of celiac disease witnessed over the past 40 years. Humans haven't changed; the wheat has changed.

Some defenders of modern wheat ask, "Isn't gluten still just gluten?" So what if a handful or a few dozen amino acids in gluten are shuffled around? It's still gluten, isn't it, the protein that allows wheat to become dough with its unique viscoelastic properties that allows the pizza maker to toss his dough in the air to mold into

"I've witnessed an incredible range of conditions reverse with removal of all wheat, the majority of which I did not expect."

this phrase, "traditional breeding methods," and "no genetic modification" as a smokescreen to conceal the extreme genetic changes introduced into the plant.

Among the many changes introduced into the modern, high-yield, two-foot-tall semi-dwarf strains of wheat that now dominate the wheat market are alterations in the amino acid structure of the gluten proteins. Celiac disease researchers have proposed that these changes in the genetic and biochemical

pizza? The nature of immune responses is based on just such small changes in protein structure, and a few amino acids is more than enough to amplify or reduce immune and inflammatory responses in susceptible individuals. Changes in gluten structure may also explain the recently described increases in inflammatory and autoimmune conditions like rheumatoid arthritis, inflammatory bowel diseases (ulcerative colitis and Crohn's disease), and even type 1 diabetes in children.

BW: I am particularly interested in the gluten proteins in wheat and similar grains because they trigger celiac disease and gluten sensitivity. I have found that many people with difficult-to-treat health conditions have underlying gluten sensitivity, a condition not well recognized by mainstream medicine, but one that is thought to be a possible precursor to celiac. Are you aware of gluten sensitivity and how it can be detected through blood and stool tests?

WD: Let me first make the point that gluten sensitivity is only one aspect of adverse reactions to modern wheat. There are other components of wheat that have nothing to do with gluten that can still exert undesirable, sometimes devastating, health effects on humans. What I am advocating is not gluten elimination for the gluten sensitive. I am advocating wheat elimination for everybody.

Nonetheless, reactions to gluten, "gluten sensitivity," can of course be expressed as celiac disease. This can be identified by measuring high levels of antibodies in the bloodstream, such as anti-gliadin antibodies, and transglutaminase and endomysial antibodies. Other practitioners advocate salivary gliadin antibodies (not as reliable) or recovery of antibodies in stool (probably more reliable). Most gastroenterologists diagnose celiac disease with biopsy of the small intestine (which I do not advocate).

However, there is a growing appreciation that reactions to gluten can occur in people without

any of these tests proving positive. Inherited genes that predispose to this situation, such as variants of HLA-DQ2 and HLA-DQ8, for instance, can account for reactions to gluten but with negative gliadin, transglutaminase, and endomysial antibodies, and negative biopsy. Unfortunately, people who have negative antibody tests are often dismissed as having "irritable bowel syndrome" or some other condition, when it is truly some reaction to wheat, such as gluten sensitivity.

Not having an antibody or genetic marker prove positive does not necessarily mean that the reaction is benign or harmless. I've seen life-threatening levels of wheat and gluten sensitivity, such as colon hemorrhage, recede and disappear with removal of wheat and gluten in people with all negative blood markers and negative intestinal biopsies. At present, the most confident way to identify wheat and gluten sensitivity, however, is not stool examination, biopsy, antibody tests, salivary tests, or even HLA tests, but complete removal of wheat and gluten.

BW: You have put more than 2,000 patients on a wheat-free diet. Have you seen conditions other than those related to heart disease risk improve?

WD: I've witnessed an incredible range of conditions reverse with removal of all wheat, the majority of which I did not expect. Even today, I am still learning new lessons on what happens when you remove all wheat.

Nearly everybody who eliminates wheat reports a reduction in hunger. The rolling, rumbling hunger that commonly occurs two hours after, say, a bowl of Shredded Wheat cereal that makes snacking necessary, and again and again in two-hour cycles, all goes away. Instead, people who eat a wheat-free breakfast at, say, 7 A.M., are satisfied until noon, or are not hungry at all. Hunger also feels different, more of a soft reminder that eating something might be a good idea, not the sharp and even painful hunger of wheat consumption.

Among the most common experiences is complete relief from the common gastrointestinal conditions of acid reflux and the cramps and diarrhea of irritable bowel syndrome. People with inflammatory bowel diseases, Crohn's disease and ulcerative colitis, report fewer flare-ups, much reduced symptoms like diarrhea and cramps, and many are able to reduce or stop medications.

By the way, relevant to the probiotic world, it is my suspicion that wheat consumption is associated with marked shifts in intestinal bacteria type and quantity, followed by pancreatic dysfunction; removal of wheat corrects these phenomena in most people, but I suspect there are people who have suffered so much intestinal damage that further steps, such as probiotics and pancreatic enzymes, are required to make a full recovery of bowel health.

Relief from arthritis and joint pain is also very common. The most responsive form of joint pain is that in the fingers and hands, followed by other joints. Leg swelling—i.e., edema—also commonly improves or resolves entirely. People who have inflammatory arthritis conditions such as rheumatoid arthritis report fewer joint pain and swelling, and are frequently able to reduce medications with fewer flare-ups.

In the area of mood and mind function, improved energy and fewer mood swings, along with improved sleep, are frequent experiences. Although variable, I've witnessed dramatic improvement in people who have been diagnosed with bipolar illness, depression, anxiety disorders, and other behavioral conditions; typically, symptoms are improved markedly, occasionally completely. Migraine headaches can be dramatically improved; I've witnessed several people who, having suffered headaches nearly daily for decades, obtain total relief within 72 hours of stopping wheat.

There are benefits that are magnified by the weight loss that results from wheat elimination. People who lose, say, 30 pounds and three inches from their waist experience even greater relief from joint pain, especially from the knees, and further improvement in energy and mood.

BW: Your message is similar to mine; what is needed is not simply the removal of refined sugars from the diet, but also refined carbohydrates like those found in breads, pastas, cereals, etc. Cutting out only refined sugars is not enough. Your patients have responded very well to a wheat-free diet. Explain what improvements you've seen.

WD: I agree: Removing sugars from the diet is only part of the solution.

People often regard sugars as the primary problem and "healthy whole grains" as part of the solution. Let me tell you what I see. When people eliminate wheat from their lives, it means they've eliminated the gliadin protein that drives appetite. People then lose their desire for sweets and can pass them up without difficulty. And, usually after a few weeks to months, most people experience a heightened sensitivity to the sensation of sweetness, and sweets start to taste sickeningly sweet. Avoiding or minimizing them then becomes easy.

in the exorphins. I know about exorphins from my research into the effects of gluten on autistic children. Tell us how exorphins are keeping us addicted to wheat.

WD: No other food exerts addictive properties on us like wheat.

The gliadin protein unique to wheat is degraded in the human gastrointestinal tract to small polypeptides (proteins) that have the unique capacity to bind to the human brain and exert peculiar effects. In children with ADHD and autism, it provokes behavioral outbursts, inattention, and other behavioral problems, while in people with schizophrenia

"No other food exerts addictive properties on us like wheat."

So avoiding sweets does not eliminate the real cause of the problem. Eliminating wheat eliminates the cause and is followed by unexpected improvements in appetite control, impulsiveness, and food choice.

BW: One main hurdle to overcome when taking wheat out of the diet is the addictive properties of wheat. This is also one good reason why wheat is making us fat. The addictive properties you mention are found

it provokes auditory hallucinations (hearing voices) and social detachment. It can also provoke the manic phase of bipolar illness. In people with binge eating disorder, it provokes binges—i.e., eating, eating, and eating—far beyond physiologic need, typically followed by a "purge." In people without behavioral disorders, however, it provokes appetite.

Make no mistake: The food industry knows this. It explains why you will find wheat flour or other wheat-derived products in nearly every processed food on the shelves. Is wheat flour really necessary in Campbell's tomato soup or Twizzlers? Putting wheat flour into anything and everything has become a useful way for the food industry to increase revenues. Inclusion of wheat increases calorie consumption, on average, 400 calories per day. Let's do some arithmetic: 400 calories per day times 365 days

But there's only one food that yields substantial quantities of opiate-like compounds that needs to be blocked: wheat.

So we have the odd situation of the food industry feeding us wheat products at every turn to stimulate appetite, while we have a drug industry coming to our rescue. Or we can avoid the whole mess and eliminate wheat.

"I would estimate that, of a hundred people on a statin drug, maybe three need it."

per year times 300 million Americans . . . that's a lot of food; that's a lot of money.

Removal of wheat results in reduced calorie intake of 400 calories per day. This develops even in people who are not instructed in limiting any other calories. In other words, even if we were to say "eliminate wheat but it's okay to eat ice cream and candy, provided it contains no wheat," calorie consumption still goes down

One way to eliminate the addictive properties of wheat is to eliminate wheat, of course. Another way is to take an opiate-blocking drug such as naltrexone. And, in fact, a drug company recently applied to the FDA for use of naltrexone for weight loss; in their clinical trials, participants lost 22 pounds in 6 months.

BW: I especially found interesting the fact that the same drug used to block the action of heroin in the bodies of drug addicts also blocks the binding of exorphins to the brain. Think about how many people crave carbs. This is part of the reason. How do your patients get over this craving?

WD: It requires removal of all things wheat in the diet. This process of removal is accompanied by a withdrawal syndrome in about a third of the people who do this. As you'd expect with any withdrawal from an opiate-like compound, such as wheat gliadin–derived exorphins, people can experience marked fatigue, mental "fog," occasionally depression. Thankfully, the process rarely lasts more than five days and is physically harmless. People emerge on the other side of their withdrawal with renewed energy, faster weight loss, and improved sense of well-being.

Removing wheat removes carbohydrate cravings. Cutting back carbohydrates without entirely removing wheat, by the way, does not work very well. This is a common reason for low-carbohydrate diets to fail or to yield unsatisfactory results. Someone cuts carbs but maintains a modest intake of "healthy whole grains," since we are bombarded with this message every day. As a result, they cannot control appetite or impulse, and they fail to achieve weight loss goals. As long as wheat is still in the picture, losing weight and controlling appetite is impossible for most people.

BW: Do you think anyone benefits from taking a statin drug?

WD: I would estimate that, of a hundred people on a statin drug, maybe three need it. There are genetically determined abnormalities where people really do benefit from statin drugs, such as familial heterozygous hypercholesterolemia, in which people have extremely high LDLs and tend to get heart disease at a young age. Also, some people with the gene known as ApoE4 need to take statins.

People with the ApoE4 gene are incredibly efficient at survival in the wild: They're resistant to malaria and other tropical infections, and they tolerate periods of starvation very well. Put them in a modern environment, with overexposure

to processed foods, and they are efficient at absorbing many dietary components. Twenty-five percent of ApoE4 people overabsorb dietary cholesterol and fats. They tend to have higher LDL and total cholesterol levels.

ApoE4 people also have increased carbohydrate sensitivity. The way I look at it is that the ApoE4 person is carbohydrate sensitive, but the abnormalities are magnified by fat intake. So that person should be, first of all, low carbohydrate; second of all, somewhat limited in fat exposure.

But the conventional notion of ApoE4 is: Cut the fat. These people become diabetic. Their bellies grow. They get hypertensive. They get small LDL. They get all the phenomena we see from carbohydrate overconsumption.

Statin drugs treat high LDL cholesterol, a value that is not actually measured—it's calculated. It's a calculated LDL value from something called the "Friedewald equation," based on observations made in the 1960s. I call it fictitious LDL; 27 billion dollars a year in statin prescriptions for a fictitious number. What if the equation is deeply flawed? What if the assumptions built in the equation are deeply flawed because they come from 1963 technology and understanding? Fictitious LDL has very little resemblance to genuine numbers when you do real testing, such as lipoprotein testing.

BW: In this book, I talk about the role of the gut in relation to the development of heart disease. Certainly, because all food is absorbed through the gut, food is one main gut connection to heart disease. I also talk about how gut dysfunction contributes to inflammation, which affects most all of the factors contributing to heart disease. There is a gut connection to it all. Whether it's from an imbalance in the gut bacteria, intestinal permeability, constipation, poor digestion of food, or any of the many digestive disorders, they all affect what enters our body. Do you find digestion improves in patients on a wheat-free diet?

WD: Absolutely. In addition to relief from acid reflux and irritable bowel symptoms, people report improved bowel regularity and the notion of needing wheat fibers disappears. Nutrient absorption is also improved. It is not uncommon that, upon eliminating wheat, vitamin B12, folate, and zinc levels increase without supplementation. Note that at least some of the fortification required for wheat products may be due to the impaired bowel health from wheat consumption.

I worry about the people who, on eliminating wheat, experience improvement but are left with a residual bowel problem, such as some continued symptoms. These are people I suspect have managed to do damage to their small intestine that provides the signals for pancreatic enzyme production, or have caused disruption in the intestinal bacterial type and number (e.g., bacterial overgrowth). I have limited experience in this area, but I suspect these are the people who should seriously consider probiotics, prebiotics, and pancreatic enzyme supplementation.

BW: Do you think wheat is the only refined carbohydrate implicated in leading to obesity, or do you focus on wheat because it's so widely consumed? I ask this because what I see is more and more people substituting wheat breads, muffins, and cakes with wheat-free breads, muffins, and cakes. But since these are still refined grains, and still break down quickly to sugar in the body, it seems like we're trading one bad thing for another. Would you agree?

WD: Yes, absolutely.

We don't want to eliminate wheat but substitute the lost calories with jellybeans and soft drinks. But that's the mistake many people make when they substitute wheat products with gluten-free products. Most gluten-free products, such as gluten-free multigrain bread, are made with cornstarch, rice starch, tapioca starch, or potato starch. These dried starches are among the very few foods that increase blood sugar higher than even wheat! They are terrible for metabolism, leading to insulin resistance that leads to diabetes, and add to visceral fat accumulation. (Gluten-free belly?)

Beyond the generally awful gluten-free processed foods now sold, carbohydrates in general have become a major problem in the American diet. Eliminating wheat eliminates the worst of the worst in the form of carbohydrates, since eliminating wheat eliminates gliadin, which stimulates appetite. Lose the wheat, appetite drops. Many people do just fine just by doing so, while concentrating on eating real, healthy foods like nuts, eggs, cheeses, vegetables, etc. However, so many Americans are diabetic or prediabetic, overweight or obese, that a full unraveling of the metabolic mess created will occur faster and more effectively with cutting back other carbohydrates as well.

This is an individual issue. A slender, athletic 30-year-old woman already at ideal weight with no blood sugar issues, for instance, may experience improved intestinal and joint health by eliminating wheat but is otherwise fine just following a healthy diet. But a 60-year-old, 295-pound obese male on the verge of converting from prediabetes to diabetes will do better with a reduction in total carbohydrates along with wheat elimination to facilitate weight loss and reduction in high blood sugar and insulin resistance. For someone like this, overall carbohydrate restriction, even of foods that are ordinarily considered healthy, such as fruit and non-wheat grains like millet and quinoa, is very helpful and is most likely to yield benefits like full reversal of excess weight and prediabetes.

BW: Why do so many people believe the low-fat/high-carbohydrate diet is a heart-healthy diet?

WD: If you go from eating a standard American diet of fast food burgers and French fries to a low-fat/high-carbohydrate diet, the arteries will relax, showing an apparent improvement in blood flow. You may even lose a few pounds at first. Basically, you are going from a poor diet to a better diet, so you will see some improvement in endothelial normalization and other measures, sure, but it does not mean that diet is the best diet. Low-fat, high-carbohydrate diets eventually yield undesirable effects, such as a drop in HDL cholesterol, a rise in triglycerides, and prediabetic blood sugar levels.

BW: My viewpoint is that we should be getting our carbs from plenty of vegetables. That way, not only do we get a huge array of phytonutrients, but the fiber found in vegetables helps break down the carbs slowly, helping to regulate blood sugar. From what I've learned, this diet leads down the pathway to health—lean proteins, healthy fats, and plenty of vegetables. You have put many patients on a similar diet. How successful has this been for regulating heart disease risk, especially weight loss?

WD: I agree: Vegetables should be the cornerstone of a truly healthy diet. This dietary approach is exceptionally effective in correcting the causes of heart disease.

Unfortunately, most people will not see the degree of metabolic improvement that develops from this diet because they make the crucial mistake of allowing their doctor to rely on misleading cholesterol, or lipid, testing. I call this the "kindergarten version" of assessing heart disease risk. The "college version," the more advanced level of testing, or lipoprotein testing (I use NMR lipoprotein testing offered by Liposcience, Inc.), reveals

"I now advocate total wheat elimination not just for gluten-sensitive or overweight people, but for everybody."

the full extent of metabolic transformation. It will show, for instance, that this diet causes small LDL particles—the number one cause for heart disease in the United States, not "high cholesterol"—to plummet. Along with reduction in small LDL, triglycerides drop dramatically and HDL ("good") cholesterol goes up. Because many, if not most, people reduce or entirely reverse insulin resistance, prediabetic or diabetic patterns, and inflammatory markers like C-reactive protein, risk for heart disease is markedly reduced.

Note that this approach is essentially the opposite of that advised by "official" agencies, i.e., cut your fat, cholesterol, and eat more "healthy whole grains." The diet advised for people to follow after heart attack, for instance, makes the situation worse, not better. I restrict fats only for people who buy conventionally raised, "factory farm" meats, not if they are purchasing free-range organic meats, as well as in some genetically determined exceptions (e.g., ApoE4 genetic type).

In my heart disease prevention practice (I converted my practice from an angioplasty and stent practice to a preventive practice,

since there is nearly no need for heart procedures in my practice anymore), I rarely see heart attacks. In fact, heart attacks only occur in the noncompliant, disinterested, or people who I've just met who haven't yet had sufficient time to follow this diet. An essential part of the transformation from high-risk for heart disease to low- or no-risk is weight loss. This diet approach is wonderfully effective for achieving weight loss, especially from the "wheat belly," the metabolically active fat that surrounds the abdominal organs. Loss of two to three inches just in the first few weeks of following this dietary approach is common.

BW: Eating a diet high in wheat results in high blood sugar, high insulin, high triglycerides, more small dense LDL cholesterol, expanding waistline, high blood pressure even—it's amazing more people don't realize all this. We are faced with aisles upon aisles of wheat at the supermarket, thinking the foods we put into our basket are healthy because they contain whole grains. What inspired you to go head-to-head with wheat, educating the public about its dangers?

WD: Yes, exactly: Wheat consumption makes the situation far worse, not better.

Just the simple fact that two slices of whole wheat bread raise blood sugar higher than table sugar and many candy bars, all plain as day for everyone to see in tables of glycemic index, was enough to get me started on asking people to eliminate wheat. But those who did so experienced such an incredible spectrum of other health benefits and weight loss that it spurred me on to apply this approach to a broader population. Once I witnessed the spectacular health transformations occur, there was no turning back. I now advocate total wheat elimination not just for gluten-sensitive or overweight people, but for everybody.

BW: **What about non-wheat grains? Are those healthy?**

WD: Putting aside the issue of gluten in rye, barley, and bulgar, non-wheat grains don't have the gliadin protein of wheat, they don't have the lectins that disrupt intestinal barriers, and they don't have the amylopectin A that is responsible for the extravagant high blood sugars of wheat, but they still have carbohydrates. So if I overconsume, say, millet bread, or a dish made of quinoa, I'm going to have high blood sugar.

BW: **What else do you recommend for heart-health support?**

WD: In addition to diet and exercise, I recommend omega-3 fish oils and I recommend normalizing vitamin D levels. I also recommend that people monitor blood sugar levels with a glucose meter. Pre-meal and one hour post-meal tests will give you a good idea of what your peak blood sugar levels are after eating. I actually recommend looking for no change. For example, if your pre-meal blood sugar level is 90, then you want to aim for a one-hour post-meal blood sugar level of 90. If you go from 90 to 140, find out what food did it and get rid of the food, or cut the portion size.

This is particularly helpful in people who can't seem to lose weight no matter what they do. They finally lose weight because they aren't triggering insulin, which is triggered by blood sugar. They begin to mobilize fat instead of storing it. They also begin to see changes in metabolic patterns, such as a rise in HDL levels, reduction in HbA1c blood glucose, reductions in small LDL, and reductions in triglycerides. That little trick is extremely effective for managing metabolic distortions.

BW: **Thank you so much, Dr. Davis, for talking to me about how wheat plays a major role in the development of cardiovascular disease. It is inspiring to see a mainstream medical doctor taking much more than the standard cookie-cutter approach to medicine. You are at the cutting edge of medicine. We will all stand around ten years from now saying, "I told you so." In fact, we even do that today as more and more science supports our message. Thanks again.**

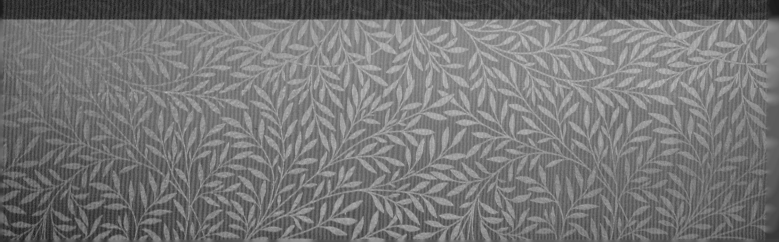

"Healthy citizens are the greatest asset any country can have."

—Winston S. Churchill

Chapter 5
The Fattening of America

Obesity rates in the United States are so high and have increased so much since 1980 that obesity is now considered an epidemic. More than one-third of U.S. adults and 17 percent of U.S. children are obese.[1] From 1980 to 2008 obesity rates for adults doubled, and for children tripled. In addition to this, 34 percent more of U.S. adults are overweight but not yet obese. That means two-thirds of U.S. adults are overweight or obese. This is truly an epidemic.

Obesity refers to an excessive amount of body fat, and overweight is the state of being over normal weight, but not yet obese. Obesity is measured using the body mass index (BMI) calculation: weight (in kilograms) divided by height (in meters) squared. Categories of obesity and overweight as calculated with BMI follow.

BMI	Weight Status
< 18.5	Underweight
18.5–24.9	Normal
25.0–29.9	Overweight
30.0–30.9	Obese
> 40.0	Extreme obesity

Similar to the categories developed for high cholesterol, high blood pressure, and high blood sugar, the BMI range for overweight has been lowered from over 27.3 for women and over 27.8 for men, to 25 or more for both men and women. Further, a study published in 2001 found that people with a BMI in the upper range of normal (22.0 to 24.9) were still at increased risk of developing chronic diseases, suggesting that adults should try to maintain a BMI between 18.5 and 21.9 to minimize their risk.[2]

BMI is not a direct measure of fat, however, so it may not always represent an accurate picture of obesity. BMI underestimates fat percentage in people with less muscle mass, and overestimates fat percentage in people with high muscle mass. At a similar BMI, women have more body fat than men.[3] Further, BMI alone is not the most reliable measure to determine risk for obesity-related diseases such as heart disease.[4]

Myth:

A little meat on your
bones is healthy.

_____

Fact:

Even people who are overweight, but not obese, are at increased risk of heart disease.

_____

For these reasons, two other measures are available: waist circumference and waist-to-hip ratio. Waist circumference, as the name indicates, measures the circumference of the waist. With a measuring tape, waist circumference is measured just above the hip bone, while the belly is relaxed. Patients are asked to exhale during measurement to achieve the most accurate measure. Risk categories based on waist circumference follow.

High-Risk Waist Circumference

Men: Waist circumference > 40 inches
Women: Waist circumference > 35 inches

Waist-to-hip ratio measures the waist about one inch above the navel, and the hips at the widest portion of the buttocks. These measures are calculated to identify people with "apple-shaped" bodies, who accumulate abdominal fat and are at increased health risk compared to people who accumulate fat around the hips, characteristic of "pear-shaped" bodies. Waist-to-hip ratio can be useful, but it may be misleading, because it can identify both an obese and a lean person with the same ratio. Risk categories based on waist-to-hip ratio follow.

High-Risk Waist-to-Hip Ratio

Men: > .90
Women: > .80

Measuring waist circumference is now regarded as a reliable measure of accumulated abdominal fat, and, thus, risk for obesity-related diseases. It is also the easiest to obtain, requiring only a tape measure and no calculations. Although use of BMI has traditionally been the standard measure for obesity, additional measurement of waist circumference and waist-to-hip ratio gives a better picture of overall health risk.[5,6,7,8]

Obesity and Heart Disease

Obese individuals are more likely to develop a number of health problems, including high cholesterol and triglycerides, type 2 diabetes, high blood pressure, metabolic syndrome, heart disease, stroke, cancer, sleep apnea, depression, gallbladder disease, infertility, non-alcoholic fatty liver disease, osteoarthritis, and skin problems, to name just a few. Notice how many of these conditions are related to heart disease. Obesity on its own is a major risk factor for the development of heart disease,[9] and as we see here, it is also related to many other risk factors for heart disease. Prevention of heart disease should begin by addressing obesity and excess weight.

Disorders Associated with Obesity:[10]

- Asthma
- Breathing difficulties
- Cancer
- Complications of pregnancy
- Coronary heart disease
- Dyslipidemia
- Elevated insulin
- Gallbladder disease
- High blood pressure

- Increased surgical risk
- Insulin resistance
- Menstrual irregularities
- Osteoarthritis
- Premature death
- Psychological distress
- Sleep apnea
- Stroke
- Type 2 diabetes

Obesity—Let's Break It Down

We know that obesity is the accumulation of body fat. Now let's look at what drives this fat accumulation. The conventional thought on fat accumulation is that it is the result of an imbalance between the amount of energy consumed (as food) and energy exerted (as physical activity). This idea becomes complicated when we factor in type of diet, hormonal influences, certain medical conditions and medications, age, environmental toxins, and even gut function. All of these factors can affect metabolism, complicating the "calories in, calories out" equation.

Traditionally, body fat was thought to be simply a storehouse for triglycerides, the storage unit of fat. It is now understood, however, that fat tissue, or adipose tissue, is an endocrine organ that plays a major role in metabolism.[11] Fat tissue secretes a variety of molecules, known as adipokines, which send signals to distant systems of the body. Fat cells also contain receptors that receive signals from different systems of the body. Together these functions classify fat tissue, or adipose tissue, as an organ.

Of the many molecules secreted by fat tissue—most being inflammatory in nature—one stands out as a beneficial adipokine: adiponectin. Adiponectin regulates insulin sensitivity and fat oxidation, and may even lower the risk of heart attack.[12] Levels of adiponectin are lowered in obese people, while inflammatory adipokines, such as TNF-alpha and interleukin-6 (IL-6), are raised.

Location of body fat determines its effect on metabolism. Abdominal fat, also known as visceral adipose tissue (VAT), is considered the most metabolically active of all body fat. This explains why people who have accumulated belly fat are most at risk for metabolic diseases. If you have VAT, you are at higher risk of developing insulin resistance, high blood sugar, blood lipid abnormalities, high blood pressure,

Body fat is now considered an organ.

blood clotting, and systemic inflammation,[13] all risk factors for heart disease.

The Role of Inflammation

Obesity is associated with chronic, low-grade inflammation, much of which is triggered by the fat cells themselves. Many of the adipokines and immune cells found in fat tissue produce inflammation.[14] In an intricate web of inflammation, insulin resistance, and fatness (or VATness, if you will)—each fueling the other in a vicious cycle—metabolic abnormalities arise, leading to heart disease.[15] For more information on insulin resistance, see chapter 4.

Inflammation initiates atherosclerosis, as well as plays a role throughout the entire atherosclerotic process. One example of this is seen in people with inflammatory conditions such as rheumatoid arthritis and lupus, who are more likely to have atherosclerosis than healthy individuals.[16] Further, systemic inflammation resulting from infections such as periodontal disease is also associated with increased risk of cardiovascular disease.[17] The gut also contributes to systemic inflammation.[18]

Another important factor contributing to systemic inflammation is the ratio of omega-6 to omega-3 fatty acid in the body. Omega-3 and omega-6 fatty acids are considered essential because the body cannot produce them on its own—they must be obtained from the diet. The ideal omega-6/omegas-3 ratio is anywhere from 1:1 (closer to what our primitive hunter-gatherer ancestors ate) up to 4:1. Western diets are deficient in omega-3 fatty acids, however, yielding a ratio more like 15:1 (high omega-6 and low omega-3).[19]

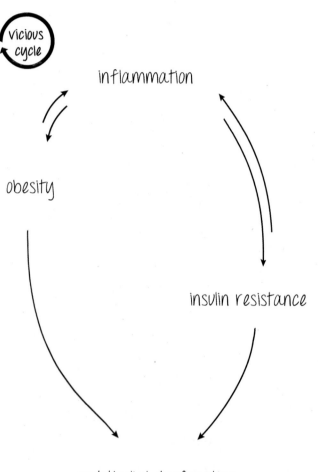

Both omega-3 and omega-6 are essential to life, but too much omega-6 increases inflammation in the body. As a general rule, omega-6 fatty acids increase inflammation and omega-3 fatty acids decrease inflammation.[20] The omega-3 to omega-6 imbalance created by the Standard American Diet is a major contributor to inflammation in the body. A diet high in oily fish, or a high-quality omega-3 fish oil supplement, can help improve the ratio of omega-3 to omega-6.

Studies have found that higher prenatal fish and omega-3 intake in pregnant women is associated with decreased obesity rates during early childhood.[21] Omega-3 fatty acids are particularly beneficial during prenatal development and childhood. These studies illustrate the influence of nutrition as early as in the womb. See chapter 15 in the Love Your Heart section for more information on omega-3s.

HEART DISEASE

Similar to the inflammation associated with other risk factors of heart disease such as high cholesterol, high blood pressure, and high blood sugar, high blood levels of the inflammation marker high-sensitivity C-reactive protein (hs-CRP) are found in obese people (and these levels are reversed with weight loss), suggesting a web of metabolic abnormalities with inflammation found throughout.[22] Even in young adults, being overweight or obese was found to be associated with elevated levels of hs-CRP, suggesting a state of low-grade systemic inflammation in these people.[23] For more information on inflammation, see chapter 6.

Weight loss is the best way to reduce the systemic inflammation triggered by fat. Whether by diet, exercise, or even surgery, all methods of weight loss have been found to reduce systemic inflammation.[24] Indeed,

Western diets are deficient in omega-3 fatty acids.

weight loss in obese people can improve or prevent many of the obesity-related risk factors for heart disease.[25]

We know that accumulation of belly fat is a trigger of inflammation involved in heart disease, but keeping in line with the nature of looking for the root cause of heart disease, we must ask the question: Why does belly fat trigger inflammation? For a possible answer, we can look to the gut.

Gut Connection to Obesity

Due to the considerable number of gut bacteria, and their ability to ferment nutrients and produce biologically active compounds, the gut microbiota affect the metabolism of the host (the human or animal in which the bacteria reside), particularly when it comes to obesity and metabolic disorders.[26] The first studies to uncover this gut connection have found that bacterial diversity is decreased, the number of gut bacteria in the Firmicutes phylum (a bacterial taxonomic category) is increased, and the number in the Bacteroidetes phylum is reduced in obese mice and humans, compared to lean individuals.[27,28,29] In these studies, weight loss was found to reverse the changes in gut microbiota to that of lean individuals.

Obesity-related gut bacteria are able to harvest more energy from food than are the gut bacteria of their lean counterparts.[30] This was discovered when lean mice were colonized with gut bacteria from obese mice, and rapidly gained weight within the next 10 to 14 days despite a decrease in food consumption.[31] This is thought to occur due to increased harvest of and absorption of monosaccharides and short-chain fatty acids produced during the bacterial fermentation of nondigestible carbohydrates by the obese gut bacteria, their conversion to fats in the liver, and to microbial influences on genes that regulate fat accumulation.

A main question about this gut-obesity connection is: Which comes first, the obesity or the gut imbalance? One study involving children found that a change in the gut microbiota preceded weight gain.[32] Numbers of gut bacteria of the genus *Bifidobacterium* were found to be higher during infancy in children who remained normal weight at seven years compared to overweight children. This study suggests that high numbers of *Bifidobacterium* during infancy are protective against becoming overweight. Indeed, bifidobacteria are the most prevalent gut bacteria in healthy, breastfed infants.[33] And the likelihood of being overweight or obese during childhood has been found to be 13 to 22 percent lower in those children who were breastfed during infancy.[34] Further, overweight pregnant women have been found to have lower numbers of bifidobacteria than normal-weight women.[35] And overweight mothers give birth to infants with lower numbers of bifidobacteria, suggesting the obesity-related microbiota is inheritable.[36]

Another study highlighting the gut origin of inflammation in obesity involved 120 pregnant women.[37] Of these women, concentrations of bacterial toxins, or endotoxins, in the blood were twice as high as in lean pregnant women. The high endotoxin levels were associated with increased inflammation in fat tissue, and an increase in C-reactive protein and interleukin-6 levels, both markers of inflammation. This study demonstrates that low-grade endotoxemia (bacterial toxins in the blood) is associated with low-grade inflammation in fat cells of obese women. The researchers of this study suggest that bacterial pathogens contribute to this inflammation found in fat tissue. Thus, the gut connection to obesity.

Bacterial toxins enter the bloodstream through an increase in intestinal permeability, a condition known as leaky gut. This is how gut bacteria can contribute to systemic inflammation: by entering the bloodstream through a leaky gut. Indeed, even in healthy people, increases in intestinal permeability have been found to be associated with increased abdominal and liver fat, suggesting the gut is the source of excess belly fat and metabolic dysfunction.[38]

Most people know someone (or are that someone) who very carefully counts calories but cannot seem to lose weight at the same rate as other people.

Administration of probiotics has been suggested as a way to modify the harmful metabolic effects of imbalanced gut flora, a condition known as dysbiosis. In one study, the probiotic *Lactobacillus acidophilus* was found to prevent a loss of insulin sensitivity after endotoxin injection in people with diabetes or glucose intolerance compared to a placebo group.[39] In another probiotic study, *Lactobacillus gasseri* was found to reduce body weight, BMI, waist and hip circumference, and abdominal and subcutaneous fat in overweight or obese individuals compared to those receiving a placebo.[40] More studies investigating the beneficial effects of probiotics on obesity are under way. See chapter 15 in the Love Your Heart section for more information on the benefits of probiotics.

How Sugar and Carbs Affect Obesity

Evolutionarily, humans have consumed a diet high in omega-3 fatty acids, vitamins, minerals, phytonutrients, and fiber, all from whole foods. With the advent of agriculture, the diet became more grain-based but was still high in whole foods. With the Industrial Revolution, the diet has shifted to processed, grain-based foods, refined sugars, and flours, and is now low in phytonutrients, omega-3 fats, and fiber. The result of this change in diet has been an increase in obesity, now reaching epidemic proportions.

Body fat accumulation is established by the balance between lipogenesis (the construction and storage of fat molecules in the body) and lipolysis (the breakdown of fats). Although you might think that dietary fat is the primary source of fat buildup, it is actually dietary

MYTH:
Dietary fat makes you fat.

FACT:
Carbohydrates have more of an effect on fat storage than dietary fat.

carbohydrates that stimulate fat storage[49] more than dietary fat itself.[50] Dietary carbohydrates raise blood sugar and blood insulin levels, both of which increase the production of triglycerides, the storage unit of fat. As you recall from chapter 2, a high blood triglyceride level is a risk factor for heart disease.

Simply put, a diet high in grain-based and refined carbohydrates, starches, and simple sugars triggers insulin resistance, inflammation, production of triglycerides, and other blood lipid abnormalities, all increasing the risk of obesity.[51] When you continue down this pathway, metabolic syndrome, type 2 diabetes, and heart disease develop.

Following a low-carbohydrate diet has been found in many studies to not only induce weight loss but to favorably affect blood lipid abnormalities and blood sugar control compared to a conventional, reduced-fat, low-carbohydrate diet.[52,53,54] See the Love Your Heart section for more information on a successful eating plan for heart health.

TIP:

Gut bacteria contribute to systemic inflammation by releasing toxins into circulation through a leaky gut.

Childhood Obesity

The childhood obesity rate in the United States has more than tripled since 1980.[41] More than 30 percent of children in the United States are overweight or obese. For this reason, it is thought that today's children will be the first generation to actually have a shorter lifespan than the previous generation.[42]

Obesity in childhood affects many systems of the body. Health conditions that were once thought to only occur in adults are now showing up in childhood. In fact, arteries of obese children have been found to resemble the arteries of a 45-year-old.[43] The metabolic syndrome, which leads to type 2 diabetes and heart disease, is increasingly being found in obese and overweight children as young as five years old.[44] And the problem is not going away. Heart disease rates are predicted to increase among young and middle-aged adults over the next twenty years due to current childhood obesity rates.[45]

Factors contributing to childhood obesity include poor diet and not enough physical activity, increased stress,[46] prenatal exposure to chemicals,[47] and lack of breastfeeding,[48] implicating a gut imbalance as a factor leading to obesity.

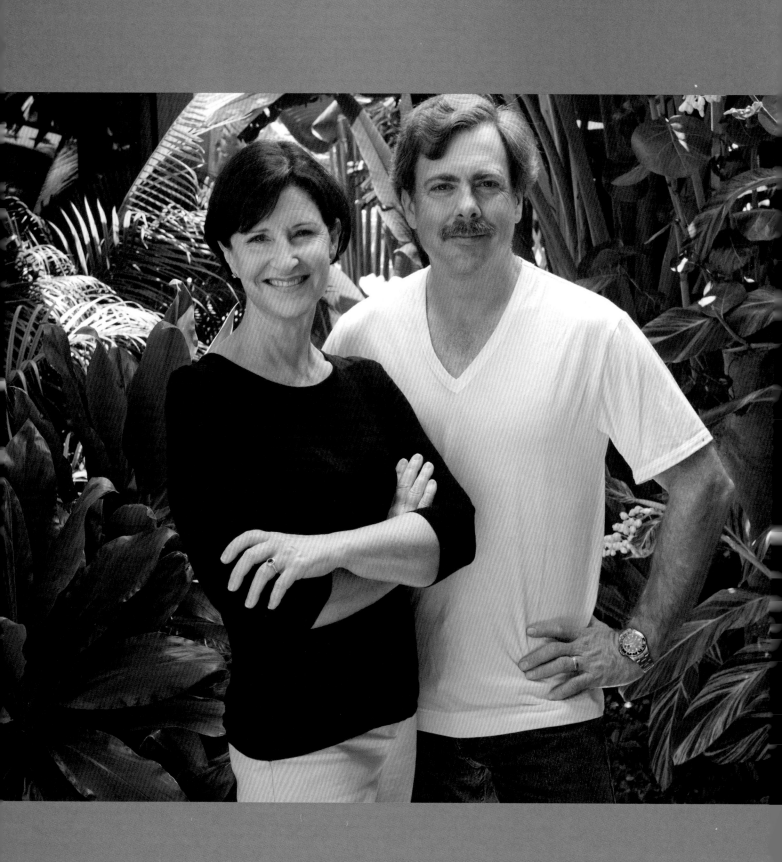

Obesity—the Final Answer for Stan and Sandee

The reduction of cardiovascular risk by lowering cholesterol and blood sugar in my husband, Stan, and by lowering blood pressure in my sister Sandee, comes down to a few necessary changes. Both had to reduce the amount of fat on their bodies, remove sugar from their diets, and address inflammation with dietary supplements. So how did they do?

After going to the doctor and getting on a weight-management program, Stan began to have success. Once he lost an initial 10 to 15 pounds, he became very motivated. I could see in him the lightbulb come on, saying: I can do this!

Stan had spent at least 10 to 15 years of his life like a yo-yo. He would lose ten pounds, his cholesterol would go down, and six months later—triggered by stress or a lot of travel—the weight came back on, he'd stop his supplements, and the cycle continued. Stan's biggest obstacle was sugar. Each time he returned to unhealthy eating habits, his sweet tooth was to blame. He really felt that diet and exercise did not work for him. What he didn't realize is the role sugar played in his health.

After addressing his weight gain by removing sugar and taking the right supplements, Stan was very inspired. His food program consisted of very exact ways of eating by measuring the amount and kind of foods he ate. Instead of counting carbs, he counted teaspoons of sugar. So he could eat six to seven teaspoons of sugar from fruits and vegetables a day. That's right—all sugars were counted in teaspoons, and they came from fruits and vegetables. No added sugar, bread, pasta, or anything white. His diet consisted of protein, dairy, vegetables, and fruits, in portion control, and he ate six times per day.

I didn't know how well he would adapt to the diet, as his sugar addiction was so strong, but he really loved being in control of his health. He bought measuring cups and little glass containers that were the exact size of a portion of protein, veggies, or fruits. (See the Love Your Heart Eating Plan for more information.) Over the course of nine months he lost 40 pounds.

Adding omega-3 fish oils, fiber, and a liver detox supplement to Stan's diet program helped him lower his cholesterol from as high as 780 down to 180. Because Stan does not get at least 35 grams of fiber from his diet, he adds a supplement to support healthy elimination and help lower cholesterol.

The biggest surprise and blessing of all has been how this diet has changed our relationship. When Stan became interested in his health in this way, it really brought us together. We planned our meals together, and he even started to cook and go to the grocery store! The outdoor grill has been a big part of cooking our meals. Men like fire and the outdoors, it seems. Stan's experience with weight, cholesterol, and blood sugar has been a success not just in how he feels and looks but in the joy it brings our marriage.

As for Sandee, my sister, remember that she was diagnosed with high blood pressure and prescribed medication. Her goal was to get her blood pressure under control and get off the medication within three to six months. After seeing Stan's progress, she was impressed.

Sandee decided to follow Stan's footsteps in diet, supplements, and lifestyle. She began counting teaspoons of sugar and portion size. She increased omega-3s and fiber. Because she has struggled with sugar addiction her whole life, taking sugar out of her diet was one of the biggest steps in achieving her goal. I think sugar addiction is similar to alcohol addiction. Both have a similar effect on brain chemistry. I see children of alcoholics, as well as recovering alcoholics, turn to sugar as their substance of addiction.

In the last year, Sandee has lost 40 pounds and is off all medication. She feels she is finally free from the addiction to food. Her saving grace has been protein. Coming from a diabetic family, she recognizes the value of healthy protein sources as a great alternative to sugar and carb cravings.

If I had not seen it with my own eyes, I wouldn't believe the effect sugar and carbs have had on my family's heart health. I hope this book's Love Your Heart Program, which sets out achievable goals that work, will be an inspiration for others. ∎

Standard Treatment

A combination of diet modification and increased physical activity is the best lifestyle approach to reduce obesity. Ironically, a reduced-calorie, low-fat, high-carbohydrate diet is the most commonly recommended diet for obesity. This diet tends to be very difficult to follow, and may not be effective long term. Thus the yo-yo effect of dieting, in which weight is lost, only to be gained again once the diet is stopped. While it is certain that calories play a role in the accumulation of weight, there is more to the story than simply calories in, calories out.[55] Most people know someone (or are that someone) who very carefully counts calories but cannot seem to lose weight at the same rate as other people. As we have learned, there are factors other than calories that affect metabolism and that can interfere with weight loss.

Weight-loss medications may be prescribed for people who are unsuccessful at losing weight with diet and exercise alone. These drugs work by either creating feelings of fullness, reducing appetite, or by limiting the absorption of fat. Only four drugs have been approved by the FDA for weight reduction:[56] sibutramine, phentermine, diethylpropion, and orlistat. An over-the-counter version of orlistat, which limits fat absorption, is also available. These drugs are not without side effects.

There are many surgical procedures for obesity that are now performed by surgeons trained in bariatric surgery. These procedures are costly and associated with a small amount of risk. When considering these operations, it is important to know all the options and to find a surgeon who has done many of these procedures.

Tips for Helping Reduce Obesity

See the Love Your Heart section for a complete program to support heart health.

- Eat a diet low in grain-based, refined, and starchy carbohydrates and sugars, and high in vegetables, healthy fats, and lean proteins, nuts, and seeds.

- Increase your amount of physical activity. Find an activity you enjoy and get moving!

- Support healthy digestion and balance your gut with probiotics to help reduce inflammation.

- Take an omega-3 fish oil supplement to increase the omega-3/omega-6 ratio.

- Optimize your vitamin D level. (Achieve an optimal level between 50 and 70 ng/mL.)

"But for one's health as you say, it is very necessary to work in the garden and see the flowers growing."

—*Vincent van Gogh*

Chapter 6

Inflammation—You Might Not Know You Have It

Myth:
When you have inflammation, you feel pain.

Fact:
Inflammation can be present in such a way that you might not even know it's there.

When most people think of inflammation, they think of joint pain, cuts, or something that hurts. But inflammation cannot always be felt. In fact, inflammation can be present in such a way that you might not even know it is there. This kind of inflammation—chronic, low-grade inflammation—is also known as silent inflammation because it can be present without being felt.

We have already seen that inflammation is closely related to high cholesterol, high blood pressure, high blood sugar, and obesity. And we have learned that inflammation is involved in the entire process of heart disease—from initiation of artery damage to the blockage of arteries by blood clots, which leads to stroke and heart attack.[1] As if that's not bad enough, inflammation plays a role in most, if not all, chronic diseases. Autoimmune disease, arthritis, diabetes, depression, dementia—inflammation plays a big role in each one.[2]

Despite its involvement in so many disease processes, inflammation is a necessary process in the body. It plays an essential role in immune function. It is inflammation that drives the elimination of foreign invaders from the body. We could not live if it weren't for inflammation.

Inflammation—Let's Break It Down

Inflammation is sometimes described as a fire—an apt analogy due to the many different fuels that can feed the fire of inflammation. Think of the inflammation of heart disease as a big fire, like a forest fire, damaging the arteries and leading to heart attack and stroke. Think of chronic, low-grade inflammation as a small fire, like a campfire, found throughout the body in many different forms, silently fueling the larger fire of chronic disease.

Think of chronic, low-grade inflammation as a small fire, like a campfire, found throughout the body in many different forms, silently fueling the larger fire of chronic disease.

The body is under constant surveillance by the innate immune system, the primitive branch of the immune system. When a foreign invader or injury is detected, the innate immune system responds immediately with inflammation—the fire that destroys the invader. Foreign invaders include microbes (bacteria, fungus, or virus), undigested food particles, allergens, or environmental toxins.[3] When detected, the immune system triggers the release of a number of immune cells and chemicals, sparking the fire of inflammation.

In general, inflammation should occur in response to a foreign invader, an injury, or some sort of malfunction, working to destroy and eliminate foreign substances or abnormalities, and to resolve in due time. Inflammation resolution is crucial for the body's return to homeostasis, or balance.[4] When inflammation does not properly resolve, when the trigger of inflammation is constant, the result is chronic, low-grade inflammation. This type of silent inflammation essentially resets the body's point of homeostasis—it creates a new normal, resulting in suboptimal function in the body.[5] It is this long-term, suboptimal function that leads to chronic disease.

How Is Inflammation Measured?

Inflammation in the body can be detected by measuring the amount of C-reactive protein (CRP) in the blood. CRP is produced by the body in response to inflammation. It is a general marker for systemic inflammation, and it is a stronger predictor for cardiovascular disease than even high cholesterol.[6] Specifically, the high-sensitivity CRP test (hs-CRP test) should be used for the proper assessment of cardiovascular risk. Cardiovascular risk is found at levels of inflammation lower than that of other acute conditions, making the hs-CRP test the accurate measure of risk.[7] Risk categories based on measured hs-CRP are as follows.

High-Sensitivity C-Reactive Protein

< 1 mg/L	Low cardiovascular risk
1–3 mg/L	Moderate cardiovascular risk
> 3 mg/L	High cardiovascular risk

If CRP levels over 10 mg/L are obtained, the test should be repeated a few weeks later because it may mean an infection is triggering the high CRP levels.[8] For this reason, it is recommended that the hs-CRP test be done when you are feeling well. This test can easily be added to regular blood tests evaluating blood lipids.

C-reactive protein is not only a marker of inflammation; it is also involved in the inflammatory process and the development of atherosclerosis.[9] CRP stimulates the release of inflammatory cytokines from the artery lining. This is one of the first steps in the development of atherosclerosis—a process known as endothelial dysfunction. See chapter 9 for more information on this process and what can be done about it.

Another test that evaluates inflammation levels in the body is a lipid peroxide test. This test measures cell membrane fatty acid oxidation, which indicates the body's level of free radical damage. When free radicals damage the fatty acids of cell membranes by oxidizing them, lipid peroxides are produced. High levels of lipid peroxides are associated with cancer, heart disease, stroke, and aging.[10,11] Metametrix Clinical Laboratory offers a lipid peroxide test to help detect this inflammatory process in the body.

There are many fuels feeding the fire of inflammation.

Inflammation Triggers

To control inflammation in the body, we need to understand what triggers it. What fuels the fire of inflammation? There are in fact many fuels feeding the fire. Let's take a closer look at these triggers.

ACUTE INFLAMMATION

Infection The most obvious trigger of inflammation is infection. Infections are full-blown pathogenic invasions of bacteria, fungus, or virus. Think of the common viral cold or flu infection and you can easily see that inflammation runs rampant. Red, swollen nose and throat, fever, pain—these are all obvious symptoms of an inflammatory process that is ridding the body of foreign invaders, a process that eventually brings the body back to balance.

Injury When you cut your finger, sprain an ankle, or even hit your head on a hard object, the inflammatory process is activated. During the inflammatory process normal cells and tissues are damaged, triggering an inflammatory cascade that brings in more blood and cells to clean up the damage and initiate the healing process.

SILENT INFLAMMATION

Poor Diet The Standard American Diet (SAD) is high in inflammation-promoting foods: processed, refined grains, chemicals and additives, and unhealthy fats (too many omega-6 fats); and low in anti-inflammatory foods: vegetables and fruits, fiber, healthy fats (omega-3, omega-9, and medium-chain triglyceride saturated fats as found in coconut oil), lean proteins, nuts, and seeds.[12] The nutrient-poor, calorie-dense SAD is a major contributor to inflammation, and thus to the modern epidemic of obesity and diabetes, and to most chronic diseases today, certainly including heart disease.

TIP: A diet high in healthy omega-3 oils, vegetables, fiber, lean proteins, nuts, and seeds helps to reduce inflammation in the body.

Omega-6 to Omega-3 Ratio Excess consumption of omega-6 fatty acids produces inflammation, whereas increased omega-3 consumption decreases inflammation. The omega-6/omega-3 imbalance created by the SAD diet promotes an inflammatory state in the body. This is one of the major contributors to silent inflammation, and it is associated with heart disease.[13] Low levels of omega-3 fatty acids in the blood are associated with increased levels of inflammation,[14] while high intake of omega-3 has been found to reduce CRP and IL-6 (another inflammatory marker) in healthy adults.[15] Omega-3 fatty acids help to bring about the resolution of inflammation[16]—allowing inflammation to occur only as much as it is needed for the body to heal, and then resolving the inflammation before too much damage is done. See chapter 15 in the Love Your Heart section for more information on omega-3s.

Carbohydrates and Sugar The Standard American Diet (SAD) is high in grain-based, processed, and starchy carbohydrates and sugar, and low in vegetables and fruits. This diet increases chronic inflammation.[17] One well-known culprit is the sugar-sweetened beverage, consumed in high amounts by Americans. Even low to moderate consumption of sugar-sweetened beverages in healthy young men over a period of just three weeks was found to increase inflammation.[18] One way in which sugar and carbohydrates increase inflammation is by increasing insulin resistance, which, as we learned in chapter 4, is a major factor in the perpetuation of inflammation in the body.

Omega-6 to Omega-3 Ratio: The Standard American Diet is high in omega-6 fatty acids and low in omega-3 fatty acids. Although both types of fat are essential, meaning **they can't be produced by the body and must be obtained through the diet,** the ideal ratio of omega-6 to omega-3 in the diet is between 1:1 and 4:1. Our hunter-gatherer ancestors consumed a diet with a 1:1 ratio of omega-6 to omega-3. In contrast, the SAD ratio is about 20 to 25:1 (very high in omega-6 and very low in omega-3).[19]

The Standard American Diet (SAD) is high in grain-based, processed, and starchy carbohydrates and sugar, and low in vegetables and fruits. This diet increases chronic inflammation.

The Standard American Diet (SAD) is high in grain-based, processed, and starchy carbohydrates and sugar, and low in vegetables and fruits. This diet increases chronic inflammation.

Even whole grain foods have the potential to increase blood sugar, leading to inflammation. Carbohydrates break down into sugar in the body, creating similar effects as sugar. In contrast, a low-carbohydrate diet has been found to decrease markers of inflammation in overweight and obese men who are otherwise healthy.[20]

Low Fiber Intake The Standard American Diet is very low in fiber. Most Americans consume less than half of the recommended 25 to 35 grams of daily fiber intake. Foods high in fiber include vegetables and fruits, whole grains, legumes, and nuts and seeds. These foods are lacking in the SAD. Diets high in fiber have been found to be protective against high levels of inflammation[21] and are healthy for the heart.[22] See chapter 15 in the Love Your Heart

section for more information on the benefits of fiber.

Stress Our modern lifestyle is wrought with stress. Deadlines, making ends meet, lengthy to-do lists, and keeping up the pace are all considered normal in today's world. Not only does stress trigger inflammation, but inflammation triggers stress, creating a vicious cycle that ends in heart disease.[23] Inflammation due to stress may account for the 40 percent of people with atherosclerosis who have no other risk factors.[24] Stress itself is an important part of maintaining a healthy heart. See chapter 8 for more information on the link between stress and health.

Obesity As we learned in the previous chapter, body fat is an organ of its own, producing an array of metabolically active chemicals, many of which are pro-inflammatory. Belly fat is particularly to blame when it comes to fat-induced inflammation. Belly fat, or visceral abdominal fat (VAT), is a main risk factor for heart disease and diabetes, largely due to the

←——————————— inflammation spectrum ——————————→

ACUTE INFLAMMATION

→ injury

→ infection

SILENT INFLAMMATION
(chronic, low-grade inflammation)

→ physiological imbalance

gut triggers {
poor diet
toxins
poor digestion
food sensitivity
dysbiosis
leaky gut
}

We are swimming in a toxic soup. All of these toxins increase inflammation in the body and interrupt many different necessary functions. Reducing toxicity is crucial.

harmful effects of the inflammation it produces.[25] See chapter 5 for more information on the link between obesity and inflammation.

Toxins Toxins come in many forms: cigarette smoke; particulate matter from air pollution; pesticides, herbicides, and chemical additives in our food; heavy metals from different sources; hormone disruptors in plastics; and fire retardants on just about everything. We are swimming in a toxic soup. All of these toxins increase inflammation in the body and interrupt many different necessary functions. Reducing toxicity is crucial. See chapter 12 for more information on the link between toxins and heart disease.

Food Sensitivities Foods sensitivities involve a reaction by the body against certain foods we eat. Normally, when food passes through the digestive system, it is recognized as a friendly passerby; the immune system leaves it alone. With food sensitivities the immune system reacts to certain foods as if they were foreign invaders. This process triggers inflammation. Sometimes the response is stronger and felt immediately, and other times the response creates an underlying silent inflammation that might not create overt digestive symptoms but that manifests in different areas of the body. Gluten sensitivity is a perfect example of this process.

Many people have underlying food sensitivities and don't know it.

Poor Digestion Incomplete digestion of food is a trigger of inflammation, and also of food sensitivities. Incomplete digestion may be the result of many factors: poor diet, poor chewing, insufficient digestive enzyme secretion, or insufficient stomach acid production. All of these processes contribute to the incomplete breakdown of foods into smaller, absorbable parts. The result is poor nutrient absorption, and inflammation due to the recognition of undigested food particles as foreign by the immune system.

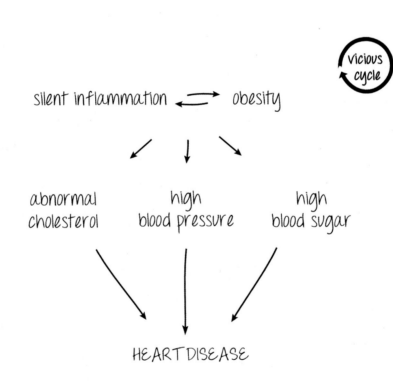

Digestive Imbalance The gut is populated with trillions of bacteria. Ideally, the balance of these bacteria favors the beneficial (probiotic) bacteria and neutral (commensal) bacteria, and minimizes the potentially harmful (pathogenic) bacteria. Unfortunately, there are many factors that create an imbalance in the gut bacteria. These include mode of delivery at birth (vaginal delivery is optimal; Cesarean birth creates imbalance), lack of breastfeeding during infancy, poor diet, antibiotic overuse, stomach acid suppression (with antacids or acid blockers), constipation, and other digestive conditions.

The gut bacteria are found throughout the digestive tract, and are particularly prolific in the intestines—where up to 80 percent of the immune system also resides. Much of the gut bacteria line the intestines, and are said to help educate the immune system.[26] When there is an imbalance in the gut bacteria, also known as the gut microbiota, the immune system reacts by creating inflammation.[27]

Leaky Gut Leaky gut, also known as increased intestinal permeability, involves damage to the intestinal lining that creates holes that allow larger-than-normal particles to pass through the intestines and into circulation. Think of the intestinal lining as a screen. Screens keep out larger, unwanted bugs, but they let in air. In a similar way, the intestinal lining keeps out large, unwanted particles and microorganisms, but it lets in smaller digested nutrients that the body needs.

TIP:
Leaky gut is one of the main ways in which gut inflammation triggers systemic inflammation, leading to heart disease. By fixing leaky gut you are addressing an underlying contributor to heart disease.

When the gut lining is compromised, as occurs with leaky gut, undigested food particles and bacterial and environmental toxins are allowed to pass through the intestines and enter circulation. Leaky gut is one of the main pathways by which gut inflammation triggers systemic inflammation, essentially creating a portal through which inflammation can access the rest of the body. Leaky gut is something you want to avoid.

When most people think of leaky gut, if they think of it at all, they associate it with digestive conditions like irritable bowel syndrome (IBS),[28] inflammatory bowel disease,[29] or celiac disease. But leaky gut has been found in many different health conditions—both digestive and nondigestive. Increased intestinal permeability has been associated with chronic heart failure,[30,31] diabetes,[32,33] fatty liver disease,[34] stress,[35] chronic fatigue syndrome,[36] fibromyalgia,[37] autism,[38] eczema,[39] asthma,[40] and more. In fact, leaky gut has been found even in healthy people and is associated with an accumulation of belly and liver fat.[41]

Many of the factors that contribute to inflammation also contribute to leaky gut. Poor diet, food sensitivities, incomplete digestion, and gut imbalance all contribute to leaky gut in an intricate web that increases inflammation and facilitates its spread throughout the body.

Chronic Infections

Recently, the case has been made for the contribution of infections to the development of heart disease. Various infectious agents have been identified as possible causative factors, and other infections have been identified as contributors to atherosclerosis through stimulation of systemic inflammation, a factor that we have seen plays a major role in the development and progression of heart disease. Even relatively minor infections have been shown to increase the risk of heart attack and stroke.[42]

Systemic inflammation can come from a number of sources, both infectious and noninfectious. Infectious bacterial pathogens that have been associated with heart disease include: *Chlamydia pneumoniae*, *Helicobacter pylori*, periodontal disease–related bacteria (*Porphyromonas gingivalis*, *Streptococcus sanguis*, *Streptococcus viridans*), *Mycoplasma pneumoniae*, and *Haemophilus influenzae*, in addition to other chronic bacterial respiratory, urinary, dental, and other infections. Infectious viral pathogens associated with heart disease include *Cytomegalovirus*, Herpes simplex viruses, Epstein-Barr virus, Hepatitis A, influenza viruses, and human immunodeficiency virus (HIV).

Pathogen Burden

Although all of these pathogens have been linked to heart disease, it appears that the total pathogen burden, rather than individual pathogens, may have the greatest effect on heart disease risk. The total pathogen burden hypothesis states that an increased burden of chronic infections leads to greater levels of inflammation, heart disease, and cardiovascular events.[43] It is possible that acute or chronic infections could cause heart disease on their own, but it is more likely that infections contribute to heart disease along with other traditional risk factors such as abnormal blood lipid levels and high blood pressure.[44]

One study reported that the presence of any chronic bacterial infection—respiratory, urinary, dental, or other—increased four-fold the risk of developing atherosclerosis of the carotid artery.[45] Another study of more than 1,000 heart disease patients found that cardiovascular death was associated with increasing infectious burden.[46] Both these studies found increased risk with higher levels of systemic inflammation.

Chlamydia pneumonia C. pneumoniae is a common cause of respiratory tract infection, infecting 50 percent of all people by age 20. C. pneumoniae has been detected in atherosclerotic plaque, especially in severe plaques.[47] C. pneumoniae has also been found to contribute to the oxidation of LDL cholesterol particles.[48] As we learned in chapter 2, oxidized LDL is especially damaging to the arteries.

Helicobacter pylori H. pylori, the organism that causes peptic ulcer disease, is another potential pathogen associated with heart disease. H. pylori infection has been found to increase C-reactive protein (CRP), the main marker for systemic inflammation, as well as promote blood clotting factors.[49] Although studies looking at blood levels of H. pylori have not found a link to heart disease, the pathogen's

contribution to systemic inflammation likely contributes to the disease.

Cytomegalovirus Cytomegalovirus (CMV) is a herpes-family virus, a common pathogen found in more than 70 percent of people with heart disease.[50] CMV has been found to increase lipoprotein(a), a risk factor for heart disease, enhances blood clotting factors, and is associated with higher rates of artery blockage occurring in people who have undergone surgery to widen atherosclerotic arteries.[51] Similar to other pathogens, increased levels of systemic inflammation increase the risk of heart disease in people with CMV infection. In patients with high CRP levels and CMV detected in the blood, the risk of cardiovascular-related death is increased, more so than in people with either high CRP or CMV alone.[52] CMV patients with high levels of IL-6 (another marker of inflammation) were also at increased risk,[53] highlighting the integral role of inflammation in conjunction with infections related to heart disease.

Periodontal disease Periodontal disease, or disease of the gums and bone that support the teeth, has also been linked to heart disease. According to the American Academy of Periodontology, people with periodontal disease are twice as likely to have heart disease as people without it. They are also more likely to experience a heart attack.[54] Two bacteria known to cause gum disease, Porphyromonas gingivalis and Streptococcus sanguis, have been found in atherosclerotic plaques.[55]

It is thought that oral bacteria and bacterial toxins enter systemic circulation, contributing to the chronic, low-grade inflammation that is the silent hallmark of heart disease.[56] These bacteria add to the total pathogenic load of the body, potentially leading to heart disease. Thus, good dental hygiene is important for heart health. Indeed, treatment of periodontal disease has been found to improve certain cardiovascular outcomes, such as blood vessel function.[57]

Since infections have been implicated as contributing factors to heart disease, treating these infections with antibiotic or antiviral medications is being studied. Clinical trials examining the cardiovascular benefits of antibiotic or antiviral therapy in people with some of the infections mentioned above have yielded mixed results, however. Total pathogen burden can be difficult to treat due to the many pathogens involved and to the difficulty of treating viral infections with antiviral drugs. Further, the risks associated with long-term antibiotic use should be carefully considered when addressing chronic infections.

Anti-inflammatory therapies may be of cardiovascular benefit for patients with chronic infections. Since chronic infections are particularly unhealthy for the heart in people with inflammation, lowering inflammation becomes especially important.

Standard Treatment

Weight loss and a healthy diet are effective methods for reducing chronic, silent inflammation.[58,59] Unfortunately, emphasis on the importance of lifestyle changes such as these is not the focus of traditional medicine. Instead, anti-inflammatory drugs are often prescribed. Aspirin is one of the most common drugs recommended for the reduction of inflammation associated with cardiovascular disease. Aspirin originates from the bark of the willow tree and is used as a pain reliever and anti-inflammatory drug. Aspirin has been found to reduce levels of C-reactive protein,[60] but overuse of aspirin can cause gastrointestinal bleeding, so its proper use should be considered under the guidance of a physician.

One class of drugs, the thiazolidinediones, has been found to improve insulin sensitivity and decrease inflammation, but some of these drugs come with severe side effects. Other drugs that have been found to reduce inflammation are COX-2 inhibitors, fibrates, ACE inhibitors, and statin drugs.[61] These drugs are also used to improve other aspects of cardiovascular disease, but their beneficial effects on inflammation illustrate the importance of inflammation to the development of heart disease and the importance of looking to the root cause of heart disease rather than treating the end results.

Tips for Helping Improve Gut Function

See the Love Your Heart Section for a complete program to support heart health.

- Eat a diet low in grain-based, refined, and starchy carbohydrates and sugars, and high in vegetables, healthy fats, and lean proteins, nuts, and seeds.

- Increase your amount of physical activity. Find an activity you enjoy and get moving! Regular exercise helps reduce inflammation.

- Support healthy digestion and balance your gut with probiotics to help reduce inflammation in the body.

- Take an omega-3 fish oil supplement to increase the omega-3/omega-6 ratio.

- Optimize your vitamin D level. (Achieve optimal levels between 50 and 70 ng/mL.)

- If you smoke, quit.

- Check hsCRP levels and lipid peroxide levels to detect underlying inflammation.

Heart Disease—Dad's Journey Continues

My dad's story began with a diet high in sugar, which led to weight gain, diabetes, and eventually bypass surgery, all conditions fueled by inflammation. Read the first part of his story on page 70. My dad relied heavily on his doctors, believing their every word. Because of this, I thought he might be more inclined to consider natural healing modalities if he heard about them from a doctor. So one day I asked him to come to Florida from North Carolina to listen to a holistic-minded MD speak on heart disease.

By this time, my dad was tired of taking so many medications (17 total!) with minimal benefit. He was tired of seeing doctor after doctor, with no end in sight to the medication. His diabetes raged on, along with many other health challenges. By this point, he was willing to hear what the holistic doctor had to say.

He came to Florida and went to the seminar. At the time I was working in a holistic health clinic practicing nutrition, colonics, and detoxification. During his visit I explained the importance of gut health and how detoxification was a key factor to good health. I actually gave my father a few colonics. Let me tell you, you have really resolved issues with your father (and I had plenty) when you can give him a colonic.

My dad was familiar with my own health challenges. By seeing me in my practice and knowing how I had turned around my own health, he could see how my health had improved as a result of my new career in holistic healing.

That, and the information he gained from the doctor's lecture on heart disease, inspired him to go back to North Carolina to begin chelation therapy (a therapy which removes heavy metals from the blood), along with a diet and exercise program.

I have to say, my dad gave it his best shot. He lost 30 pounds and within three months he was off all medication. It really was a miracle. No diabetes, no blood thinners, nothing! He was taking a lot of supplements and my mother made sure his diet changed. He enjoyed good health for the next two years.

Unfortunately, two years later they found a tumor on my dad's brain. The doctors informed him that if he did anything "natural," they wouldn't treat him. Although this was a hard message for me to hear, I understood my dad's situation. He was put on medication and lived for about another year. I truly believe the years of using NutraSweet (which contains aspartame, found to have carcinogenic properties) could have been a factor in the development of my dad's brain tumor.

My dad's health went downhill again, and he finally died of congestive heart failure. Through the ups and downs of his last year of life, we had a wonderful time. During one of the down times, I asked the cardiologist how he thought my dad was doing. Amazingly, he told me that if my dad did not have a strong gut, he would not have lasted this long. I thought to myself, what a thing for this allopathic doctor to say to me!

My dad left this world in his sleep with full mental faculties. His mind was sharp as a tack. He was a great teacher, and I am grateful to have shared his life. ■

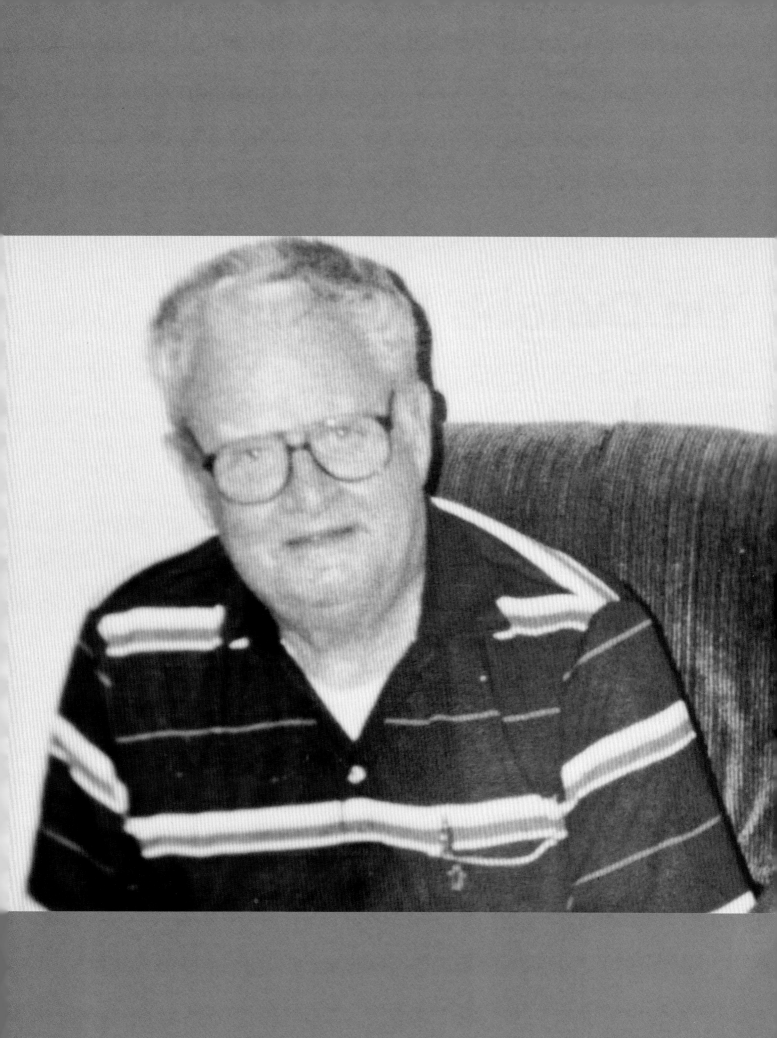

interview

Dr. Dwight Lundell

Brenda interviews cardiac surgeon and the author of *The Cure for Heart Disease: Truth Will Save a Nation*

BW: Dr. Lundell, first I want to thank you for taking the time to do this interview. As a heart surgeon, you bring an especially interesting perspective to this book. Your message is in line with my own: We must get to the root cause of heart disease (which means getting to the root cause of inflammation) to have the most positive effect on the nation's number one killer. Tell me, how did you come to recognize the role of inflammation in heart disease?

DL: The classic signs of inflammation are redness, swelling, pain, and warmth. In the operating room I could see two of these: redness and swelling around the coronary

artery, especially where the plaques were. Then I began to study the very recent research showing that microscopically there are typical changes of inflammation found in atherosclerotic arteries.

BW: Early on, you had trouble fully accepting the cholesterol-causes-heart-disease theory. Many of the patients you operated on had normal cholesterol levels. Why do so many people believe this theory?

DL: More than half of all the patients I operated on had normal levels of cholesterol. Indeed, a recent study showed that 70 percent of all patients admitted to hospitals with heart attack had normal cholesterol levels. I could never understand why a normal substance vital to so many cellular functions could cause coronary artery disease just because it was more of it than "normal."

BW: Historically, when did heart disease emerge?

DL: The prevalence of the disease emerged when humans converted to an agricultural-based society from a hunting and gathering society. The mid-twentieth century is when it became a real problem; concern really rose when it was discovered that young soldiers

DL: Every government regulation is the product of lobbying: by those groups that will be harmed, and by those groups that will benefit. When the first dietary guidelines were published food industry groups spent millions of dollars lobbying the various agencies and legislators so that the recommendations became favorable to the industries paying the lobbyists. Basically, the recommendations were exploited by the production and heavy promotion of low-fat, grain-based foods that were cheap, subsidized, and highly profitable.

BW: You also talk about how dietary fat doesn't necessarily make us fat. How is that so?

"The fact is, it is not how much we eat, but what we eat and what our bodies do with what we eat, that determines health and weight."

killed in the Korean War had evidence of significant artery disease.

BW: In your book *The Cure for Heart Disease*, you talk about the influence of food industries on dietary recommendations—particularly the Food Pyramid (now My Plate). How did these industries influence the current myth that a low-fat, high-carbohydrate diet is healthy?

DL: The simple-minded appeal that fat has 9 calories per gram versus 4 calories per gram for carbohydrates fits icely with the "calories in, calories out" mantra. But this ignores the basics of metabolism. Calories are processed in different ways and do different things. The fact is, it is not how much we eat, but what we eat and what our bodies do with what we eat, that determines health and weight.

BW: So if it's not fat that makes us fat, what is it?

DL: Ever since Banting's "Letter on Corpulence" published in 1869 and up through the 1960s scientists have documented that reducing the intake of starchy and sweet foods is the key to weight control.

BW: You recognize that a low-carbohydrate diet is a more heart-healthy option than current dietary recommendations. Why is a low-carb diet not more widely recommended?

DL: Low fat became sort of the "state religion," and those who dared question it were subjected to ridicule and professional discrimination, as in the case of Dr. Atktin's congressional hearings. It has been amazing to see the medical profession so overwhelmed by the push for low fat and cholesterol control.

BW: How do healthy versus unhealthy arteries age?

DL: Healthy arteries do not build up the plaque that obstructs them; they remain pliable and responsive to the demands placed on them. With inflammation control, we have the potential to save our own lives by maintaining healthy arteries into old age.

BW: You talk about how all cells in our bodies are connected. I think this is an important message. For my part, I want to help people realize that inflammation can come from many sources, and that an important—

though often overlooked—source is the gut. You also talk about finding the root cause of heart disease by addressing inflammation. You say, "It doesn't do us any good to just look at the heart. We've got to go back to the root of the problem. We've got to start from scratch. We've got to see where the issue truly begins in the biological process." Yes! You are so right. Could you talk more about this?

DL: We have about five liters of blood that is circulated throughout the body once every minute. This means that it takes less than a minute for a chemical in the blood to move from one spot to another. Inflammation is the response to injury, whether it is bacterial, viral, chemical, or physical. The inflammatory response triggers a cascade of chemicals called cytokines that orchestrate the inflammatory response, and these cytokines affect every cell they are exposed to. Think about the last time you had an infection, say a head cold: Why did you ache all over? It was due to the action of the inflammatory cytokines. For example, an infection in the foot will cause the arteries in the heart to be activated to fight any invader that may come along. All cells in our body are connected.

BW: What are some main sources of inflammation?

DL: We live in an environment where many things can harm us and cause inflammation. Fortunately, we have protective barriers: the skin, the respiratory system, and the gastrointestinal tract. We also have to provide the proper nutrients to allow the most efficient response to an insult.

A high-carb diet causes elevated blood sugars, which injures the blood vessels, cells in the eye, the kidney, and nerves. Think of the unique

DL: Control of blood sugar to stop the damage from a high-carb diet, natural anti-inflammatory nutrients such as omega-3 from fish oil, CLA (conjugated linolenic acid), and antioxidant foods and supplements. It is also important to exercise, because muscle cells produce lots of anti-inflammatory cytokines when active.

"We live in an environment where many things can harm us and cause inflammation. Fortunately, we have protective barriers: the skin, the respiratory system, and the gastrointestinal tract."

complications that occur in poorly controlled diabetics: blindness, kidney failure, nerve damage, and vascular disease. If we do not maintain the integrity of our natural barriers—skin, GI tract, and lung—we are subject to more injuries and inflammation. If we do not maintain proper nutrition for the inflammatory system we are subject to increased inflammation from smaller injuries.

BW: What are the best ways to quell inflammation?

BW: Thank you so much for the interview, Dr. Lundell. You are doing a great service by educating people about the importance of getting to the root causes of heart disease. Your message is an important one. Thank you for having the courage to question conventional thinking!

"The greatest wealth is health."

—*Virgil*

Chapter 7

The Gut Connection

The digestive tract, or gastrointestinal (GI) tract, which runs from the mouth to the anus, has a surface area that could cover a tennis court. Over the course of an average lifetime, more than 60 tons of food will pass through the GI tract.[1] Most people think of the digestive system as a food processor of sorts; it breaks food down into smaller nutrients so that the body can absorb them. In the process, it produces waste. This is about as far as most people go when thinking about digestion. But there is much more to the digestive tract than simply food processing and pooping.

The lining of the intestinal tract, called the epithelial lining, is a one-cell-thick layer separating the intestine—and all its contents—from systemic circulation. Think of this layer almost like that of skin, separating the inside of the body from the outside. Technically, contents passing through the digestive tract are only considered to have entered the body once they pass through the epithelial lining, officially entering systemic circulation.

We Are Outnumbered

Lining the digestive tract, especially the intestines, are trillions of microorganisms—mostly bacteria, but also yeasts and parasites. In fact, the gut harbors 100 trillion bacterial cells—that's 10 times the number of cells that make up your entire body![2] Concentrations of microorganisms in the mouth and esophagus are moderate, with a decrease in the stomach due to the presence of bacteria-inhibiting stomach acid, and then a gradual increase in the small intestine leading to the large intestine, which contains the majority of gastrointestinal bacteria.[3]

Collectively, the gut bacteria weigh four pounds. That's the weight

Myth:

The digestive system only functions like a food processor, breaking down food and assimilating nutrients.

Fact:

The digestive tract is also home to trillions of bacteria that play an important role in digestive and overall health.

---

of a brick! The collection of microorganisms in the gut is known as the gut microbiota, or gut microflora (gut flora for short). These microorganisms live in symbiosis—in a harmonious relationship—with each other and the host (that's you), and are nourished by food that passes through the digestive tract. The gut microbiota acts as an organ of its own,[4] rivaling the metabolic function of the liver.[5]

The gut microbiota acts as an organ.

The influence of the gut bacteria on health is increasingly being realized. The Human Microbiome Project is a massive research project, funded by the National Institutes of Health, with a goal of characterizing the microbial communities found in and on the human body, and of examining the role of these microbes on human health and disease.[6] The gut microbiome refers to the collective gut bacteria, including the genomes of the bacteria, containing a total of more than 100 times the genes of the human genome itself.[7] For this reason, it is thought the gut bacteria may have more control over our health than even our own genes.

In a healthy person, the gut microbiota is made up of mostly beneficial (probiotic) and neutral (commensal) bacteria, with potentially harmful (pathogenic) bacteria in the minority. When this balance is disrupted, the potentially pathogenic bacteria (and other opportunistic microbes such as yeast) gain the upper hand, increasing inflammation and leading to an array of health conditions, both digestive and nondigestive. This imbalance of gut microorganisms is known as dysbiosis.

The main functions of the normal gut flora include:[8,9]

- Fermentation of nondigestible dietary components
- Production of short-chain fatty acids
- Production of vitamins K and B
- Absorption of ions
- Protection of the intestinal lining
- Protection against, and inhibition of, pathogens
- Balance of immune response
- Regulation of inflammatory response
- Regulation of fat storage

Probiotics

Probiotics are defined as "live microorganisms which confer a health benefit on the host when administered in adequate amounts."[10] The most widely studied probiotic bacteria found to be beneficial to human health are *Lactobacillus* and *Bifidobacterium* species and the probiotic yeast *Saccharomyces boulardii*.[11] The administration of probiotics benefits the host (the person taking the probiotics) by improving the contents and action of the gut microflora.[12]

TIP:

Lactobacillus and *Bifidobacterium* are two of the most widely studied probiotics found to be beneficial to human health.

Because of the close proximity of gut bacteria to the intestinal lining, and because up to 80 percent of the immune system resides in the gut, probiotics have an immune-balancing effect. The immune system in the gut has the important job of recognizing foreign invaders and mounting an inflammatory response against them, while at the same time recognizing the wide array of food contents as harmless, and not mounting a response against food.[13]

Probiotics help balance immune response by educating the immune system on how to respond appropriately to gut contents.[14] When the gut does not respond appropriately to its contents, which usually occurs when there is an imbalance in the gut bacteria, a wide array of health conditions, both digestive and nondigestive, may result. Maintaining digestive balance with probiotics has a range of health benefits,[15] largely due to their influence on the inflammatory response of the immune system.[16] Probiotics help to counteract inflammation by helping to break down undigested food in the gut, reducing inflammatory compounds secreted by the immune system in the gut, and promoting a healthy balance of gut bacteria.[17]

What Can Go Wrong?

Dysbiosis As mentioned previously, the gut flora can become imbalanced, a state of dysbiosis that favors the potentially pathogenic bacteria and suppresses the growth of beneficial bacteria. Dysbiosis involves an alteration from the normal, established gut flora. Because of the complexity of the gut microbial composition, dysbiosis can take many forms. A general dysbiosis may occur, with excessive amounts of potentially harmful bacteria and/or lowered amounts of beneficial bacteria. Or dysbiosis may show up as a particular condition.

One manifestation of dysbiosis is known as small intestinal bacterial overgrowth (SIBO), a condition in which the bacteria from the colon back up into the end of the small intestine, growing in high numbers as they do in the colon. This creates digestive discomfort and symptoms such as gas and bloating. SIBO is

Up to 80 percent of the immune system resides in the gut.

commonly found in people with irritable bowel syndrome (IBS), the most commonly diagnosed digestive condition.[18]

Another form of dysbiosis involves an overgrowth of the yeast *Candida albicans*, an organism that normally populates many areas of the body—nose, throat, mouth, digestive tract, and genito-urinary tract—in small amounts, but can gain the upper hand under certain conditions, such as after antibiotic treatment or steroid medication; during periods with high estrogen levels from pregnancy, birth control pills, estrogen replacement, or obesity; when the diet is high in carbohydrates, sugar, yeast foods, molds, or fermented foods; or in people with diabetes.[19] *Candida* overgrowth creates gut inflammation and nutrient deficiencies, and is associated with many different health conditions and symptoms.[20]

Dysbiosis, or the alteration of gut bacteria, is associated with a host of conditions, both digestive and nondigestive. When the gut flora is out of balance, harmful organisms gain the upper hand and produce an array of harmful toxins that trigger inflammation, damage the intestinal lining, and can lead to poor health. In fact, Hippocrates himself, the father of Western medicine, stated in 400 B.C., "death sits in the bowels" and "bad digestion is the root of all evil."[21] Today this message rings true as science is working out the intricacies of the effects of the microbiota on human health.[22] As a result of the powerful impact the gut flora have on the immune system, dysbiosis can have far-reaching effects.

The most common trigger of dysbiosis is antibiotic use.[23] The word *antibiotic* means, literally, "against life." Antibiotics kill bacteria; they don't distinguish between the good and bad bacteria— they kill them all. Normally the good bacteria keep the harmful bacteria in check, but suppression of good bacteria by antibiotics makes it easy for potentially harmful bacteria to thrive. This is what creates dysbiosis. Some of our friendly flora never fully recover after antibiotics, and in fact, antibiotic overuse has been blamed for the increase in conditions such as obesity, type 1 diabetes, inflammatory bowel disease, allergies, and asthma.[24]

> Hippocrates himself stated in 400 B.C., "death sits in the bowels" and "bad digestion is the root of all evil."

Stress is another contributor to dysbiosis. Stress has the effect of shutting down digestion. This is known as fight-or-flight mode. When under stress, your body is in fight-or-flight mode. The body's physiology diverts its energy from digestion to those functions most useful in life-or-death situations, like increased heart rate, acute senses, and so forth. The production of stomach acid is reduced, digestive motility slows, and there is a reduction in the amount of beneficial gut bacteria.[25] In life-or-death situations, this is useful, but in today's world, stress has become a normal aspect of everyday life, and it's affecting our digestion.[26]

Another major contributor to dysbiosis is diet. A high-sugar diet has been found to slow the intestinal transit time of food (essentially promoting constipation) and increase gut bacterial fermentation and concentrations of bile acids in the colon, indicating an alteration in gut bacterial activity.[27] Slow gut transit time increases the production of potentially harmful bacterial toxins that can have negative consequences on health.[28] Think about it—the longer waste sits in your colon, the more it putrefies, producing toxic by-products. This is why regular bowel elimination is so important.

A change from a healthy diet to the Standard American Diet (SAD), a diet high in carbohydrates and sugar, unhealthy fats, and processed foods, and low in vegetables, fiber, lean protein, and healthy fats, impairs the balance of healthy gut flora. In fact, the SAD diet has been found in an animal model to alter the gut microbiota after just one day.[29] Two weeks into the SAD diet came an increase in fat storage. A high-fiber diet, on the other hand, helps support the growth of beneficial gut bacteria, which is thought to be an important contributor to the management of metabolic syndrome.[30]

Dysbiosis induced by the SAD diet leads to immune dysregulation, and thus the production of inflammation. In contrast, when the gut is balanced, the immune system is regulated, and homeostasis, or balance of the body's systems, is attained.[31]

TIP:
Antibiotic use, poor diet, and stress have been found to create gut imbalance. You have the ability to reverse this imbalance.

Inflammation Gut inflammation, like any inflammation in the body, may be present in an obvious form, as occurs in the inflammatory bowel diseases, diverticulitis, or gastritis; or it may occur in in a subtler, more silent form, as chronic, low-grade inflammation. Remember that chronic, low-grade inflammation exists behind the scenes—cell by cell, tissues and organs are silently damaged and body functions are eventually altered. All of this happens and you may not even know it. One major source of chronic, low-grade inflammation is the gut.

Gut inflammation often occurs in response to alterations in gut bacterial balance or activity. Frequently, it is the bacterial components or products produced by the bacteria that stimulate inflammation, rather than the bacteria themselves.[32] One major gut bacterial component thought to have an impact on metabolic factors such as obesity and insulin resistance is the bacterial toxin lipopolysaccharide (LPS).[33] Studies on this particular gut connection suggest that the gut microbiota is a causative link connecting inflammation to metabolic abnormalities.

diet, chronic stress, or any number of other factors, you are triggering a chronic, low-grade inflammatory response that is slowly, silently affecting different systems of your body. Perhaps this manifests as a skin condition, perhaps it manifests as an arthritic condition, perhaps it manifests as a neurological condition, or perhaps it manifests as a metabolic condition such as heart disease.

Generally speaking, inflammation is inflammation. It manifests as many different chronic health conditions depending on where in the body it is focused. But it can come from many different sources, one of the most prominent being the gut. This is why we look back to the gut as the root cause of poor

The gut is a major source of inflammation.

The gut is a major source of inflammation, and this inflammation not only affects the inflammatory response from the gut—remember that up to 80 percent of the immune system resides in the gut—but also enters systemic circulation through an increase in intestinal permeability induced by the gut inflammation, creating a direct connection between the gut and the rest of the body. Indeed, gut inflammation is recognized as a contributor to the development of heart disease.[34]

Think about it—if you have a gut imbalance, whether from overuse of antibiotics, poor

health, or, conversely, we look to the gut as having the potential to create good health. We begin our journey to whole body health in the gut. We build the foundation of total body health in the gut.

Food Sensitivities Inflammation may also occur in response to undigested food particles or dietary allergens.[35] Food sensitivities are more common than most people realize. Food sensitivities are a major source of silent inflammation that can lead to health conditions far removed from the gut.[36]

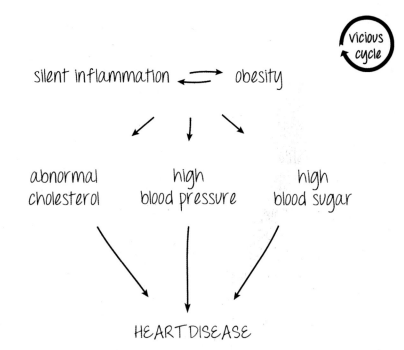

Stress Stress also induces gut inflammation,[37] and to make it interesting, gut inflammation induces stress.[38] This is one of many vicious cycles that exist in relation to the gut. See the chapter 8 for more information on stress and heart function.

Leaky gut An underappreciated gut condition affecting many people, and underlying a range of health conditions, is leaky gut, or increased intestinal permeability. In a healthy state, the gut lining allows only the smallest food particles, nutrients, and substances to pass through the gut lining into circulation. When the gut lining becomes compromised—due to inflammation, and often triggered by dysbiosis—

leaky gut results, creating a gateway into the body for toxins, undigested food particles, and bacteria to enter circulation.

Think of your intestinal lining as a screen, letting in fresh air but keeping out larger pests such as insects. When the screen has a hole, however, the unwanted insects get in. Leaky gut is like having a screen with holes—the unwanted particles leak into systemic circulation. The result of this constant influx of foreign invaders into systemic circulation is a response by the immune system that creates inflammation. Indeed, leaky gut is a major connection between the gut and the rest of the body.

Leaky Gut

Close-up view of leaky gut. In the presence of leaky gut, or increased intestinal permeability, harmful bacteria (green), toxins (brown) and undigested food particles (brown) enter through a damaged intestinal lining (pink).

Toxins and undigested food particles

Epithelial cell (intestinal lining)

Harmful bacteria

Capillary

Lymphatic capillary

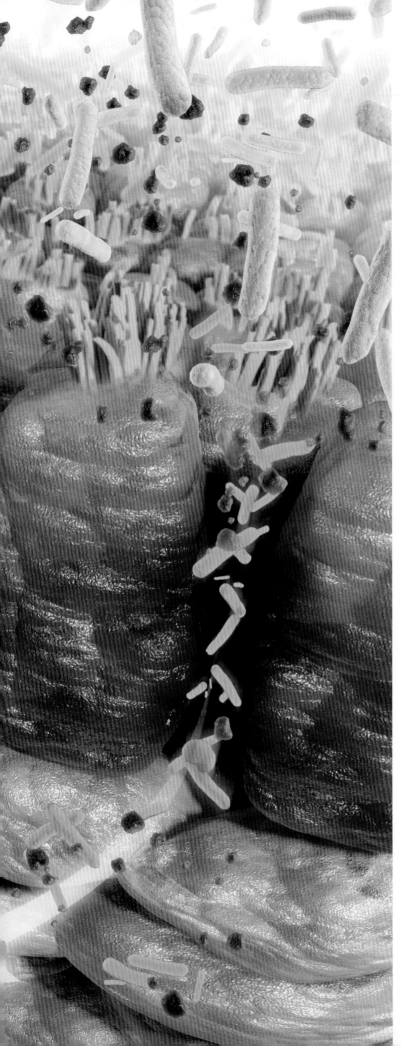

Before you think you are in the clear because you don't have a digestive condition and you are in tip-top shape, think again.

Even if your diet is impeccable, you're not under any stress, you don't take any medications, drink alcohol, or smoke—even if you are as healthy as you can possibly be, you could still have leaky gut. That's right. Most people relate leaky gut to poor digestive health, but a recent study has found that even healthy people can have leaky gut.[39] What's worse, these people were also found to have increased abdominal and liver fat storage, suggesting that leaky gut may trigger metabolic dysfunction, even in seemingly healthy people.

Low stomach acid Stomach acid, or hydrochloric acid (HCl), is normally released into the stomach in small amounts at the sight or thought of food, and it is released in larger amounts when food enters the stomach. HCl has a number of important roles in digestion. The presence of HCl in the stomach helps to untangle protein molecules so that they can be better digested, and it also triggers the production of pepsin, the digestive enzyme responsible for the digestion of protein in the stomach. Further, HCl regulates the acidity, or pH level, in the stomach. When present in adequate amounts, HCl increases stomach acidity, essentially sterilizing the stomach against pathogens that pass through the stomach with food. The presence of HCl is also necessary for the proper assimilation of certain vitamins and minerals, such as folic acid, vitamin C, beta-carotene, iron, and some forms of calcium, magnesium, and zinc.[40]

These days, when most people think of stomach acid, they associate it with heartburn and acid reflux. We have been told by doctors and pharmaceutical companies that the cause of heartburn is too much stomach acid. This is a convenient and profitable notion, as pharmaceutical companies have drugs that effectively suppress stomach acid and relieve the symptoms of heartburn.

The doctors and pharmaceutical companies are not all wrong by saying stomach acid causes heartburn. But there is more to the story. If you look back to research that dates before the advent of proton-pump inhibitors and H2 acid blockers as treatment for heartburn, you will find that the underlying malfunction involves the end of the esophagus—the lower esophageal sphincter (LES).

The LES functions as an opening that normally stays closed except when swallowing, as a way to let contents pass through the esophagus into the stomach, and to keep them in the stomach. When the LES does not close properly, stomach contents, including acid, can back up into the esophagus, irritating the delicate esophageal lining.

While most people think heartburn is due to too much stomach acid, too little stomach acid is actually a common cause of heartburn symptoms. Especially with age, up to 40 percent of people may have little or no stomach acid production.[41] Low stomach acid helps explain the symptoms of heartburn for a couple reasons.

First, if there is no stomach acid to help break down protein, which can be difficult to digest, protein foods remain undigested in the stomach for longer periods, which can create the symptoms of heartburn and belching and irritate the esophagus. Second, stomach acid triggers the release of digestive enzymes into the upper small intestine by the pancreas. Pancreatic enzymes help to digest protein, fat, and carbohydrates, playing a major role in the eventual absorption of nutrients. Low stomach acid may inhibit the secretion of these digestive enzymes,[42] resulting in malabsorption of nutrients and the incomplete digestion of food, causing digestive symptoms.

In fact, indigestion (which is as it sounds: the incomplete digestion of food) is a common condition often diagnosed instead as acid reflux because the two share similar symptoms.[43] This is another convenient and profitable misdiagnosis for pharmaceutical companies, who have the perfect solution— acid-suppressing medications. If, instead, we look to the root cause of these symptoms, we understand that poor digestion and not enough stomach acid are often the problems.

So instead of treating the symptom of heartburn with a quick fix (in the form of acid-suppressing medications), we instead look to the root cause of the problem—poor digestion and eating habits (eating too much or too fast and inadequate chewing) and low stomach acid.

Insufficient digestive enzymes

Digestive enzymes produced by the body are produced in smaller amountst in the mouth and in the stomach, and in larger amounts by the pancreas to be secreted into the upper small intestine, or duodenum. By far, however, the majority of enzymes originate in the intestinal lining.[44] If there is a dysfunction in the ability of the pancreas to produce enzymes, or if the intestinal lining is compromised, undigested food passes through the intestines, which can trigger an inflammatory response by the immune system. This is one way in which food sensitivities and allergies develop. Insufficient digestive enzyme production can occur for many reasons, including illness, injury or trauma, excessive exercise, aging, toxic exposure, genetic predisposition, or a combination of these.[45]

Gut disorders In addition to the conditions mentioned above, there are many more digestive disorders that introduce dysbiosis and inflammation, or that trigger leaky gut. Millions of Americans suffer daily from such common conditions as heartburn, gastroesophageal reflux disease (GERD), inflammatory bowel disease (IBD), irritable bowel syndrome (IBS), and more. Symptoms such as bloating, gas, constipation, diarrhea, and stomach pain are some of the most common symptoms encountered during a visit to the doctor. Unfortunately, many people are given pills to cover the symptoms, rather than given advice about how to look for the root cause of these conditions. Many of these people are even told "it's all in your head" and given antidepressants, a common practice that really misses the mark.

> **While most people think heartburn is due to too much stomach acid, too little stomach acid is actually a more common problem.**

The quote to the left highlights the intricate interrelationships of the various digestive functions, and how an imbalance or malfunction in one area has far-reaching effects that extend well beyond the digestive tract. This is the gut connection. And this is how gut function can affect even the function of the cardiovascular

The Gut Connection to Heart Disease

To quote the *Textbook of Functional Medicine*: "Loss of digestion and absorption efficiency and integrity may lead to cascading multisystem failure. Maldigestion can lead to symptoms of gas, bloating, diarrhea, pain, and/or constipation—that is, general irritability of the system. Gut irritability, left untreated, may lead to leaky gut and the development of food allergies, bacterial or yeast overgrowth, and the production of toxins. Toxins may accelerate the irritation and leakiness, resulting in toxic molecules entering the portal and then systemic circulation. This creates stress on systemic defenses, leading to immune, hormonal, or inflammatory imbalance." [46]

system. The contribution of chronic, low-grade inflammation by the digestive system—induced by an array of digestive disorders and imbalances—is an important contributing factor to heart disease[47] that is overlooked by modern medicine. Building total-body health through optimal digestive function is key. Truly, the heart of total-body health lies in the gut.

Evidence that gut bacteria are different in obese people and people with type 2 diabetes (both conditions characterized by chronic, low-grade inflammation) has led to the investigation of gut imbalance as a cause of metabolic diseases.[48,49] Indeed, the gut microbiota of obese individuals has been found to more efficiently harvest nutrients from food and increase fat storage in animal studies,[50] and has been found to induce low-grade inflammation that creates metabolic abnormalities such as obesity and insulin resistance.[51,52,53] In children, differences in gut flora during infancy were found to predict those who became overweight by age seven.[54] That is, those infants with lower levels of beneficial bifidobacteria later became obese compared to those infants with higher levels of bifidobacteria. This suggests that a lack of bifidobacteria contributed to the development of overweight. Further, increasing the amount of bifidobacteria in the gut has been found to reduce diet-induced endotoxemia, a condition that occurs when bacterial toxins leak into systemic circulation through a leaky gut, and that has

been linked to chronic, low-grade inflammation, leading to features of metabolic syndrome and endothelial dysfunction.[55]

Non-alcoholic fatty liver disease (NAFLD) A condition that deserves special mention as a gut connection is non-

The heart of total-body health resides in the gut.

alcoholic fatty liver disease (NAFLD). NAFLD is characterized by an increase in fat accumulation in the liver. NAFLD affects up to one-third of Americans,[56] though most of these people do not know they have it. NAFLD has become more common as the obesity epidemic unfolds, and it is now considered one of the components of metabolic syndrome. As we have learned, metabolic syndrome can lead to type 2 diabetes and heart disease.

Because the liver is the first stop for all things absorbed from the gut, it is considered part of the digestive system. For this reason, the gut has a major effect on liver function. Studies have found that leaky gut caused by dysbiosis is associated with NAFLD, suggesting that leaky gut plays an important role in the accumulation of fat in the liver.[57] Further, the leakage of bacterial toxins into circulation—endotoxemia—has been implicated in the development of NAFLD.[58] Again, here is a gut connection that can lead to heart disease further down the road.

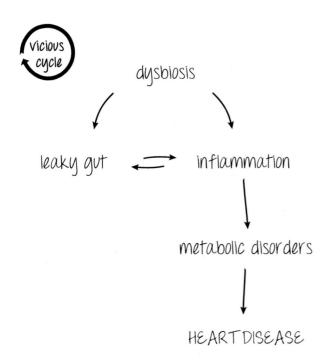

Digestive Complexity

Evaluating digestive imbalances can be complex because of the array of influences on digestive health. The physiologic processes involved in breaking down, digesting, and assimilating nutrients, removing waste from the body, defending against foreign invaders, and communicating with the immune and nervous systems are intricate and involve interconnections that require in-depth consideration.

Addressing each of these processes, and correcting imbalances by figuring out what is needed, and what is needed to be removed, is the essence of building digestive health. And

digestive health is the foundation for total-body health, upon which heart health is built. Think about what you choose to put into your body and how you choose to support its health and healing. Honor the complexity of the body's function and its ability for healing. Know that you have more influence on your health than you may think.

Digestive Evaluation

There are certain tests available that allow you to get an idea of your digestive health. Two important tests include the Comprehensive Stool Analysis (CSA) from Doctor's Data Laboratory and the Food Sensitivity Test from EnteroLab.

The CSA gives a good baseline picture of your gut health in a similar way that preventive blood work does. This test will show a gut imbalance even before symptoms develop. Because gut imbalance can lead to so many health conditions, correcting this imbalance is essential, even before health conditions arise.

The food sensitivity tests available from EnteroLab allow you to determine if you are reacting to certain foods that pass through your digestive system. Many people suffer from chronic health problems because they regularly consume foods that create an immune response in the gut that they may not feel but that occurs daily. Over time, this reaction slowly creates an imbalance in the gut bacteria, creating inflammation and leaky gut. This process introduces a chronic, low-grade inflammatory response in the body. As we have learned, this silent inflammation can trigger a host of health conditions throughout the body.

Stop looking for quick solutions for your symptoms. Instead, look to your inner terrain. You will find the real source of health in your gut. Then you can heal from the inside out.

Tips for Helping Improve Gut Function

See the Love Your Heart Section for a complete program to support heart health.

- Eat a diet low in grain-based, refined, and starchy carbohydrates and simple sugars, and high in vegetables, healthy fats, and lean proteins, nuts, and seeds.

- Increase your amount of physical activity. Find an activity you enjoy and get moving!

- Support healthy digestion and balance your gut with probiotics to help reduce inflammation in the body.

- Take an omega-3 fish oil supplement to increase the omega-3/omega-6 ratio.

- If you are not consuming at least 35 grams of fiber daily to promote regular elimination and healthy gut bacterial balance, take a fiber supplement.

- If you have digestive symptoms, try taking digestive enzymes (with or without HCl, depending on your stomach acid production) with every meal.

- Optimize your vitamin D level, between 50 and 70 ng/mL.

- If you have food sensitivities, eliminate those foods from your diet. If you think you have a food sensitivity, try an elimination diet or a food sensitivity test from EnteroLab.

- Test your gut balance with a Comprehensive Stool Analysis.

interview

Dr. Leonard Smith

Brenda discusses the gut connection to heart disease with vascular and general surgeon and co-author Leonard Smith, MD

BW: Dr. Smith, thank you for this interview. Your knowledge on the latest research as it relates to the gut, and to integrative medicine, is truly amazing. As a general vascular surgeon deeply entrenched in integrative medicine, you bring important information to this book, as you always do with my books. Tell us about your medical background.

LS: I completed the general and vascular surgery programs at both the University of Florida and University of Miami. I then stayed in Miami as codirector of the surgical ICU and taught surgery there for two years before going into surgical practice in Gainesville,

Florida. I also taught students as a member of the part-time volunteer faculty of the University of Florida. I retired from surgery and for the last six years I have been a medical advisor of the Department of Integrative Medicine, and on the volunteer surgical faculty at the University of Miami.

BW: How did you come to be interested in integrative medicine?

LS: My interest in integrative medicine began in the early 1980s. Working as a vascular surgeon I saw hundreds of vascular patients with significant amounts of hard and soft plaque material in their carotid, femoral, or coronary arteries. In fact, in many cases of redo coronary artery surgery where we had used saphenous veins to replace and bypass diseased arteries, a year or two later even the veins would be filled with hard and soft plaque material. I saw an even more graphic example of arterial disease in abdominal aortic aneurysms. They contained material that looked in every way like the gristle and fat that we find in the meat and chicken we eat. In addition, the cracked aneurysm walls were hard as rocks, at times making it very difficult to suture in new grafts.

I began to wonder about diet as the major contributor to this buildup and started to study nutrition. Around this same time, many of my patients were bringing me articles about plant-based diets and multivitamin/antioxidant supplementation. The more I read, and the more meetings I went to, the more I realized that vascular disease (like most all disease) is basically an alteration in gene function or expression brought about by epigenomic changes. The epigenome consists of molecular structures that fit around the genes (like clothes around a person), and strongly influence which genes are active and which are silent (much like the conductor of an orchestra). The epigenome (the conductor) responds to the environment (the audience) from which it receives its cues, and interacts by changing how it plays the genome. In other words, in a healthy environment you get good gene responses, and in an unhealthy environment, you get bad gene responses.

We didn't know much about epigenetics back then, but now we know that the environment we present to our epigenome determines which genes are expressed, and which are silenced, and the result is our phenotype. So it is not merely by chance that we have either a healthy muscular phenotype or an unhealthy obese phenotype. We now know that diet, sleep, elimination, toxicity, stress, malnutrition, inflammation, infections, exercise, and other lifestyle factors determine who we are—in other words, our phenotype. Thus, I began to incorporate integrative and lifestyle medicine into my surgical practice in 1982. Because I have seen it improve health in so many people, I have practiced integrative medicine ever since and now do it full time, mainly in a teaching capacity, but I still see a few patients and consult with doctors about difficult cases on a regular basis.

BW: What is integrative medicine?

LS: Allow me to expand on what I just said a little differently. To me, integrative medicine simply means combining the best of lifestyle management with the best standards of modern medical care. My definition of lifestyle includes diet, exercise, sleep, elimination, stress modification, psycho-emotional and spiritual attunements, detoxification based on challenge testing, and diagnostic testing looking at appropriate biomarkers and genomic markers. This usually leads to supplementation with vitamins, minerals, prebiotics/probiotics, antioxidants, essential fatty acids, and essential amino acids. Remember, diet includes mostly plants that are loaded with beneficial bacteria. In addition, supplementing with prebiotics and probiotics is wise, in order to maintain balance in your largest organ—your microbiome, or the 100 trillion bacteria composed of more than 1,000 species and subspecies of bacteria living in your intestinal tract.

BW: In comparison to conventional medicine, how does integrative medicine view heart disease?

LS: Integrative medicine is conventional medicine and more. Integrative medicine would still look at the traditional risk factors for heart disease, but it would also look at tests and biomarkers to determine if someone was on the pathway to developing vascular disease long before they exhibited symptoms. The testing may be based on family history, stress levels, poor diet, overweight, lack of exercise, and more.

We now know that over half of people hospitalized for heart disease have normal standard lipid levels that include total cholesterol, HDL, triglycerides, and the calculated LDL cholesterol. Unfortunately, for many people, the first and only symptom of heart disease is chest pain, cardiac arrest, and death! This is why it is so important to have the right balance of omega-6 and omega-3 essential oils. It has been shown that having the correct Omega-3 Index greatly reduces the likelihood of death following a heart attack.[1]

An integrative approach to medicine seeks to treat and prevent heart disease by addressing the underlying causes, whereas conventional medicine is generally concerned with managing symptoms through medicines, stents, or surgery. Don't get me wrong; this is often what is acutely needed. Pacemakers, medicines, stents, and surgeries have saved millions of lives, but lifestyle support is a must for long-term health and survival.

BW: What is heart disease?

LS: There are as many aspects of heart disease as there are parts of the heart. Congenital diseases, holes in the heart (VSDs and ASDs), diseases of the four heart valves, cardiomyopathy (diseases of the heart muscle often due to viruses), endocarditis (inflammation of the heart lining due to inflammation or infection), arrhythmias (diseases of the electrical system of the heart), and most common are diseases of the coronary arteries, which is what generally lead to arrhythmias, congestive heart failure, and heart attacks. However, I would like to point out that it is unusual to have diseases of the coronary arteries without also having disease in many other arteries of the body, especially in cerebrovascular, renal, peripheral (especially the lower legs), and intestinal arteries.

BW: What are the major causes of this vascular disease that affects not only the heart but the brain, kidneys, lower extremities, and all of the body?

LS: Vascular disease can, in fact, affect any blood vessel in the body. What causes it is multifactorial, with one or more of the following occurring at the same time: genetic/

epigenetic changes; lifestyle influences: diet, micronutrient deficiencies, inadequate sleep, poor bowel elimination, stress, and physical inactivity; allergies; and environmental toxicity: infections and microbial toxins, toxic minerals and fat-soluble toxins, air and water pollution, and electromagnetic pollution. These causes contribute to the biggest pathophysiologic mechanism of arterial disease: inflammation in the blood and/or arterial lining that extends into the wall of the arteries.

BW: Let's talk more about inflammation. What causes inflammation?

LS: First I would like to define inflammation as a response of all vascular tissues to harmful

foreign, an alarm reaction is created on the part of the body, beginning with the release of chemokines and cytokines (such as TNF-α, IL-6, IL-1β, and IL-17) that then upregulate (overactivate) the immune system, causing injury or destruction of tissues such as the arterial lining. Unfortunately, this immune response may also attack normal tissues in addition to the foreign antigens, as normal tissues may resemble the foreign antigens. This is known as antigen mimicry and is the underlying process involved in autoimmune disease.

BW: Why do you think many people—doctors included—do not realize the gut connection to systemic health, including heart health?

"It has been shown that having the correct Omega-3 Index greatly reduces the likelihood of death following a heart attack."

stimuli or injury that causes damage. It is the natural attempt by the body to remove the injury and to repair the damage. I think it is mainly tied in with immunity. Whether from injury or caused by antigens (matter that triggers an immune response) that come from microbes or microbial toxins, partially digested foods, allergenic or sensitive foods, and absorbed or inhaled toxins that the body identifies as

LS: It may be the out of sight, out of mind concept. I wonder how many people look at their bowel movements regularly. Most people do not realize that our bodies are made up of about 10 trillion cells, yet our gut bacteria cells number 100 trillion. These bacteria make up about 80 percent of the 3 to 4 pounds of fecal matter most people carry in their colons, and contain 100 times more DNA than our own body.[2]

"A compromised gut lining triggers an inflammatory immune response that allows toxins, bacteria, and undigested food particles to access the bloodstream, further increasing the inflammatory response in the bloodstream."

Significant changes in stool appearance, coupled with bloating, discomfort, and even minor changes in overall sense of well-being, may mean you have invited some unintended guests to lunch. These guests—the microbes that are consumed with food—dine in your intestinal "restaurant" on your partially or poorly digested food, hook up with their friends, reproduce more microbes just like them, and set up shop in your gut. This is a graphic way of saying that the bacteria you ingest with your food may not be beneficial, and may shift the microbial balance in their favor, creating what is known as dysbiosis—gut bacterial imbalance. Here the problems begin due to loss of intestinal barrier function also known as increased intestinal permeability, or leaky gut.

BW: So how does this bacterial gut connection lead to heart disease?

LS: As I mentioned, dysbiosis creates a scenario of, at the very least, low-grade inflammation (like a mild sunburn), which increases intestinal permeability and turns the immune system on high alert, triggering bodywide intravascular inflammation that heats up the arterial lining. Hot arteries are sticky and leaky arteries, attracting immune cells, thickening arteries, and eventually leading to heart attack.

So let's go back to the topic of increased intestinal permeability, or leaky gut. The gut lining is very selective. When the gut lining is healthy and intact it only lets in small molecules like digested food, and it keeps out larger molecules, bacteria, and toxins that should not be absorbed. The problem begins when the gut lining loses its selectivity due to inflammation. Leaky gut often goes unrecognized, but can be detected using the lactulose-mannitol intestinal permeability test.

According to Leo Galland, M.D., there are four vicious cycles that contribute to leaky gut syndrome (and are worsened by it): allergy, malnutrition, bacterial dysbiosis, and hepatic stress. Repairing and conserving the integrity of the gut lining is of utmost importance. A compromised gut lining triggers an inflammatory immune response that allows toxins, bacteria, and undigested food particles to access the bloodstream, further increasing the inflammatory response in the bloodstream. Endothelial dysfunction results, leading to the formation of soft plaque, and possibly rupture of that plaque, ending in heart attack.

Remember that the digestive tract begins in the mouth. In a clinic in Ft. Lauderdale, I was involved in a study of more than 1,000 patients in whom we measured hs-CRP (highly sensitive C-reactive protein) levels, an indicator of systemic inflammation. We then sent patients with high hs-CRP levels to an orthodontist to check for periodontal disease. The vast majority had gingivitis. After one or two months of treatment for gingivitis, we retested the hs-CRP levels and found that most went back down to normal levels. The presence of oral pathogens and periodontal disease has been found to be associated with heart disease. *Chlamydia pneumoniae*, one particular oral pathogen that gets between the teeth and the gums, enters systemic circulation and is associated with heart disease. In fact, *C. pneumoniae* has even been found in atherosclerotic plaque.[3]

If we know that bacteria from the mouth can enter circulation and trigger heart disease, bacteria from the gut could certainly also play a role. Indeed, studies are beginning to recognize just that. Gut bacteria upregulate inflammation through increased intestinal permeability. We know that at least 60 (some say up to 80) percent of the immune system resides in between the submucosa and the wall of the gut—the gut-associated lymphoid tissue (GALT). The GALT is highly responsive to the antigenic load being delivered to it. If the GALT doesn't like what it is presented, it will respond with a firestorm of inflammation in an effort to get rid of it. This inflammatory response is not necessarily confined to the gut. It leads to chronic, low-grade, systemic inflammation.

Studies are elucidating the relationship between intestinal permeability and metabolic disorders (like those associated with the metabolic syndrome and that lead to heart disease) by way of a phenomenon known as metabolic endotoxemia. Researchers have found that people who eat a high-fat diet experience a higher amount of bacterial toxins (a specific endotoxin known as lipopolysaccharide, or LPS, from the cell walls of gram-negative bacteria) entering the bloodstream through increased intestinal permeability when compared to those people who do not eat a high-fat diet.[4] Replacing bifidobacteria, beneficial gut bacteria, has been found to slow the absorption of LPS through the gut lining.

When the LPS travels into the bloodstream it literally sits on white blood cells—on the CD14 and TLR4 receptors—and upregulates immunity, triggering an inflammatory process that leads to insulin resistance, ending up with endothelial dysfunction. There is no question that too much inflammation in the blood, whether from bacteria or toxins, upregulates immunity—innate immunity, Th1 cellular immunity, Th2 humoral immunity, and Th17 cellular immunity—creating, basically, hot, angry blood that damages the lining of arteries.

Endothelial dysfunction is similar to intestinal permeability in that it involves a compromise in the lining of the arteries—the endothelium. White blood cells known as monocytes enter through a "leaky vessel," whereby they become known as macrophages. The macrophages engulf oxidized LDL (which became oxidized as a result of inflammation in the bloodstream) until they enlarge. Enlarged macrophages filled with LDL are known as foam cells. Foam cells, along with reactive oxygen species and other free radicals create a fire underneath the arterial lining—the characteristic soft atherosclerotic plaque with a fibrous top (like a pimple) that may rupture, triggering the clotting mechanisms, blocking arteries, and leading to heart attack.

BW: What can people do to support heart health?

LS: We know that lifestyle plays the biggest role. Proper diet, plenty of exercise, adequate sleep, regular bowel elimination, support of the body's detoxification pathways, stress management, and psycho-spiritual-emotional reorientation to elicit contentment and happiness are where it's at. I think that in the future we will have access to detox centers that are used like the fitness centers of today. These centers will offer ways to support all of the lifestyle factors listed above.

Doctors will become like health coaches, and they will set the example rather than offer advice in "Do as I say, not as I do" fashion.

Also important is supplementation with fiber, omega-3s, vitamin D, and prebiotics and probiotics. Prebiotics are the foods that feed probiotic bacteria, or the beneficial gut bacteria. Prebiotic foods include artichokes, asparagus, onions, garlic, and chicory, to name a few. Prebiotic and probiotic formulas can be taken to help change the ratio of gut flora in a beneficial way.

That is the future of medicine. People will heal themselves. All the information is available; we have only to seek it out, and then put it into practice. Keep plugging away at improving the lifestyle factors above. This is truly how to prevent, and even reverse, heart disease.

BW: Insulin resistance and inflammation go hand in hand. How can we fix this vicious cycle?

LS: We definitely have to fix insulin resistance, but it needs to be done slowly with many different interventions. It has been shown that when blood sugar is too rapidly lowered, patients may do poorly.[5] Insulin resistance is actually a protective mechanism for preventing too much sugar from entering the cells, also known as glucotoxicity. High intracellular glucose indirectly blocks ATP production in the mitochondria, which is not good. Thus, insulin resistance slows the absorption of glucose to maintain mitochondrial function, serving as a protection mechanism.

This highlights the importance of lowering blood glucose and correcting insulin resistance gradually with appropriate medications, if needed, and diet, hydration, exercise, stress reduction, sleep, exercise, and appropriate supplements, as mentioned previously. High blood sugar leads to fat storage, which

a profound effect on the food we digest and on how we digest it, and helps to produce vitamins like vitamin K and B12. Beneficial gut bacteria help to crowd out bad bacteria, fungi, and parasites, produce short-chain fatty acids (fuel for the colon lining), absorb toxins and facilitate their removal from the body, and communicate,

> "I have seen hundreds of patients improve various ailments, including bowel irregularity, psoriasis and other skin conditions, and certainly inflammatory bowel disorders, by taking probiotic bacteria."

increases inflammation. In addition, high blood sugar not only glycates hemoglobin, it glycates other serum proteins like albumin, creating major free radicals known as advanced glycation end products (AGEs), and other free radicals that can then oxidize LDL, leading to plaque formation.

BW: What do you believe is the role of probiotic bacteria to our overall health?

LS: I have seen hundreds of patients improve various ailments, including bowel irregularity, psoriasis and other skin conditions, and certainly inflammatory bowel disorders, by taking probiotic bacteria. The bacterial flora has

educate, and program our immune system so that it knows when to attack, and when to not attack, the particles that enter systemic circulation every day.

Gut bacteria affect many metabolic processes related to food. We know that the gut bacteria present in obese people are different from, and are more efficient at extracting calories from food as compared to the gut bacteria, of lean people.[6] Scientists are currently working out the details of these complex interactions. In the future, we will know a lot more about what bacterial species are beneficial for an array of different health conditions.

BW: So the good gut bacteria are on our side.

LS: Right. For example, in some people who have severe bacterial imbalance, common after antibiotic treatment, a particular pathogen—*Clostridium difficile*—takes over, causing diarrhea that can be mild or severe, and recurrent. Severe *C. difficile* infections are one of the most frightening things I have seen as a physician. It is probably one of the leading causes of emergency colectomy (colon removal) surgery today.

Even people who have mild *C. difficile* infection may experience recurrent infection that

recently talked to physicians who have used this therapy. One gastroenterologist has treated ten patients with chronic recurrent *C. difficile* with fecal bacteriotherapy using bowel movements from healthy family members. The stool is screened for pathogens and the family member's blood is screened for viral pathogens. After the patient is treated with the antibiotic vancomycin and the laxative polyethylene glycol, both to lower the pathogen load, blended and filtered stool is transplanted with a colonoscope into the terminal ileum and the colon. So far, ten out of ten of these patients have not experienced a recurrence of

"Omega-3s have important anti-inflammatory properties in the gut, as well as throughout the body."

disappears after treatment, only to reappear a few weeks later, in a vicious cycle that gradually destroys the intestinal lining and may lead to a host of autoimmune conditions. It is critical that these people get cured.

One treatment for recurrent *C. difficile* appears to be fecal bacteriotherapy, the transfer of feces from a healthy donor to the colon of the infected patient. This therapy is not new; it's been around since the 1950s. I have

C. difficile diarrhea. Some of these people get better within 24 hours. It's a remarkable therapy.

There are now many papers coming out on the benefits of fecal bacteriotherapy, especially for treatment of recurrent *C. difficile* infection.[7,8] The same gastroenterologist I mentioned above also informed me that fecal transplants are being used in patients with Crohn's disease, ulcerative colitis, and even morbid obesity. If you consider the effect certain gut bacteria have on obesity, changing the gut balance to resemble that of a healthy individual might certainly lead to weight loss. Some people have a difficult time losing weight, even with a very low calorie diet. It is important to know that it's not just what you eat, but who (your gut bacteria) are helping you eat.

Taking fecal bacteriotherapy to the next level, and relating it back to heart health, researchers in the Netherlands have found that fecal transplants from lean donors improved hepatic and peripheral insulin resistance, in addition to fasting lipid levels, in obese individuals with metabolic syndrome.[9] This is a perfect example of the gut connection to metabolic syndrome and then to cardiovascular diseases.

I think we are looking at a very different future in terms of how we will deal with all illnesses. It is a cosmic comedy of sorts—the answer to many of our health problems is as close as the bacteria that reside in our own guts. By rebalancing the gut with the right bacteria, we will probably be able to fix many of the problems in the body.

BW: Fecal transplant is not widely available, or widely applicable, yet. What is the next best thing?

LS: Probiotics. Here is a snapshot of the future: There will be available probiotic formulas— perhaps available as transplants—that contain more than 100 bacterial species that have been found to benefit human health. These will be microbiome transplants—a super multistrain probiotic, if you will, that reflects the balance of gut bacteria in a healthy human.

You see, people tend to have a balanced microbiome until something happens: an illness, or even a great deal of stress, like a death in the family. Stress lowers the beneficial *Lactobacillus* and *Bifidobacterium* species in the gut. The neutral bacteria become pathogenic, and the pathogenic bacteria really get out of hand, increasing intestinal permeability. What begins as a stressful issue turns into a health issue, and vice versa, in a vicious cycle of declining health. In the future, we will have the ideal microbiome solution for humans, which will address many different health conditions. It will be like a library of various human microbiomes that have the right number and types of bacteria for different conditions frozen and ready to go, much like we are currently doing with our cord blood stem cell banks.

BW: The gut connection to heart disease continues to unfold. Are there any other interesting studies to note?

LS: Published studies continue to elucidate the mechanisms by which gut bacteria and probiotic administration contribute to heart health. A recent study in animals has even found that a combination of *Lactobacillus* plantarum and *Bifidobacterium lactis* reduced heart attack size by reducing the amount of leptin in the blood, in a similar way as the antibiotic vancomycin.[10] The probiotics affected heart attack size as much as the strong antibiotic, which highlights a strong role of the gut microbial balance in relation to heart health.

BW: What about omega-3s? Why are they important?

LS: Interestingly, omega-3 fatty acids have been found to improve the immune effects and adhesion properties of *Lactobacillus paracasei* probiotics in the gut.[11] So taking omega-3s with probiotics may be a good idea. Omega-3s have important anti-inflammatory properties in the gut, as well as throughout the body. Omega-3 status is a fundamental determinant of health—heart health, brain health, whole-body health, really.

The omega-3 oils are essential, literally. Alpha-linolenic acid (ALA) is the omega-3 essential fatty acid that must be obtained from the diet because the body does not make it. Linoleic acid (LA) is the omega-6 fatty acid that must be obtained from the diet. Because the body cannot make these fats, they are considered essential fatty acids. But you also need EPA and DHA because although the body can convert some ALA into EPA, and to a lesser extent, into DHA, you can't make enough of it endogenously. This is why an omega-3 fish oil supplement is important.

If you really want to know your fat status, do an oil check, just like you do with your car. The red blood cell membrane essential and metabolic fatty acid blood test, or the Omega-3 Index finger prick test, will give you a good idea of the levels of different fats that are incorporated into the membrane of your red blood cells. This represents a picture of long-term fatty acid status, rather than a snapshot of one moment in time.

If you do not have enough of the omega-3s EPA and DHA, the body will produce inflammatory compounds known as prostaglandin E2 (PGE2) from the omega-6 metabolite DGLA. DGLA converts to arachidonic acid (AA), which then converts into PGE2. If EPA and DHA are abundant, the DGLA will be converted to the anti-inflammatory PGE1. Further, EPA and DHA trigger the production of another anti-inflammatory compound, PGE3. You want a balance between the anti-inflammatory PGE1 and PGE3 with the inflammatory PGE2. You get that balance by increasing omega-3 fish oil intake (high in EPA and DHA), lowering omega-6 fat intake, reducing oxidative stress, and controlling blood sugar levels.

Because animal products are higher in arachidonic acid (AA), especially fattier meat and red meat, it is important to balance animal product intake with plenty of vegetables. There are many reasons to eat plenty of vegetables. In fact, one study tested the effects of increasing daily intake of vegetable and fruit from 5 to 12 servings in healthy women. Even though these women already had a relatively high vegetable and fruit intake (especially when compared to the average American, who eats less than two servings daily), increasing to 12 servings daily significantly reduced their levels of a marker of oxidative DNA damage

(8-OH deoxyguanosine).[12] So the more vegetables and fruit you eat (low glycemic fruit in moderation), the less oxidative stress in your body, and the less damage to DNA, important for overall health.

basketball, football, track, or soccer. The cardiac stress test can pick up very minor changes, indicating a problem that could lead to tragic death, particularly in a child or teen.

"One of the hallmarks of integrative medicine (also known as preventative or functional medicine, see www.functionalmedicine.org) **is that we are doing functional testing long before diseases develop."**

BW: What are important tests people should take to determine and monitor heart disease risk, in order of importance?

LS: One of the hallmarks of integrative medicine (also known as preventative or functional medicine; see www.functionalmedicine.org) is that we are doing functional testing long before diseases develop. There are many tests available—some are expensive, and some are relatively inexpensive and covered by insurance. Most people are aware that a cardiac stress test is an important diagnostic test to determine the efficiency and health of the heart. I do recommend that everyone get this test done at some point. It is probably important even for children and teens, especially if they are playing highly aerobic sports such as swimming,

Adding heart rate variability (HRV, a measure of cardiac autonomic balance) and echocardiogram (ECHO, an ultrasound of the heart) gives considerably more information that could detect asymptomatic heart problems that could be serious. I know many would say these are expensive tests, but why not invest in your health and maybe prevent a serious problem? I also know if we got our medical economics/politics worked out many of our important tests would be less expensive.

In terms of early prevention, I honestly think the best place for everyone to start—adults and kids alike (especially if overweight)—would be the glucose/insulin stress test. This test stresses your pancreas's ability to make insulin and respond to feedback signals, and basically gives a snapshot of how the cells in your body are responding to the glucose and insulin load coming through the vascular system to cell surface receptors throughout the body.

percent of people with a totally normal standard lipid profile will have significant negative vascular event, it should be obvious that this panel alone prevents many people from becoming aware of their health risks.

"Most doctors order the standard lipid panel... this panel alone prevents many people from becoming aware of their health risks."

Typically the test first measures fasting glucose and insulin, then the person takes 75 grams of oral glucose as a drink or tablets, and glucose and insulin levels are checked at 30 minutes and again at 1 and 2 hours.[13] Many doctors only check the fasting blood glucose or maybe two-hour glucose. If the fasting and challenged insulin are not checked, the patient is done a real disservice. It is even possible that patients may have a normal fasting insulin, but the challenged insulin at 1 or 2 hours stays high (over 50 iu/ml). If this is true, they are likely to have increased fat storage, high blood pressure, and increased inflammation in the blood, which will lead to vascular dysfunction, and all the problems mentioned earlier.

Most doctors order the standard lipid panel: total cholesterol, LDL cholesterol, HDL cholesterol, and triglycerides. Since about 50

Here are some of the other valuable blood tests to add:

- 25 OH vitamin D blood test: It's very important to keep level around 50 ng/mL.

- hs-CRP: A valuable marker of inflammation; less than 1.0 is ideal.

- Hemoglobin A1C (HbA1c): A good indicator of high blood sugar during the 3 months prior to the test; should be <5.7%, ideal is 4%–5.4%. Glycated hemoglobin is the percentage of sugar stuck to hemoglobin producing a free radical, thus lower is better in general.

- Homocysteine: A marker of inflammation related to B vitamin deficiencies; ideal is less than 10.

- Fibrinogen: An inflammation marker.

- Iron and ferritin levels: Major inflammation if they are too high; many people have genetic variations (hereditary hemochromatosis, or HHC) that cause their iron to be quite high and they should donate blood about every 2 months to prevent cardiovascular disease.

- LDL particle size: Small and dense are bad, large are good.

- Oxidized LDL: The dangerous form of LDL.

- Apolipoprotein A1: Attaches to HDL and helps remove cholesterol from vessels.

- Apolipoprotein B: High levels of ApoB can lead to plaques and could cause vascular disease; it is associated with LDL and takes cholesterol to cells.

- ApoB/ApoA1 ratio: Should be <.8.

- HDL particle size: Ideal would be increase in total number, size, and amount of HDL. We now know total HDL number is not as important as HDL function. Function tests are being developed to access the true value of HDL in a given patient.

- Adiponectin: Usually low when insulin is high, and when it rises (as with exercise), it tends to reverse insulin resistances.

- C-peptide: A C-peptide test measures the level of this peptide in the blood. It is generally found in amounts equal to insulin because the two are linked when insulin is produced in the pancreas. Basically, it is a biomarker for insulin.

- Proinsulin: If proinsulin is elevated in the blood, it means beta cell function is poor due to inability to make insulin from proinsulin.

For more information on functional testing see page 277.

There are actually many more, but this would be a good start. Possibly the simplest and cheapest test would be to measure VAT (visceral adipose tissue, or belly fat), using a tape measure around the waist just above the hip. Men need to be 40 inches or less and women 35 inches or less.

Another option would be to see an integrative practitioner who can do what is known as bioimpedance analysis. This is a quick and easy noninvasive test in which small electrical leads are placed on a hand and ankle (much like an electrocardiogram), and information is obtained that will give you your total fat mass, lean mass (muscles, bones, tendons, organs, etc.), total body water, and intracellular and extracellular water. These approximate numbers are very informative about one's state of hydration, inflammation, and whether they have enough muscle mass compared to fat, as a marker of true health. Usually this is a call for getting back to exercise—aerobic, resistance training, and stretching—and for staying well hydrated.

BW: Thank you so much, Dr. Smith, for talking to me about the gut connection. You are a walking encyclopedia, and your contribution to this book has been eye-opening, for sure. Your ability to keep up with the latest studies, and to apply them from an integrative standpoint, is commendable. Thank you for always keeping me up to date on this cutting-edge research.

"No matter what, remember to breathe."

—*Dave Ellis*

Chapter 8
Stress

When most people think of stress, they think of it as a bad thing. Simply put, stress is the feeling that arises when life's demands exceed a person's ability to handle those demands. The feeling of stress is often associated with a negative event or emotion, but there are actually two types of stress: distress and eustress.[1] Distress is the negative-type stress, the characteristic feeling associated with a job loss, an argument with a friend, or an unexpected traffic jam. Eustress is the feeling experienced during events such as a raise, a marriage, or when winning a race. Eustress is an important part of many pleasurable activities. All these events place stress on the body and mind, but not all are perceived as negative.

Homeostasis—Total Body Balance

The human body has an amazing capacity for finding balance, or what is called homeostasis. The many physiologic processes in the body all have the overall intention of returning the body to homeostasis. When stress is felt, whether it's emotional, mental, or physical, the body responds by increasing the production of stress hormones in an effort to return the body to a homeostatic balance. This function falls under the direction of the autonomic nervous system, the part of the nervous system that controls the involuntary functions of the body such as heart rate, metabolism, and digestion.

Autonomic Nervous System

The autonomic nervous system is comprised of two parts: the sympathetic and parasympathetic nervous systems. The sympathetic nervous system activates heart rate, increases blood pressure for increased blood flow, and releases stress hormones such as adrenaline (epinephrine) and cortisol. Essentially, the sympathetic nervous system controls the fight-or-flight response, the body's reaction to stress. During fight-or-flight, fat is mobilized from fat cells and nutrients are carried throughout the body, especially to the brain and muscles, decreasing reaction time. Short term, this is a very useful physiologic response to a stressful situation.

Evolutionarily, the fight-or-flight response was essential for survival in life-or-death situations; it prepares the body to meet the demands of stress. In today's world, the stressors we encounter are usually not a matter of life or death, but instead are encountered in a mild form on a regular basis. Our ability to cope with stress has not changed much over the past several thousand years,[2] however. Challenging situations in today's world trigger the fight-or-flight response just as the dangerous situations our ancestors faced did. Chronic stress, as experienced by so many people in our modern world, has the effect of resetting the body's point of homeostasis to a new, not-quite-balanced set point,[3] which has long-term effects on our health—physically, mentally, and emotionally.

The parasympathetic nervous system regulates calmer actions in the body such as digestion. The sympathetic and parasympathetic nervous systems work in a push-pull manner. When the sympathetic nervous system is activated, the heart speeds up, adrenaline courses through the body, and digestion is slowed. When the sympathetic nervous system calms down, the parasympathetic nervous system is activated and digestion begins again. Think about how when you get upset you lose your appetite or get a stomachache. These are the manifestations of the autonomic nervous system at work.

——————— Sympathetic nervous system

——————— Parasympathetic nervous system

The Autonomic Nervous System

The autonomic nervous system is made up of the parasympathetic (green) and sympathetic (blue) divisions, which work in a push-pull manner. When the sympathetic nervous system is activated, the parasympathetic nervous system is slowed, and vice versa.

TIP:

Chronic stress has
long-term effects on
our health—physically,
mentally, and emotionally.

Physical – Asthma • Back pain • Change in appetite • Cold, clammy hands • Constipation • Coughing • Cramps • Diarrhea • Dizziness • Dry mouth • Facial tics • Facial tightness • Fatigue • Headaches • Heartburn • Heart palpitations • Indigestion • Muscle aches, stiffness, tension • Nausea • Skin disorders • Sleep disturbances • Stomach pains • Sweating or facial flushing • Tapping or drumming fingers **Emotional** – Anger • Anxiety • Confusion • Depression • Difficulty concentrating • Excessive crying without obvious cause • Fear • Feeling of time pressure • Forgetfulness • Frustration • Impatience • Irritability • Lack of emotional feeling • Overreaction to events • Panic • Withdrawal **Behavioral** – Chain smoking • Excessive drinking • Hair twisting • Nail biting • Pacing • Picking at skin • Rapid speaking • Restlessness • Teeth grinding

Signs and Symptoms of Mental Stress[4]

Stress and Heart Disease

Stress is one of the most common patient complaints. Many studies evaluating stress have found it to be as important a risk factor for cardiovascular disease as high cholesterol, high blood pressure, and smoking.[5,6] The physiological response to stress, by increasing blood pressure and heart rate, increases turbulence in the bloodstream, which puts pressure on the walls of the arteries, damaging the artery lining.

In countless studies, stress has been linked to cardiovascular disease. In middle-aged men, stress is a risk factor for cardiovascular disease, and particularly for fatal stroke.[7] Work stress, in particular, not only plays a role in the development of heart disease but has also been associated with a higher risk of metabolic syndrome and obesity, two conditions that can lead to heart disease.[8] People with chronic work stress have twice the odds of developing metabolic syndrome than those people without stress.[9] And in women, stress from marital relationships has been found to seriously affect heart disease outcomes.[10]

Depression, social isolation, and lack of quality social support—all of which involve stress—are particularly strong risk factors for heart disease.[11]

Myth:

Only major symptoms of stress require attention.

Distressed patients with heart disease are more likely to be re-hospitalized within six months of their main cardiovascular hospitalization.[12] Reduction of psychological distress has been found to reduce death after heart attack in patients participating in stress interventions.

Age becomes a factor when considering the heart disease risk of stress. Older adults are less resilient to stress and illness than younger adults, leaving them more susceptible to develop heart disease.[13] Abdominal fat also plays a role in a person's vulnerability to stress. In one study in premenopausal women, those with higher waist-to-hip ratios had higher cortisol levels and reported more chronic stress.[14] This study also suggested that the stress-induced cortisol secretion may contribute to the accumulation of belly fat, highlighting the important role of stress in the development of chronic disease.

Depression and Heart Disease

Depression deserves special recognition as it relates to heart disease. Depressed individuals have a decreased ability to return to a normal heart rate after a stressful event. This dysfunctional stress response can contribute to heart disease risk.[15] Further, up to 15 percent of patients with heart disease

In countless studies, stress has been linked to cardiovascular disease.

and up to 20 percent of patients who have undergone coronary bypass surgery experience major depression.[16]

Depression has been found to be such an important risk factor in heart disease that the American Heart Association recommends that all heart disease patients be screened for depression.[17] Depression can lead to heart disease for two main reasons. One, people who are depressed are more likely to engage in activities that increase heart disease risk, such as smoking, drinking alcohol, or avoiding exercise, and two, depression contributes to the same metabolic abnormalities as stress. This is because depression is a form of stress. Addressing depression is crucial in people with heart disease.

Fact:

Even mild, seemingly "normal" stress can take a toll on your health, especially heart health.

The Dalai Lama, when asked what surprised him most about humanity, answered, "Man. Because he sacrifices his health in order to make money. Then he sacrifices money to recuperate his health. And then he is so anxious about the future that he does not enjoy the present; the result being that he does not live in the present or the future; he lives as if he is never going to die and then he dies having never really lived."

Heart Rate Variability

Repeated activation of the autonomic nervous system, as occurs with chronic stress, lowers heart rate variability, a condition associated with stress.[18,19] Heart rate variability is a measure of the naturally occurring, beat-to-beat changes in heart rate. Deep inhalation should increase heart rate, which shortens beat-to-beat variability, and exhalation lengths the variability, or slows heart rate. The greater the variation between the shortening and lengthening heart beat patterns during breathing, the lower the cardiovascular risk.[20]

Think of heart rate variability as the balance between the two branches of the autonomic nervous system. The sympathetic nervous system should increase heart rate upon inhalation, and the parasympathetic nervous system should decrease heart rate upon exhalation. Again we see the push-pull relationship of the autonomic nervous system—parasympatheic with sympathetic.

Essentially, heart rate variability is a measure of a person's ability to respond to stress. A decrease in heart rate variability indicates an imbalance in autonomic nervous function, likely induced by stress. Heart rate variability can be measured by echocardiogram, and also by the emWave device, available from the Institute of HeartMath.

Inflammation and Stress

There are many contributing factors to stress, and to the release of stress hormones. Stress hormones are regulated by the hypothalamus gland, considered the master gland of the neuroendocrine system. During stress, the hypothalamus stimulates the pituitary gland, which in turn stimulates the adrenals to secrete more of the hormone cortisol. This is known as the HPA axis. Cortisol increases blood sugar, suppresses the immune system, increases fat deposition, and breaks down muscle. Elevated levels of cortisol are found in people with both acute and chronic stress.[21,22]

The hypothalamus also stimulates the sympathetic nervous system to release the hormones adrenaline (epinephrine) and noradrenaline (norepinephrine) from the adrenal glands.

Adrenaline increases heart rate, constricts the blood vessels to increase blood flow, and dilates airways for improved breathing capacity. Noradrenaline increases heart rate, triggers the release of glucose from energy stores, increases blood flow to muscle, and increases the brain's oxygen supply.

Inflammation in the body has a major effect on the HPA axis, acting as a potent trigger of the stress response.[23] Conversely, stress increases inflammation in the body.[24] This vicious cycle is an important one to address, because of the many sources of both stress and inflammation. The stress-inflammation cycle can lead to an increase in abdominal fat, insulin resistance, and abnormal blood lipid levels, all contributors to heart disease.[25]

A passage from the *Textbook of Functional Medicine* highlights the far-reaching effects of stress: "The current conceptualization is that chronic dysregulation of the HPA axis, the autonomic nervous system, and the immune system contributes to chronic alterations in metabolism and inflammation, which then interact with other influences (e.g., nutrition, genetics) to cascade into specific diseases such as the metabolic syndrome, hypertension, cardiovascular disease, and even depression and cancer."[26]

TIP:

Address sources of inflammation as a way to reduce the body's stress response, and vice versa.

People vary in their ability to respond to stress. Some people do well under short-term stress, riding on the adrenaline and utilizing the increased blood flow to their advantage. Other people do not perform well under stress, instead feeling overwhelmed. Not many people do well under chronic stress, however. Over time, chronic stress wears on the body and mind, leading to mental fatigue, emotional instability, and physical illness.

The Gut Connection to Stress

It is well known that stress can affect gut function. Stress shuts down the parasympathetic branch of the autonomic nervous system, slowing digestion, reducing motility, and halting digestive secretions. Think about how you lose your appetite when you get in an argument, how your stomach turns when you are nervous, or how your stomach hurts when you're upset. These are all manifestations of stress on the gut.

The gut houses its own branch of the nervous system, the enteric nervous system, made up of about 100 million nerves connecting the gut to the brain by way of the autonomic nervous system. We already learned that

the autonomic nervous system is responsible for the stress response. Now we can see how closely tied the gut is to this system. This is known as the gut-brain connection.[27]

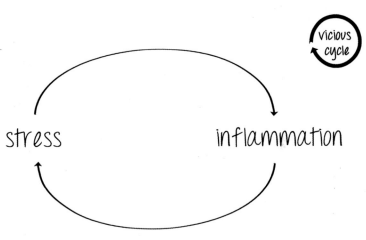

One of the main ways stress alters gut function is by increasing leaky gut, or intestinal permeability.[28] Remember from chapter 7 that leaky gut is like having holes in the screen of your intestinal lining. Normally, the intestinal lining should let in small nutrients, but with leaky gut, the intestinal lining is damaged and leaks larger-than-normal food particles and toxins into systemic circulation. Leaky gut is one of the main pathways triggering chronic, low-grade inflammation, and stress is one

TIP:

Gut bacteria have been found to regulate the body's stress response.

cause of this. Both chronic stress and acute stress have been found to increase leaky gut.[29]

Stress also changes the gut bacterial balance. Decreases in the beneficial bacteria *Lactobacillus*, and increased susceptibility to infections have been demonstrated in animal studies evaluating the effects of stress on the gut.[30] Researchers have also found shifts in the proportions of some gut bacterial species in people experiencing stress from anger or fear.[31] Recent studies support the role of probiotics in alleviating stress-induced alterations of gut function, particularly by reducing intestinal permeability, or leaky gut.[32] Indeed, the gut microbiota has been found to regulate the HPA stress response.[33]

The gut itself can be a source of stress for many people. It is estimated that one in four people in the United States has frequent gastrointestinal problems that can severely disrupt a normal lifestyle.[34] This is another vicious cycle—stress increases gut dysfunction, and gut dysfunction increases stress.

The Gut-Stress-Heart Connection

stress

abdominal fat

gut dysfunction

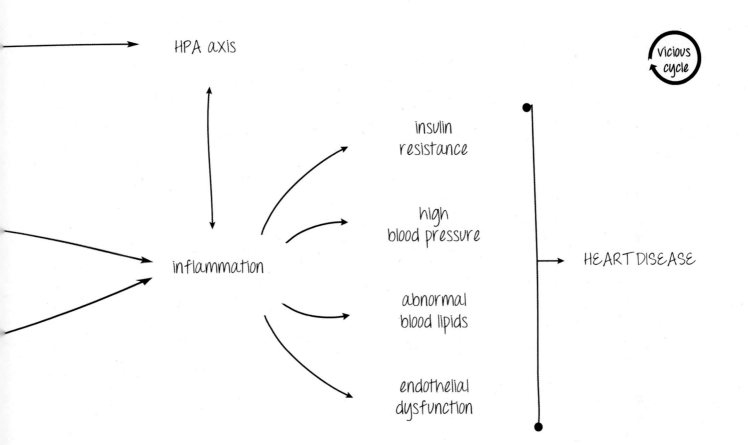

HPA axis

inflammation

insulin resistance

high blood pressure

abnormal blood lipids

endothelial dysfunction

HEART DISEASE

vicious cycle

Stress Reduction

Looking at the many adverse effects that result from stress, or that are intertwined with the stress response, it becomes clear that stress management is crucial. This chapter has only touched on the many negative outcomes of stress on the body and mind, and particularly on the heart. In today's world, stress is virtually unavoidable, highlighting the importance of stress relief. Fortunately, there are many ways to relieve stress. The following is a summary of stress management techniques and practices.

Lifestyle balance An imbalance between work, family, and personal time is a common cause of stress. Evaluate your relationship to each of these facets of your life, and try to bring about more balance among them.

Healthy diet Adopt a healthy diet as a way to maintain optimal total-body health. What you eat affects your health and mood, so choose the healthiest foods to put into your body so that you have the proper fuel to get you through your day.

Exercise Get moving to reduce stress! Find a physical activity that you enjoy and get to it. Try to exercise at least five days per week, and include strength training, aerobic activities, and stress-relieving exercises. Exercise releases endorphins, the body's euphoric neurotransmitters, and helps to balance the stress response. Yoga and tai chi are particularly beneficial stress-relieving forms of exercise because they address physical, mental, and emotional fitness.

Support A good support system goes a long way to helping relieve stress. Having someone to talk to when you need it is one of the most important ways to relieve stress. Support could come from family, friends, a counselor, or support groups. Build your support system so it's there when you need it.

Sufficient sleep Lack of sleep is often the result of stress, but it also contributes to stress, creating yet another vicious cycle that leads to poor health. Adopting other stress-relieving techniques from this list can be helpful, as well as simply making enough time for adequate sleep. Most people need at least seven to eight hours of sleep so that the body can function optimally.

Mindfulness-based stress reduction (MBSR) This technique involves the practice of mindfulness, or being aware of what happens on a moment-to-moment basis, as a way of improving physical and emotional well-being. The program was developed by Jon Kabat-Zinn, and has been well studied for its stress-relieving benefits.

Cognitive behavioral therapy (CBT) This psychotherapeutic approach utilizes goal-oriented, systematic, present-moment-based methods to address a variety of disorders, including stress. The CBT program helps to change thought patterns as a way to reduce stress.

Relaxation methods There are many different relaxation methods, all of which can help to relieve stress. Deep breathing, progressive muscle relaxation, meditation, biofeedback, and massage are a few relaxation methods that may be helpful.

Acupuncture Stress may be the result of energetic imbalances in the body that can be corrected with acupuncture, a traditional Chinese medical procedure using small needles lightly placed into certain points on the body as a way to stimulate the flow of energy, correcting imbalances. Both emotional and physical manifestations of stress can be treated with acupuncture, usually over several treatment sessions.

The Dalai Lama, when asked what surprised him most about humanity, answered,

"Man. Because he sacrifices his health in order to make money. Then he sacrifices money to recuperate his health. And then he is so anxious about the future that he does not enjoy the present; the result being that he does not live in the present or the future; he lives as if he is never going to die and then he dies having never really lived."

Tips for Reducing Stress

See the Love Your Heart section for a complete program to support heart health.

- Eat a diet low in grain-based, refined, and starchy carbohydrates and sugars, and high in vegetables, healthy fats, and lean proteins, nuts, and seeds.

- Increase your amount of physical activity. Find an activity you enjoy and get moving!

- Find a stress-relieving activity, such as yoga, tai chi, massage, breathing, relaxation, or another activity that eases stress. Find time to do this activity regularly.

- Use HeartMath's emWave to measure and improve heart rate variability.

- Support healthy digestion and balance your gut with probiotics to help reduce inflammation, which may be contributing to your stress, and improve gut function.

- Take an omega-3 fish oil supplement to increase the omega-3/omega-6 ratio.

- If you are not consuming at least 35 grams of fiber daily to promote regular elimination and healthy gut bacterial balance, take a fiber supplement.

- If you have digestive symptoms, try taking digestive enzymes (with or without HCl, depending on your situation) with every meal.

- Optimize your vitamin D level at 50 to 70 ng/mL.

"Health nuts are going to feel stupid someday, lying in hospitals dying of nothing."

—Redd Foxx

Chapter 9
Endothelial Dysfunction

Endothelial dysfunction is the very initiation of atherosclerosis, and it continues throughout the entire atherosclerotic progression. It is a condition in which the cells of the inner lining of the blood vessels, which make up the endothelium, do not function normally. The endothelium is a one-cell-thick inner lining of blood vessels, separating the bloodstream from the blood vessel itself. Maintaining the integrity of the endothelial lining is of utmost importance when it comes to protecting against cardiovascular disease.

Endothelial dysfunction can lead to an impairment of the relaxation and constriction properties of the arteries, which can lead to the deterioration of the endothelial lining. Normally, arteries experience both relaxation and constriction, depending on many factors. When arteries are too constricted, or not relaxed enough, pressure is exerted on the artery lining, causing damage. Nitric oxide is one of the body's most potent vasodilators,[1] or artery relaxers, and when it is decreased, endothelial dysfunction results. In addition, endothelial dysfunction involves excess inflammation, cell growth, and blood clotting, all promoting the development of atherosclerosis.[2]

TIP:

A high-antioxidant diet includes plenty of deeply-colored vegetables and fruits.

Oxidative Stress

In endothelial dysfunction, oxidative stress is one of the main drivers of inflammation. Oxidation also reduces nitric oxide. Remember the analogy from chapter 3 illustrating the destructive properties of oxidation: Oxidation is like a punch thrown from a bully (the oxidant), and it can easily lead to a full-blown fight if enough molecules get involved. Oxidation occurs when there are not enough antioxidants (the peacekeepers) around. The body produces its own antioxidants, and we also obtain antioxidants from the diet. A diet high in antioxidants helps to quell oxidative stress in the body. Oxidative stress is a main contributor to endothelial dysfunction.[3] It triggers inflammation and destruction of the endothelial lining.

Myth:

Atherosclerosis is simply the accumulation of cholesterol and fats in the artery wall.

Fact:

Atherosclerosis involves endothelial dysfunction and chronic inflammation in the artery wall, progressing to the buildup of plaque, and eventual heart complications such as heart attack and stroke.

Atherosclerosis

When the endothelial lining is deteriorated, it begins to attract white blood cells and small, dense, oxidized LDL particles (remember, these are the harmful carriers of cholesterol) that easily slip under the endothelial lining, due to their small size. Once under the lining, the white blood cells begin to consume the oxidized fat proteins (as a way of destroying them), and the white blood cells are then considered foam cells. This process triggers an inflammatory response that perpetuates the accumulation of more cholesterol, immune cells, fats, minerals such as calcium, and free radicals, collectively comprising atherosclerotic plaque. This is the beginning of atherosclerosis. Over time, as we learned in chapter 1, atherosclerosis leads to complications of heart disease such as heart attack and stroke.

Healthy artery

Foam cells emerge

Fatty streak develops

Atherosclerosis Progression

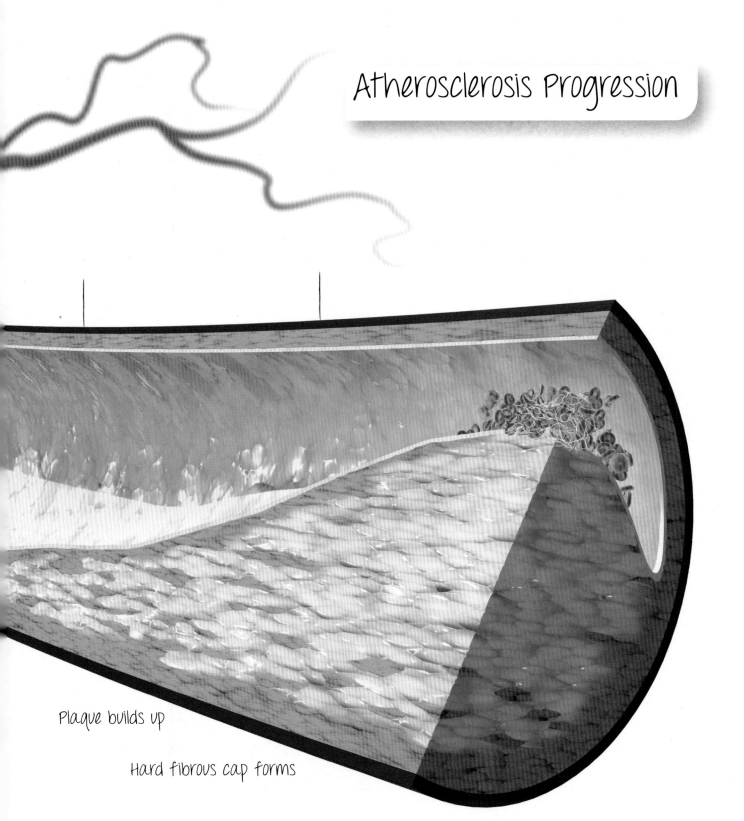

Plaque builds up

Hard fibrous cap forms

Lining ruptures and blood clot forms

The risk for developing endothelial dysfunction increases with the number of risk factors present in an individual.[4] Particularly, the combined risk factors of metabolic syndrome (abnormal cholesterol, high blood pressure, high blood sugar, abdominal fat, and high triglycerides) may have a greater impact on endothelial function than other combinations. Because of the many contributors to endothelial dysfunction, maintaining a healthy artery lining involves maintaining a balance of all cardiovascular risk factors and protective factors.

Ways to Trigger Endothelial Dysfunction

- Abnormal blood lipids
- Aging
- Alcohol
- Belly fat
- High blood pressure
- High blood sugar
- High homocysteine
- High-carbohydrate diet
- High-sugar diet
- Infection
- Inflammation
- Insulin resistance
- Low-fiber diet
- Omega-3/omega-6 imbalance
- Oxidative stress
- Physical inactivity
- Processed meats
- Smoking
- Stress
- Toxins
- Trans fats

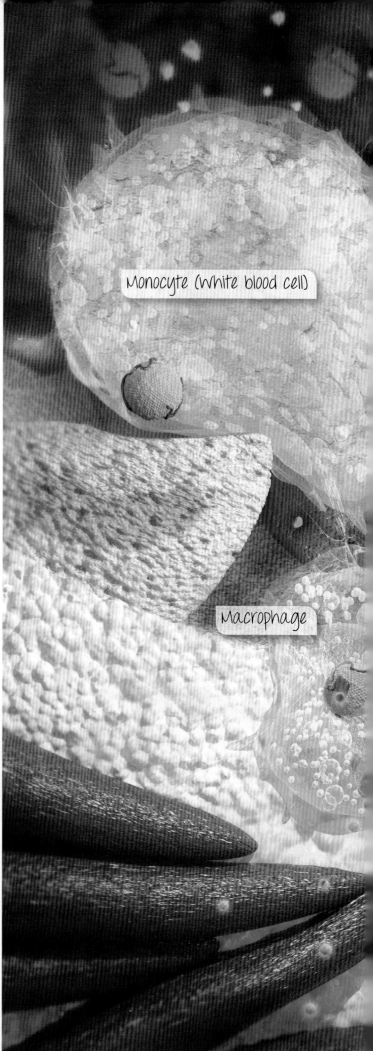

Monocyte (white blood cell)

Macrophage

Endothelial Dysfunction

Close-up view of atherosclerosis. When the endothelial lining is deteriorated, it begins to attract white blood cells and small, dense LDL particles that easily slip under the endothelial lining. Once under the lining, the white blood cells are considered macrophages, and they begin to consume oxidized LDL (as a way of destroying them). The macrophages are now considered foam cells. This process triggers an inflammatory response that perpetuates the accumulation of more cholesterol, immune cells, fats, minerals such as calcium, and free radicals, collectively comprising atherosclerotic plaque.

Red blood cell

LDL cholesterol

Endothelial cell (artery lining)

Smooth muscle cell

Fibrous cap

Plaque

Inflammatory cytokines

Foam cells

HEART DISEASE RISK FACTORS
high cholesterol,
high blood pressure,
high blood sugar

↓

oxidative stress/inflammation

↓

endothelial dysfunction

↓

HEART DISEASE

Homocysteine

Homocysteine is an amino acid that is normally found in the bloodstream, but when blood levels are elevated, it can damage the endothelial lining and other cells of the body. Excess homocysteine promotes oxidative stress, inflammation, blood clotting, endothelial dysfunction, and cell growth, all factors involved in atherosclerosis.[5] The following highlights measured blood levels of homocysteine.

Blood Homocysteine

Normal Range	High Range
< 11–15 µmol/L	> 15 µmol/L

The Life Extension Foundation recommends an optimal blood homocysteine range of 7 to 8 µmol/L, based on studies showing that heart disease risk is increased in people with homocysteine levels above 9 or 10 µmol/L.[6,7] Folic acid and vitamin B12 help to lower homocysteine levels.[8] Some people have a genetic polymorphism, or genetic alteration, that prevents them from converting folic acid into its active form, the bioactive 5-methyltetrahydrofolate (5-MTHF), which is necessary for lowering homocysteine levels in the body.[9] Up to twenty percent of people have this genetic alteration, and should take activated folic acid, or 5-MTHF, for homocysteine regulation.[10]

Testing for Endothelial Dysfunction

Endothelial function is not normally assessed, but can be using the acetylcholine test, which determines whether artery dilation or constriction predominates. Artery constriction is an indication of endothelial dysfunction. Another method of detecting endothelial dysfunction uses high-resolution ultrasound to measure the diameter of the brachial artery (the main artery in the arm) in response to an excess of blood in the artery. This measures flow-mediated dilation (FMD), an index of vasomotor function. Further, endothelial function decreases as blood levels of C-reactive protein (CRP) increase, so CRP can be used as an indirect measure of endothelial dysfunction.[11]

Tips for Reducing Endothelial Dysfunction

See the Love Your Heart section for a complete program to support heart health.

- Quit smoking.
- Reduce stress.
- Eat healthy fats.
- Improve omega-3/omega-6 ratio (more omega-3, less omega-6).
- Stop eating sugar.
- Stop eating starches and grain-based carbohydrates.
- Eat more vegetables.
- Eat more fiber.
- Reduce alcohol consumption.
- Avoid processed meats.
- Eat dark chocolate.
- Lower high blood sugar.
- Normalize blood lipids.
- Lower high blood pressure.
- Lower homocysteine with folic acid and B12.
- Treat infection.
- Reduce inflammation.
- Reduce toxin exposure.
- Increase antioxidants.
- Exercise.
- Lose weight if overweight.

interview

Dr. Thomas E. Levy

Brenda interviews cardiologist and author of *Stop America's #1 Killer: Reversible Vitamin Deficiency Found to Be Origin of All Coronary Heart Disease*

BW: Dr. Levy, first I want to thank you for taking the time to do this interview. As a cardiologist, you bring an especially interesting perspective to this book. In your book *Stop America's #1 Killer*, you make the case for vitamin C deficiency as the origin of heart disease. Throughout the book you illustrate the many different ways in which vitamin C is related to heart health, and in which vitamin C deficiency is related to atherosclerosis and heart disease. In a similar way, I have done the same thing with gut health—highlighted the many ways in which gut dysfunction can lead to heart disease, or the risk factors associated with heart disease. You also recognize gut function as a vital part of total-body health. Could you talk about that?

TL: Sure. How healthy anyone is depends on whether there exists excess oxidative stress in one or more areas of the body, and whether important antioxidant stores, highlighted by vitamin C, are significantly depleted as a result of that. All infections and all toxins—with no exceptions—cause increased oxidative stress where they are found. The malfunctioning gut, which is often constipated at least to a degree, begins to favor putrefaction of food over digestion the longer the foodstuffs remain unmetabolized and/or uneliminated.

Constipation is a very common finding due to the lack of attention to proper food combining, excess food intake, and deficient digestive enzyme function seen with so many individuals. When this occurs, a proliferation of many of the same anaerobic bacteria, such as *Clostridium* species, that produce highly potent toxins is facilitated. When this situation is chronic and never properly addressed, the continual infection/toxin presence places an

naturally occurring antioxidant. How does vitamin C help reduce the body's toxic burden, and how does that affect heart health?

TL: Toxins all deplete electrons from nearby biomolecules, resulting in their oxidation. Vitamin C can block this effect of a toxin by directly contributing its electrons to it, or vitamin C can promptly contribute its electrons to the oxidized biomolecules, restoring them to a state of normal function. When this process occurs in and around the endothelial layer of the coronary artery, atherosclerosis can be prevented and even reversed.

> **"How healthy anyone is depends on whether there exists excess oxidative stress in one or more areas of the body, and whether important antioxidant stores, highlighted by vitamin C, are significantly depleted as a result of that."**

enormous drain on the antioxidant stores in the body, leaving it exceptionally susceptible to the development of any of a wide number of acute and chronic diseases.

BW: Vitamin C is the body's most powerful

BW: You have called atherosclerosis "arterial scurvy." Could you explain?

TL: All of the common risk factors for developing atherosclerosis share the final common denominator of a pronounced deficiency of vitamin C in the arterial wall. The scientific literature supports the conclusion that none of these risk factors is able to promote atherosclerosis until this vitamin C deficiency, or arterial scurvy, is already present in the arterial wall.

BW: How does vitamin C help reverse atherosclerosis?

TL: The vitamin C deficiency in the arterial wall directly promotes the chronic inflammation that initiates and propagates the

BW: You have related vitamin C deficiency to all the major, and some minor, risk factors for heart disease development. The recognition that inflammation is a major initiator, and propagator, of heart disease is relatively recent. The gut connection to heart disease is very much tied to inflammation, just as vitamin C deficiency is. How does vitamin C relate to inflammation?

TL: In a nutshell, inflammation is increased oxidative stress with increased free radical generation by a number of different immune cells. When inflammation is a short-term and

"All of the common risk factors for developing atherosclerosis share the final common denominator of a pronounced deficiency of vitamin C in the arterial wall."

atherosclerotic process. When enough vitamin C can be effectively delivered to neutralize the oxidative stress generated by this inflammation, atherosclerosis can be slowed, stopped, and actually reversed if this vitamin C delivery is sufficient.

self-limited process, it can have very healthy consequences, as the inflammatory effect can help initiate the healing process. However, when it becomes a chronic process, inflammation nearly always leads to any of a number of different chronic degenerative diseases. Vitamin

C is basically the opposite of inflammation, and inflammation simply cannot exist where levels of vitamin C are sufficiently high.

BW: How do you recommend people take vitamin C?

TL: Any form of supplementation can be beneficial. However, when one wants to optimize the potential effects of vitamin C on any given condition, I recommend my Multi-C Protocol:

ONE: 3 to 5 grams of liposome-encapsulated vitamin C orally daily, for optimal intracellular support (www.livonlabs.com)

TWO: Multigram doses of sodium ascorbate powder taken several times daily in juice or water up to or reaching bowel tolerance, to neutralize the commonly present toxins in the gut and flood the extracellular spaces with vitamin C

THREE: Several grams daily of ascorbyl palmitate orally daily, as a form to reach fat-soluble areas (www.lef.org)

FOUR: 50 to 150 grams of vitamin C IV to "kick start" the suffusion of C into the body, several times weekly at first; this can further be optimized with 5 to 10 units of Humulin insulin mixed into the IV bag

The liposome-encapsulated vitamin C is especially effective as monotherapy, especially when there might be difficulty in finding and/or affording repeated IV administrations. However, all four prongs of the protocol are important and work synergistically.

W: What are your recommendations for optimal gut function?

TL: Proper food combining, minimal liquid with meals, digestive enzyme supplementation, smaller and more frequent meals versus larger and less frequent, complete chewing/mastication of foods, and intermittent sodium ascorbate supplementation to initiate a "C-flush," preferably a few times monthly.

BW: Do you see a link between a high-sugar or high-carbohydrate diet and heart disease? Does vitamin C play a role in this relationship?

TL: Absolutely. Glucose and vitamin C directly compete for uptake inside cells. When vitamin C supplementation is inadequate, more advanced glycosylation of biomolecules eventually takes place, and chronic degenerative diseases of all kinds, including heart disease, can take hold and progress.

BW: Thank you for your time. Your work is very important and I am honored that you shared your knowledge with me. You have been an inspiration to me for many years, and you were instrumental to my own healing when I was dealing with Lyme disease.

"The secret of health for both mind and body is not to mourn for the past, worry about the future, or anticipate troubles, but to live in the present moment wisely and earnestly."

—Siddhartha Gautama

Chapter 10

Hormones and the Heart

Heart disease is uncommon in young women, but after menopause a woman's risk for developing heart disease rises considerably. It is therefore thought that estrogen plays a protective role against heart disease in women, as estrogen levels decrease after menopause.[1] Further, early observational studies looking at hormone therapy use in women have found a link between hormone replacement therapy and reduced risk of heart disease. These observations led to the use of hormone replacement therapy as a common treatment for the prevention of heart disease in women.[2]

Myth:

All hormone replacement therapy increases risk of heart disease.

Fact:

Bioidentical hormone replacement therapy, under the right administration by an experienced doctor, can be a heart-healthy treatment.

All this prompted the Women's Health Initiative (WHI), a group of studies including two clinical trials evaluating the effects in women of two different conventional hormone therapies on heart disease, bone fractures, and colorectal cancer.[3] In one trial, women with a uterus were given progestin (a synthetic progesterone) in combination with estrogen (derived from horse urine), a treatment known to be protective against endometrial cancer. In the second trial, women without a uterus were given the estrogen only.

In 2002, these two clinical trials were stopped because preliminary data showed that, instead of being protected from heart disease, the women in the estrogen plus progestin trial were at increased risk of heart attack, stroke, blood clots, and breast cancer; and the women in the estrogen only trial were at increased risk of blood clots, stroke, and dementia. The results of these trials prompted millions of women to stop taking conventional hormone therapy.

Later evaluation of data from the WHI divided the women into age groups and determined that the women who had begun hormone therapy soon after menopause (those women aged 50 to 59) may have been at decreased risk of heart attack when compared to the women who began therapy at a later age,[4] and they had less heart disease and were less likely to die of any cause than the women taking a placebo. As a result of these findings, current recommendations for conventional hormone therapy suggest that it begin soon after menopause and that it be used at the lowest possible dosage for the shortest possible time to relieve symptoms of menopause. It is no longer recommended for heart disease prevention.

The WHI studies used conventional hormone replacement. The estrogen used in the study is an estrogen derived from horse urine. Yes, it is considered natural, and is even sometimes referred to as bioidentical (to a horse, not a human), but this form of estrogen is not found in the human body, and there are concerns that it may interfere with hormone function rather than improve it.

Further, progestin, as used in the study and commonly prescribed, is a synthetic form of progesterone 10 to 100 times more potent than natural progesterone, and does not exist in the human body. Further, in these trials, all the women received the same dosage of hormones. This assumes that all women need the same amount of hormones. These forms of hormone replacement are not recommended by most practitioners in the integrative medicine field.

Bioidentical Hormone Replacement Therapy

Holistic-minded doctors take a completely different approach to hormone replacement therapy. They tailor hormone therapy to the individual, based on symptoms and regular blood testing of hormone levels. They also use bioidentical hormones, which are natural forms of hormones that are biologically identical (bioidentical) to those hormones in the human body. Bioidentical hormone replacement therapy is a better option for perimenopausal

TIP:

Proper hormone balance is key to healthy aging.

and postmenopausal women who are concerned about the effects of hormone imbalance and heart disease risk.

Bioidentical hormone replacement involves the restoration of the sex steroid hormones, sometimes referred to simply as sex hormones: estrogens, progestagens, and androgens. These hormones are found in both men and women, but estrogens and progestagens are higher in women, and androgens are higher in men. All are essential to health, however, and hormone balance is key. The estrogens include estradiol, estriol, and estrone. Progestagens are mostly represented by progesterone. Androgens include anabolic steroids, androstenedione, dehydroepiandrosterone (DHEA), dihydrotestosterone, and testosterone.

> **An experienced doctor will look at the whole picture of health by assessing hormone levels along with symptoms and health history.**

medroxyprogesterone, is also backed by evidence that it improves cardiovascular function.[6]

Bioidentical progesterone, which can be derived from plants such as yams or from animals, or can be made synthetically, has been found to have fewer side effects and to be more bioavailable than medroxyprogesterone (Provera), the synthetic form.[7] Further, bioidentical progesterone does not have a negative effect on blood lipids or blood vessels as do synthetic progestins.[8,9] And when compared to non-bioidentical preparations, bioidentical estrogens and progesterone may help reduce risk of blood clots.[10,11]

The androgens are not always considered when it comes to hormone replacement, but this is a mistake.

Estrogen's heart-healthy qualities include beneficial changes in blood lipid levels (increased HDL cholesterol and decreased LDL cholesterol), increased vasodilation to increase blood flow, and a reduced response of blood vessels to injury.[5] Natural progesterone, in contrast to synthetic

Androgens are not only male hormones. Both women and men have androgen hormones, and they must be balanced along with estrogen and progesterone. The androgen dehydroepiandrosterone (DHEA) is the most prevalent hormone in the body, produced by the adrenal glands and the ovaries. It is a precursor for estrogen and testosterone, and it begins to decrease after age 30. There is some evidence that DHEA may help to protect against cardiovascular disease in men with higher levels of androgens, likely due to DHEA's influence on estrogen production.[12] In women, higher DHEA and androgen levels were associated with lower carotid artery atherosclerosis.[13]

Both high and low levels of the androgen testosterone have been linked to heart disease in men,[14,15] highlighting the importance of androgen hormone balance. Although the role of testosterone replacement for cardiovascular benefit is not completely understood, testosterone replacement has been found to slow or halt the progression from metabolic syndrome to type 2 diabetes and cardiovascular disease by regulating insulin, lipid levels, and blood pressure in men with low testosterone levels.[16]

Estrogen Metabolites

The effects of estrogen are being elucidated by studies of estrogen metabolites, or breakdown products. In the body, estrogens are broken down into metabolites that have been found to be associated with certain health outcomes. The estrogen estradiol is converted into estrone (which can also be converted, to a lesser extent, back into estradiol). Estrone is converted irreversibly into two main metabolites: 2-hydroxyestrone and 16α-hydroxyestrone. Another noteworthy metabolite, though found in lesser amounts, is 4-hydroxyestrone.

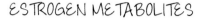

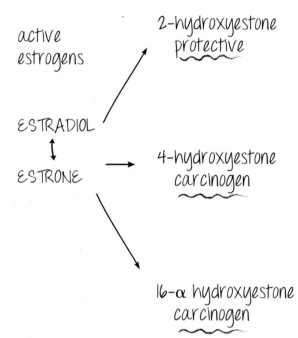

As it turns out, estrogen metabolites have significant biological activity. These metabolites play an important role in the prevention, or development of, certain diseases. The ratio of 2:16α-hydroxyestrone is particularly helpful in identifying disease risk. A high 2:16α ratio (high 2-hydroxyestrone and low 16α-hydroxyestrone) is the most protective against estrogen-related cancers: breast, endometrial, and cervical cancer, as well as prostate cancer, neck cancer, systemic lupus erythematosus, and recurrent papillomatosis.[17] Blood and urine tests are available to determine estrogen metabolite levels. 2-hydroxyestrone is considered the good estrogen metabolite, having protective effects, and 16α-hydroxyestrone and 4-hydroxyestrone are the bad estrogen metabolites, having carcinogenic effects.

Estrogen metabolites may also play a role in heart disease risk. The ratio of 2:16α-hydroxyestrone has been shown to be a significant predictor of systolic blood pressure in postmenopausal women.[18] 2-hydroxyestrone exhibits protective effects on blood vessels, which may explain the heart-healthy effects of higher concentrations of this metabolite.

the recirculation of estrogens that occurs when levels of bifidobacteria are low, in addition to liver detoxification, will all help to support healthy metabolism of estrogens. In addition, consumption of cruciferous vegetables, soy, and omega-3s from flaxseed will help to improve the ratio of 2:16α-hydroxyestrone ratio. Exercise[19] and weight loss[20] will also help to improve the estrogen metabolite ratio.

Hormone balance, in both men and women, is an important factor to consider with age. It is crucial to find a doctor who is very experienced with natural hormone replacement therapy so that you can fully understand the possible benefits of natural hormone therapy. Due to the

Estrogen is metabolized primarily in the liver, highlighting the importance of maintaining healthy liver function, a function that is dependent on digestive function.

Estrogen is metabolized primarily in the liver, highlighting the importance of maintaining healthy liver function, a function that is dependent on digestive function. Regular bowel elimination to encourage the timely release of waste will help reduce buildup of toxic estrogen metabolites. Furthermore, maintenance (or restoration) of gut bacterial balance to reduce

fluctuation of hormone levels on a regular basis, regular hormone testing with blood and saliva tests, along with careful consideration of symptoms, are both necessary parts of natural hormone therapy. An experienced doctor will look at the whole picture of health by assessing hormone levels along with symptoms and health history.

interview

Dr. Rick Sponaugle

Brenda sits down with Marvin "Rick" Sponaugle, MD, founder and medical director of Florida Detox and Sponaugle Wellness Institute about the link between toxicity, the gut, hormone dysfunction, and the heart

BW: Dr. Sponaugle, your background includes board certification in addiction medicine and anesthesiology. Your ability to correct brain chemistry patterns associated with addiction led to your finding the connection between underlying toxicity and an array of chronic health conditions. Could you expand on that?

RS: If I may provide a historical perspective, in 1998 I used my intensive care skills to design a relatively painless detox. Patients loved my detox, but too many of these patients still relapsed. Their brain chemistry was such that they felt more normal on drugs like OxyContin and Xanax. Hence, I began performing addiction research that compared changes seen on SPECT (single-photon emission computed tomography) brain imaging with brain chemistry patterns and drug craving patterns. Amazingly, no one had ever performed this practical research. My research quickly proved that patients use some drugs to stimulate their underactive brain regions and other drugs to calm overactive brain regions.

Additional research proved that gut toxicity is the number one cause of the threefold increased prevalence of depression, anxiety, insomnia, and panic disorder that has occurred since 1980. The more severe the gut toxicity, the more inflammation and the more overelectrified the brain. Gut-toxic patients are sitting in rehabs throughout America because they use OxyContin and Xanax to calm their anxious brains.

BW: What toxicities do you commonly find in people facing chronic illness?

RS: Fifty percent of my patients are non-addicted patients who suffer with a chronic illness. They typically suffer from a combination

in addition to mold toxins from water-damaged buildings, all working to shut down the immune system, decreasing their ability to defeat pathogens like *Borrelia* and *Mycoplasma*.

We diagnose gut toxicity in 90 percent of our patients. Gut toxicity causes a multitude of autoimmune diseases: psoriasis, arthritis, multiple sclerosis, and more. We also diagnose mold toxicity in 80 percent of our patients. Gut toxicity and mold toxicity cause symptoms of depression, chronic fatigue, fibromyalgia, anxiety, insomnia, and panic disorder.

Mold toxicity is an emerging illness that was much less common just fifty years ago. It wasn't until the 1970s that we began producing airtight, energy-efficient homes and office buildings. When buildings suffer water damage, mold begins to grow rapidly on cellulose material

"The more severe the gut toxicity, the more inflammation and the more overelectrified the brain."

of gut toxicity, mold toxicity, industrial toxicity, and, less often, toxicity derived from intracellular bacteria like *Borrelia* (Lyme disease) and *Mycoplasma*. The pattern we see in these chronic illness/chronic fatigue patients is a combination of yeast and bacterial gut toxins

such as drywall. Prior to 1970, walls were made out of plaster and plywood, on which mold grows slowly. The advent of the use of drywall and the production of energy-efficient homes that can't breathe has left many Americans living in what is essentially a toxic gas chamber.

"The FDA does not require that cities filter antibiotics or any other medications from drinking water, suggesting they have already approved these medications for human safety."

Various molds grow in water-damaged buildings, and most produce toxic gases.

One out of four Americans has specific genetics that leave them unable to produce antibodies to mold toxins. It's interesting that 85 percent of my patients have the mold genetics: HLA-DRBQ genetics. Mold toxicity can cause a multitude of brain disorders, neurological disorders, intestinal dysfunction, and more. Mold toxins can destroy every cell in the body.

American universities, with the exception of Michigan State and Texas Tech, appear to be at least ten years behind European medical centers with regard to knowledge of mold toxicity. I see approximately 40 new patients every month. Alarming is the fact that I am diagnosing so many mold-toxic patients with multiple sclerosis. I have diagnosed five women, ages 38 to 51, with multiple sclerosis in the last two months. Most of these patients thought they were coming to my clinic simply for addiction treatment. As it turns out, patients suffering significant mold toxicity often use

drugs like OxyContin to calm their toxin-induced anxiety.

BW: From your perspective, where do you think this gut toxicity is coming from?

RS: Since 1980, anxiety, depression, obsessive-compulsive disorder (OCD), insomnia, and panic disorder have tripled. It is my opinion that the increased prevalence of these psychological disorders is mostly derived from the ever-increasing number of Americans suffering from gut toxicity, which results from intestinal dysbiosis, or an imbalance of gut bacteria. To understand from a historical perspective why so many Americans are suffering from intestinal dysbiosis, we have to ascertain the origin of modern-day antibiotics.

In the late 1930s, a British scientist named Fleming proposed that we could make an antibiotic out of *Penicillium* mold. Ultimately the first mass production of penicillin occurred in 1944, and when the war ended in 1945, penicillin was touted as a miracle drug.

Unfortunately, by 1945 poultry farmers had moved their turkeys and chickens into poultry houses instead of raising them free range. Because of this, when one chicken developed pneumonia, hundreds died. American poultry farmers embraced penicillin with great fervor. And thus our poultry has been tainted with antibiotics for 65-plus years. Milk farmers followed suit. They discovered that milk cows produce more milk when given antibiotics. Beef farmers were next. They found they could get more money for a tender steak—meat with more fat and less muscle. To accomplish this, they began penning their cattle in Kansas City stockyards so crowded the cattle couldn't move. Standing in stockyards in their own manure, if they were not given antibiotics, they developed hoof rot. In summary, since the post–World War II days, Americans have been regularly imbibing antibiotics from their food supply.

> ## "When people drink the water in most major cities, they are readily drinking antibiotics."

Today city water is often pulled from ground water contaminated with antibiotics from farm runoff and reclaimed irrigation water runoff. The FDA does not require that cities filter antibiotics or any other medications from drinking water, suggesting they have already approved these medications for human safety. Therefore, when people drink the water in most major cities, they are readily drinking antibiotics. A recent study found that Philadelphia city water had significant levels of amoxicillin, azithromycin, and trimethoprim/sulfamethoxazole. Americans no longer need antibiotic prescriptions to develop gastrointestinal dysbiosis; antibiotics in the water and food supply constantly destroy the good bacteria that prevent overgrowth of pathogenic *Candida* yeast and bacteria like *Bacteroides*, *Klebsiella*, and Enterobacteriaceae.

BW: How does gut toxicity play a role in poor health?

RS: Pathogenic bacteria in the gut make an enzyme called urease, which hydrolyzes urea from dietary protein into ammonia, raising the intestinal pH and causing even more overgrowth of potentially harmful yeast and bacteria. The endogenous production of ammonia by these pathogenic bacteria is extremely problematic for the brain. Ammonia itself is a neurotoxin and destroys brain tissue. When excessive ammonia levels break down the blood brain barrier, the brain becomes inflamed.

In addition, the liver works diligently to conjugate estrogenic toxins in bile acids so they will be expelled from the body, yet pathogenic bacterial enzymes such as beta-glucuronidase undo this work by the liver, hydrolyzing the conjugated estrogens in bile acids. Deconjugated bile acids are extremely toxic to the colonic epithelium (colon lining), causing increased permeability, or leaky gut syndrome. Destruction of colonic epithelium also plays a role in ulcerative colitis and increased prevalence of colon cancer.

potassium with it, all causing more anxiety and, in the worst cases, panic disorder.

Serotonin deficiency is first a gut problem before it becomes a brain problem. With knowledge that 98 percent of the pre-serotonin precursor 5-hydroxytryptophan (5-HTP) is manufactured in the small intestine,

"Serotonin deficiency is first a gut problem before it becomes a brain problem."

My research has proven that gut toxicity causes excessive electrical activity in the brain via toxin-induced deficiencies of two calming brain chemicals: serotonin and taurine. Gut toxicity also causes deficiencies of magnesium and potassium, both of which relax the brain.

When the intestinal tract is overgrown with Candida, metabolism of the Candida proteins yields another brain toxin, beta-alanine. Beta-alanine inhibits brain development growth factor, a particular concern in younger children who are still in the brain development stage. Beta-alanine also competes for reabsorption of taurine in the kidneys. When taurine is wasted in the urine, it drags magnesium and

we can better understand how gut toxicity can cause severe serotonin deficiency. Pathogenic bacteria also produce a bacterial enzyme called tryptophanase, which converts tryptophan into a carcinogenic phenol, preventing the normal conversion of tryptophan into 5-hydroxytryptophan, the amino acid that becomes serotonin in the brain.

Patients who suffer from gut toxicity will initially derive some benefit from serotonin-enhancing antidepressants. However, the SSRI (selective serotonin reuptake inhibitor) antidepressants do not increase production of serotonin; they simply sit on the serotonin recycle wagon and prevent serotonin from returning to serotonin storage units in the brain. Gut-toxic patients ultimately end up with minimal serotonin in their brain and thus have no serotonin for the SSRI medications to work with. This explains the poor efficacy of these medications in many Americans.

My research has proven that serotonin and taurine deficiency derived from a toxic gut will drastically change a patient's brain scans. The gut-toxic brain exhibits an overactive emotional center called the deep limbic system, and an overactive anterior cingulate, which causes excessive worry; they become extremely anxious about life in general. They also become stubborn, unforgiving, and hyperfocused on the negative. In severe cases, patients develop symptoms of OCD (obsessive-compulsive disorder). Also, the autistic children I have personally treated have all suffered from antibiotic-induced gut toxicity. They all had excessive electrical activity in these two brain regions. When we correct their brain chemistry and, ultimately, their gut toxicity, they respond extremely well to our treatment.

Excessive electrical activity in the emotional center, or the deep limbic system, can cause severe depression and myriad symptoms. The deep limbic is called our "emotional center" because it stores our emotionally charged memories. This brain region is saturated with GABAergic (gamma-aminobutyric acid) neurons. Serotonin and taurine actually enhance GABA receptivity, or the ability of GABA to activate GABA brain receptors, which has a

calming effect. Serotonin and taurine deficiency derived from gut toxicity produces the following symptoms: depression, moodiness, irritability, negativity, hopelessness, excessive guilt, social anxiety, and the tendency to become easily offended. Many Americans suffering from gut toxicity use drugs like OxyContin and Xanax to calm these overactive brain regions. After we "fix" their gut-toxic brain, they no longer crave these drugs.

Based on my practice, I believe all Americans suffer some level of gut toxicity. It's interesting that we often hear people say that America is the most overfed and yet undernourished country in the world.

BW: Yes, it's so true! How is food addiction related to drug or alcohol addiction?

RS: The ever-increasing prevalence of neurotoxicity (brain toxicity) in Americans is a fundamental cause of the obesity epidemic in America. Let me explain the domino effect regarding the role of toxicity as the underlying causation of America's battle with obesity. The dopamine D2 receptor located in the brain's hunger center must undergo activation or we do not experience satiety, or the feeling of fullness.

Dopamine receptivity, or the ability of dopamine to activate the D2 receptor, is controlled by thyroid hormone and testosterone. When these hormones are at suboptimal levels, patients experience diminished activity in their hunger center. This makes them overeat in their attempt to reach satiety. Eating triples D2 activity in the hunger center for approximately 90 minutes. Every bite of food gives our reward center another dopamine "hit." In neurotoxic patients, gut toxins, mold toxins, and environmental toxins down-regulate the pituitary stimulation of the ovaries, testicles, and thyroid; hence, neurotoxic patients suffer reduced D2 activity. As a result, they often binge on food in their attempt to raise D2 activity to normal. Patients suffering diminished D2 activity often eat something every 90 minutes attempting to reach a state of satiety. They may say they are eating out of boredom. Furthermore, toxin-induced hypothyroidism disallows effective calorie burn, explaining why neurotoxic patients can often eat much less than others yet are unable to lose weight.

BW: How else are hormones related to this toxicity?

RS: Neurotoxicity causes global hormonal suppression. *Candida* mycotoxins, mold toxins, bacterial endotoxins, industrial solvent toxins, and pesticides induce slowing of electrical impulses in the brain's hypothalamus, which causes a reduction in pituitary hormonal output and, subsequently, diminished stimulation of

downstream glands: the thyroid gland, adrenal glands, and sex organs.

Because my medical practice is inundated with neurotoxic patients, I have treated many women in premature menopause. Toxin-induced growth hormone deficiency prevents the repair of every cell in the body, thus causing premature aging. Every decade we are seeing younger American women suffer from early menopause. It is not uncommon in my practice to see 35-year-old women who have stopped menstruating. Many of these neurotoxic women have needlessly spent thousands of dollars on infertility treatment.

> "Fat-soluble toxins migrate to, and deposit in, the fattiest organ in the human body: the brain.

Neurotoxic patients suffer inadequate production of the pituitary hormone ACTH, which stimulates the adrenal glands, causing severe chronic fatigue. Eighty percent of the female patients treated at Sponaugle Wellness Institute suffer from neurotoxin-induced TSH (thyroid-stimulating hormone) deficiency. Their brains are too toxic to produce TSH, and therefore they develop toxin-induced hypothyroidism.

Fat-soluble toxins migrate to, and deposit in, the fattiest organ in the human body: the brain.

When these lipophilic toxins deposit in brain tissue, they displace good fats, such as the omega-3s, thus weakening the integrity of brain tissue. Myelin, the insulation on brain nerves, has an 80 percent fat content. When brain myelin becomes inflamed—or worse, destroyed from toxin infiltration—patients develop multiple sclerosis. Loss of myelin results in a slowing of electrical impulses in the brain.

The pan-global suppression of hormones in neurotoxic patients causes severe chronic fatigue, depression, insulin resistance, and, essentially, decreased function of every cell in the body. The pituitary gland in the brain produces a multitude of hormones; some target an end organ, and some stimulate production of hormones in the downstream glands such as the thyroid, the adrenal glands, and the gonads (testicles and ovaries).

Testosterone deficiency in neurotoxic patients causes depression and overeating. As we discussed earlier, the hunger and reward center, the nucleus accumbens, runs on dopamine; specifically, the activation of the D2 receptor. Dopamine cannot activate dopamine receptors in the brain without optimal levels of testosterone and thyroid hormone. Testosterone deficiency derived from neurotoxicity also causes insulin resistance in both men and women because testosterone is required for optimal insulin receptivity.

Testosterone deficiency in both men and women results in elevated cholesterol and triglyceride levels; thus, neurotoxicity leads to metabolic syndrome. Premature testosterone deficiency in men and women has causation in depression and in reduced mental performance. Testosterone deficiency causes diminished D1 dopamine receptor activity in the prefrontal cortex of the brain, causing subsequent focus issues, brain fog, and, often, a misdiagnosis of ADHD.

Neurotoxicity is the common denominator in the majority of Americans who suffer with chronic fatigue and fibromyalgia. The brain becomes "too sick" from neurotoxicity to respond to falling hormone levels. Patients suffer thyroid insufficiency, adrenal insufficiency (cortisol deficiency), and testosterone deficiency. Dopamine and its two first cousins, norepinephrine and epinephrine (adrenaline), require thyroid hormone, cortisol hormone, and testosterone to activate their respective receptors throughout the brain and the body.

> **When these lipophilic toxins deposit in brain tissue, they displace good fats, such as the omega-3s."**

Inadequate activation of these three catecholamines (dopamine, epinephrine, and norepinephrine) precipitates the symptoms of chronic fatigue. Chronic fatigue is frequently diagnosed by traditional medical doctors and even physicians at more progressive anti-aging wellness centers as a primary adrenal issue. They fail to comprehend the concept that the neurotoxic brain is too sick to properly stimulate the adrenal glands. This explains why these patients do not respond to prescribed "adrenal fuel."

I frequently see chronic fatigue and fibromyalgia as codisorders because neurotoxicity also causes excessive glutamate production. Glutamate is the most powerful excitatory, or electrifying, neurotransmitter. Hence, patients who suffer from neurotoxicity experience excessive electrical current running through their brain and their body, characteristic of fibromyalgia.

Deficiency of the hormone DHEA (dehydro-epiandrosterone) is also extremely common in neurotoxic patients because the toxic brain is, again, too sick to stimulate the adrenal glands, which are responsible for the production of DHEA. DHEA deficiency is another cause of chronic pain and fibromyalgia because DHEA is required for the production of our natural opiates, the endorphins, which decrease pain. Neurotoxic women suffer deficiencies of FSH (follicle-stimulating hormone), the brain hormone that stimulates ovarian production of estradiol. Estradiol deficiency causes significant depression in women because estradiol enhances the activity of tyrosine hydroxylase, the enzyme that converts dietary tyrosine into dopamine. In addition, estradiol blocks the activity of MAO (monoamine oxidase), the enzyme that metabolizes dopamine. Women who suffer neurotoxicity suffer more depression than men because both estrogen and testosterone modulate dopamine activity in the female brain.

BW: What have you seen as far as the contribution of toxicity to conditions related to the heart?

RS: Let's first discuss gut toxicity. When patients suffer severe gastrointestinal dysbiosis, they can subsequently suffer severe malnutrition. Nutritional deficiencies can lead to high blood pressure. For example, arginine deficiency is extremely common in my toxic patients, and it plays a primary role in the causation of hypertension because arginine is a precursor to nitrous oxide. Nitrous oxide dilates the arteries and capillaries, thereby reducing what we call systemic vascular resistance—the resistance the heart must pump against in the blood vessel. Arginine is an essential amino acid. We must obtain it from food, but that is not enough; the intestine must also absorb it. When toxins destroy the intestinal lining, we cannot move the amino acids from our gut into the bloodstream.

Taurine is another essential amino acid. Toxin-induced taurine deficiency is common

"We were taught nothing about gut toxicity and how it can cause cardiac arrhythmias, but we were taught how to prescribe various drugs to reduce cardiac irritability. Amazing, isn't it?"

in my patients, especially those who suffer from excessive intestinal overgrowth of *Candida.* Taurine is the number one amino acid used by the heart. It accounts for 50 percent of the active amino acids in cardiac tissue. Taurine decreases electrical voltage in the heart's electrical system; therefore, taurine deficiency causes what we call increased cardiac irritability, and in some patients, cardiac arrhythmias.

The triple jeopardy in patients suffering *Candida* gut toxicity is that intestinal overgrowth of *Candida* also causes magnesium and potassium deficiencies. Magnesium competes with calcium for entry into the calcium channel of the cardiac nerves. When calcium enters cardiac cells, the cardiac muscle contracts. Magnesium therefore relaxes cardiac muscle; hence, magnesium deficiency causes increased "cardiac irritability," as does *Candida*-induced potassium deficiency. Potassium blocks sodium from entering electrical neurons that stimulate the heart.

We were taught nothing about gut toxicity and how it can cause cardiac arrhythmias, but we were taught how to prescribe various drugs to reduce cardiac irritability. Amazing, isn't it? In my practice, we often see young women who suffer cardiac arrhythmias because they suffer toxicity-induced deficiencies of all three nutrients—taurine, magnesium, and potassium.

Mold toxins are actually more lethal mycotoxins than intestinal *Candida* mycotoxins. European studies have proven that the trichothecene T2 toxin produced by *Stachybotrys* (black mold) decreases the electrical action potential in the cardiac cells. I doubt many American cardiologists are aware of this.

The trichothecene toxin inhibits the membrane action potential in individual cardiac myocytes by interfering with the trans-membrane movement of calcium and potassium. It can prolong the action potential by 50 percent and increase what is called the repolarization phase by 90 percent. In my practice I had a 37-year-old bodybuilder who went into heart failure the day after he cleaned out the black mold infestation in his 30-foot-long fish tank.

Trichothecene toxicity can also cause extreme heart rate variability, whereby the

glutamic acid decarboxylase, the enzyme responsible for converting glutamate, the brain's strongest electrifying chemical, into GABA, the brain's strongest relaxing brain chemical. Excessive glutamate activity subsequently causes excessive electrical voltage throughout

> **"Another mechanism by which toxicity causes havoc in the cardiovascular system is toxin-induced inflammation. Excessive toxin levels stimulate the production of pro-inflammatory messengers called cytokines. Thus, toxic overload induces an up-regulation of inflammatory chemicals throughout the body."**

patient experiences a rapid heart rate followed in just minutes by a very slow heart rate. These patients can experience constant changes in heart rate throughout the day. They frequently suffer from what is called autonomic dysfunction.

In addition, when the brain becomes saturated with mold toxins, glutamate levels surge. My research has proven that mold toxins inhibit

the brain and body. This stimulates increased vascular tone and excessive vasoconstriction. Increased activation of the muscular tone surrounding arteries and capillaries produces stiff arteries and elevated blood pressure.

Another mechanism by which toxicity causes havoc in the cardiovascular system is toxin-induced inflammation. Excessive toxin levels stimulate the production of pro-inflammatory messengers called cytokines. Thus, toxic overload induces an up-regulation of inflammatory chemicals throughout the body. Toxin-induced inflammation stimulates the blood-clotting cascade to produce excessive levels of clotting factors such as fibrinogen, a phenomenon known as hypercoagulability.

Fifty percent of my patients are at double risk for a heart attack or stroke because they suffer toxin-induced hypercoagulability. Ironically, the clotting tests I was taught to use in my intensive care training will not diagnose the hypercoagulable state in these patients.

BW: How do you treat toxicity?

RS: My toxicity protocol is very comprehensive. First, I perform an extensive evaluation of more than 300 biochemicals, including brain chemicals, hormones, nutritional factors, and biomarkers for toxicity that include various infectious agents.

After determining what the various causes of toxicity are in a specific patient, we begin using both oral and intravenous modalities of treatment to restore multiple biochemicals and hormones to their optimal level. I have designed a proprietary intravenous protocol that greatly accelerates the healing process and toxin removal above and beyond what we could achieve using the quality oral medications and herbals we used for years. Our simultaneous removal of toxins and intravenous restoration of nutritional factors produces great results within just two to four weeks, depending on the level of toxicity the patient is suffering from.

Because the mold toxins, particularly the trichothecene toxins, suppress multiple components of the immune system, our mold-toxic patients typically need treatment for undiagnosed Lyme and Mycoplasma infections. We have developed an all-natural protocol for killing these bugs with mega-dose intravenous vitamin C and oral herbal medications that optimize the patient's kill power. We effectively treat Lyme disease in many patients who have been on five or more years of antibiotics that didn't kill their Lyme.

BW: What conditions have you seen improve by treating underlying toxicity?

RS: Depression, anxiety, insomnia, panic disorder, bipolar syndrome, chronic fatigue, fibromyalgia, multiple sclerosis, Parkinson's disease, neuropathy, adult-onset diabetes, hypertension, Crohn's disease, ulcerative colitis, liver cirrhosis, and cardiovascular disease.

BW: Thank you for the interview, Dr. Sponaugle. You are a pioneer in the field of medicine, and you bring an important perspective on the importance of eliminating underlying toxicities that contribute to chronic disease. Your ability to dig deeper when assessing an array of biological imbalances is astounding. Your contribution to this book is invaluable.

"Our bodies are our gardens – our wills are our gardeners."

—*William Shakespeare*

Chapter 11

Toxins and Heart Disease

Toxins are everywhere; there is no doubt about it. In the air we breathe, in the water we drink, in the food we eat, in our homes, in most products we use—even in the most pristine places on earth—toxins are ubiquitous.

The Centers for Disease Control (CDC) performs ongoing analyses of the levels of environmental chemicals in the U.S. population. Currently, they measure 212 different toxic compounds. In the majority of people tested, the following compounds were found: acrylamides, cotinine, trihalomethanes, bisphenol A (BPA), phthalates, chlorinated pesticides, triclosan, organophosphate pesticides, pyrethroids, heavy metals, aromatic hydrocarbons, polybrominated diphenyl ethers (flame retardants), benzophenone from sunblock, perfluorocarbons from nonstick coatings, and a host of polychlorinated biphenyls (PCBs) and solvents.[1] And that only accounts for 212 of the more than 80,000 chemicals currently in use. Each year the CDC adds new chemicals to test for, but they will never be able to detect them all.

Myth:

Nothing can be done about toxin exposure.

Fact:

Supporting the body's seven channels of elimination—colon, liver, lungs, lymph, kidneys, skin, and blood—will help improve the body's natural detoxification abilities.

All of the toxins listed on the previous page have been found to interfere with normal functions in the body, and most have been associated with adverse health effects. Many of these contribute to cardiovascular disease—either directly, or indirectly through an increase in oxidative stress or systemic inflammation. For example, lead, carbon disulfide, arsenic, ozone, cadmium, vinyl chloride, fluorocarbons, Freon, and pesticides have been found to produce high blood pressure and irregular heartbeat in most studies, by way of a number of mechanisms: (1) damage to the artery lining, or endothelium, (2) promotion of excess blood clotting, (3) arterial plaque formation, (4) increase of inflammation, and (5) damage to heart and blood vessel tissue.[2]

Air Pollution

Air pollution is another major source of toxic exposure leading to, or complicating, heart disease. Both short- and long-term exposure to air pollution have been associated with increased risk for cardiovascular events like heart attack and stroke.[3] The air pollutants carbon monoxide, nitrogen oxides, sulfur dioxide, ozone, lead, and particulate matter (a mixture of solid and liquid particles suspended in air) have been associated with increased hospitalization and death from cardiovascular disease. Sources of air pollution are many: power generation, industrial combustion, metal processing, agriculture, construction and demolition, wood burning, windblown dust, pollen and molds, forest fires, volcanic emissions, vehicle exhaust, gas-burning appliances, secondhand smoke, and more.[4]

Although the Clean Air Act legislation was passed in 1970, improved air quality since

Air pollution levels do not need

then has failed to have a big enough impact on death and disease associated with air pollution, as air pollution is continually linked with human illness.[5] Both short-term and long-term studies have found air pollution linked with increased death from cardiovascular disease.[6,7,8] Air pollution is thought to contribute to systemic inflammation, which, as we have learned, is a major factor for the development of heart disease. Air pollution also affects blood pressure[9] and heart rhythm, contributing to heart arrhythmias that lead to cardiac arrest.

Levels of air pollution do not need to be very high to cause harm. Even levels considered acceptable by the Environmental Protection Agency (EPA) have been found to cause blood vessel injury, leading to heart disease–related hospitalizations and death.[10] For local air quality information about particulate matter air pollution, visit the AIRNow website.

Cigarette smoke is a major contributor to cardiovascular disease. It affects all phases of heart disease—from the initial stages of endothelial dysfunction all the way through heart attack and cardiovascular death. Both direct cigarette smoking and exposure to secondhand smoke increase heart disease risk by way of increasing oxidative stress and directly oxidating LDL cholesterol particles, increasing inflammation, worsening blood clotting factors, increasing fat oxidization, and contributing to blood vessel dilation dysfunction.[11] Children exposed to secondhand smoke are at increased risk of later developing heart disease.[12]

to be very high to cause harm.

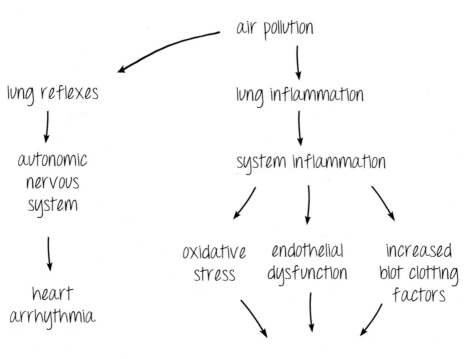

Persistent Organic Pollutants

Persistent organic pollutants (POPs) are chemicals that persist in the environment, bioaccumulating in the food web, and adversely affecting human health and the environment. Some common POPs include PCBs, DDT, dioxins, and some pesticides. POPs have

TIP:

If you smoke and you're concerned about heart disease, you've got to quit.

even been found in areas of the world where they have never been used or produced, highlighting the widespread contamination of these pollutants.[13] Elevated blood levels of POPs have been associated with high blood pressure, obesity, diabetes, metabolic syndrome, heart attack, and atherosclerosis.[14] Even at low doses of POPs similar to current exposure levels, diabetes risk is increased.[15]

Heavy Metals

Increased levels of heavy metals, particularly mercury and lead, have been found to be associated with heart disease risk factors. Lead is known to increase blood pressure, and may also decrease heart rate variability.[16] Mercury exposure has been found to inhibit the production of an enzyme involved in the protection of LDL and HDL cholesterol against oxidation.[17] Thus, high levels of mercury may increase the oxidation of LDL cholesterol particles, which, as we have learned, is a major risk factor for heart disease.

Lead exposure comes from lead pipes and lead-based paint still present in many older houses. Older individuals may have substantial lead accumulation as a result of past exposure to leaded gasoline, as well as paint and lead pipes. Heavy metals are stored for many years in the body's tissues, including bone. It is thought that bone loss, as occurs with age, may be one source for the release of heavy metals back into circulation.[18] Mercury exposure comes from consumption of certain fish, dental amalgams (silver fillings are about 50 percent mercury), and air pollution. Interestingly, silver fillings are considered hazardous waste when it comes to disposal, but there are no regulations against putting them into people's mouths.

Treatment

There is no standard treatment for toxin exposure as it relates to heart disease. Most doctors do not even consider toxins beyond cigarette smoke as being a causative factor for the development of heart disease. Most holistic-minded doctors, however, have a different viewpoint. They are very aware of the negative impact toxins have on human health.

One treatment for heart disease utilized by many integrative doctors is IV EDTA chelation therapy. IV chelation therapy involves the administration of the chelating chemical EDTA (ethylenediaminetetraacetic acid) into the bloodstream. EDTA acts as a binding agent to metal ions such as lead. It also readily binds with calcium, zinc, iron, copper, cadmium, and aluminum.

The original discovery that EDTA chelation therapy positively affects heart disease occurred in 1955 when Norman Clarke observed that patients treated for lead toxicity who also had atherosclerosis displayed improvements in their arterial disease after chelation.[19] Clarke then went on to successfully treat chest pains and vascular disease with EDTA treatment. After other researchers confirmed these beneficial effects, off-label use of IV chelation therapy for heart disease became popular among alternative medicine practitioners.

IV chelation therapy has been found in studies to improve blood flow to the brain, increase cardiac output, and improve peripheral vascular disease.[20] One interesting study found that 58 of 65 patients waiting to have cardiac bypass surgery no longer needed the procedure after having IV chelation therapy during their wait.[21]

EDTA chelation therapy is usually administered in conjunction with other nutrients delivered intravenously, particularly vitamins E, C, and B.[22] This treatment aims to remove harmful levels of aluminum, iron, copper, and toxic heavy metals. It is also thought to contribute to the removal of calcium buildup in arterial plaque, either by directly chelating it or by promoting hormone function that removes the calcium.[23]

Support of the body's seven channels of elimination—colon, liver, lungs, lymph, kidneys, skin, and blood—is an important part of reducing the toxic body burden to which we are all exposed. For more information on a comprehensive program to help improve your own detoxification pathways in the body, read my book *Detox Strategy*.

interview

Dr. R. Ernest Cohn

Brenda discusses chelation with Dr. R. Ernest Cohn, Director of the Holistic Medical Clinic of the Carolinas

BW: Dr. Cohn, thank you for taking time for this interview. You are a conventionally trained medical doctor, a doctor of naturopathic medicine, as well as a doctor of chiropractic. You have more than 35 years of clinical practice during which you have gained a deep understanding of the importance of the doctor-patient relationship. You also have a lot of experience with chelation therapy. Can you explain the origin and definition of chelation therapy?

REC: The word *chelation* is derived from the Greek words *chele*, which means "to claw," and *cation*, which means "metal ion." In other words, *chelation* means "to grab and hold onto metals" so they can be removed. Initially chelation therapy began as a method for removing excess lead in people who were exposed to it and showed high blood levels of lead. Chelation has been used for more than 50 years as an effective way to remove lead from people exposed to toxic amounts. Today chelation can be applied to the removal of lead, mercury, cadmium, aluminum, iron, copper, and many other metals.

BW: How does patient therapy fit into the treatment of cardiovascular and other metabolic diseases?

REC: There are two primary uses for therapeutic chelation: treatment of the cardiovascular system and toxic metal removal. Both of these treatments are essential in the maintenance of proper health. The primary agent used for both treatments is EDTA (ethylenediaminetetraacetic acid), in different forms. The primary types of EDTA include disodium EDTA and calcium disodium EDTA. The two forms differ in how they work within the body, binding to specific elements and causing them to be released from the body, primarily in the urine.

The disodium form of EDTA helps to displace elements, including calcium, from within the arteriosclerotic plaque, theoretically softening the plaque, and in effect improving circulation. Improvement of circulation may occur within the arteries of the heart, vessels within the brain, or elsewhere in the peripheral blood vessels of the body and extremities.

The calcium disodium form of EDTA has less affinity for calcium because it already contains it. As a result, it seeks out and binds with specific metals that have been shown to produce free radicals within the body. Free radicals can be produced by toxic metals, plastics, pesticides, radiation chemotherapy, medications, and even common, everyday substances often considered safe. While calcium disodium EDTA does not bind to most of these free radicals, it does effectively bind with many toxic metals, some of which are now found in our environment and have been associated with chronic metabolic diseases including cancer, cardiovascular disease, diabetes, and many other chronic conditions.

In addition to treating patients with chelating agents, integrative physicians (medical doctors, osteopaths, chiropractors, and naturopaths) are trained to identify agents of free radical damage and to assist and educate patients in proper dietary management, exercise, lifestyle changes, and reduction of toxin exposure.

BW: What nutrients are used during the process of chelation therapy for cardiovascular disease?

REC: Chelation therapy has been utilized by integrative physicians safely and effectively for more than 50 years. Doctors do not simply chelate their patients. Prior to the consideration of chelation therapy it is important that a patient discuss his or her medical history with an integrative physician. Patients with a history of cardiovascular disease, cerebrovascular disease, peripheral vascular disease, kidney or liver disease, or other conditions should make sure that proper laboratory testing and diagnostic procedures are performed prior to any form of treatment. This is routinely done by integrative physicians who chelate, as it should be done prior to any type of treatment performed by a physician. For example, if

> **"It is important for the patient to be willing to commit to lifestyle changes, including the removal of processed, high-carbohydrate, and highly refined foods, and to some form of exercise."**

a patient has kidney or liver disease, kidney and liver function must be assessed so that appropriate dosing of chelating agents can be applied. While chelating agents like EDTA are extremely safe, some patients require longer duration or reduced dosage of the chelating agents, at least initially. This is particularly true with more severe cardiovascular disease. Even those with congestive heart disease may be treated when proper precautions are taken.

Prior to doing chelation, integrative physicians will commonly perform a chemistry panel, essential element testing, specific cardiovascular tests, and often pre- and post-toxic metal challenge tests. With all of this information, if there is any vitamin or nutrient deficiency, it can be identified and then replaced during treatment. The physician will typically add to the IV supplements such as pyridoxine, thiamin, riboflavin, niacinamide, dexpanthenol, hydroxocobalamin, and folic acid, along with magnesium, zinc, manganese, selenium, and molybdenum. If a patient has a known allergy to any of these, the practitioner should be informed prior to treatment.

In addition, oral supplementation of a multivitamin, along with specific nutrients such as zinc, vitamin B6, and other trace elements, as well as vitamins or minerals the patient may be deficient in will likely be recommended before and after chelation. Specific agents such as CoQ10, vitamins B, C, D, and E, and free radical eliminators such as white pine bark, green tea extract, or resveratrol may be recommended.

BW: Are there any risks or contraindications involved with chelation therapy?

REC: While chelation therapy is extremely safe and many hundreds of thousands of treatments are performed annually, there are some necessary precautions, as is the case with any form of therapy. The primary concern is for patients who have impairment in kidney function, because EDTA and the toxins bound to it must pass through the kidney as they exit the body. For this reason it is important that kidney function be evaluated—including tests of serum creatinine and estimated GFR at a minimum—before chelation therapy is given.

Patients with diabetes on older diabetes medications may experience lower glucose during the therapy. For these patients it is recommended that chelation be administered at a slower speed, and after consumption of a proper meal. If necessary the patient can snack during the treatment.

While it is quite rare for large amounts of calcium to be removed during the treatment process, those who have low levels of serum calcium may experience transient lowering of these levels. Patients who are taking seizure medications need to discuss this with the practitioner.

At the site of administration it is possible to get a local irritation during administration. This is commonly controlled with the use of a small amount of heparin or by buffering the solution with bicarbonate to reduce discomfort.

Because EDTA can affect hormones like the parathyroid (which controls the absorption and release of calcium) it could trigger the parathyroid to increase the release of parathyroid hormone. People with hyperparathyroidism (not to be confused with hyperthyroidism) would need to be monitored.

People who know that they have the following conditions should advise their physician prior to treatment: tuberculosis, cardiac arrhythmia, congestive heart failure, severe liver disease, or any other serious condition.

BW: What type of results have you seen in your practice using chelation therapy for cardiovascular disease?

REC: Chelation is only part of the treatment process. Chelation therapy for cardiovascular or peripheral vascular disease should be considered for people who have a history of elevated cardiovascular markers, people who have been overweight for a significant period of time, who have high blood sugar or diabetes that is controlled, and people with a family history of arteriosclerosis or other metabolic diseases.

Before deciding on chelation therapy as part of a patient's treatment protocol, thorough examination, extensive laboratory testing, and a lengthy consultation with the patient about the findings is essential. It is important for the patient to be willing to commit to lifestyle changes, including the removal of processed, high-carbohydrate, and highly refined foods, and to some form of exercise. In our clinic, we have found that altering the patient's lifestyle and diet is essential, and produces much better results than utilizing any one protocol, such as chelation, by itself. With the addition of a proper chelating protocol over a period of time, most all of our patients do extremely well and are very satisfied with their outcomes.

BW: In the scientific community concern has been raised about the scientific evidence for chelation therapy. Can you comment on this?

REC: Actually, there is no real question of the scientific validity of chelation therapy at all. In fact,

FDA standards regarding the use of chelation for heavy metal detoxification have been in place for more than 50 years. Practitioners who are appropriately taught the standards and protocols of chelation therapy can effectively treat patients with great success. As it relates to cardiovascular disease, there have been many articles written on benefits and the comparisons of utilizing chelation therapy for cardiovascular and peripheral vascular disease. Just like many things in the health-care field, research can be done and performed when there is money applied to do the research. There has been little money made available by large pharmaceutical or health-care companies to do these expensive and potentially life-saving research studies.

BW: How does appropriate chelation therapy along with nutrition affect a person with cardiovascular or other chronic diseases?

REC: Since chelation can remove toxic metals, and many of these metals have been shown to cause chronic degenerative diseases, the combination of removing metals and then replenishing the body with proper nutrition is the best way to approach the improvement of a patient's health. Many patients have been diagnosed with cancers, and many cancers have been shown to have a link to environmental toxins. Lead, mercury, aluminum, cadmium, uranium, and many other environmental carcinogens can be removed with chelation. Vitamin C, alpha-lipoic acid, N-acetyl cysteine, glutathione, and vitamins E and D are just a few nutritional agents used by integrative practitioners via IV therapy to induce pro-oxidant

effects and help improve apoptosis (normal cell aging and destruction). Many people for whom conventional therapies have failed or are no longer considered effective have used these forms of therapy to improve their outcomes. Cardiovascular disease, bowel diseases, chronic fatigue syndrome, and cancers are but a few conditions that can benefit. Together with a diet high in raw foods, juicing, colonic irrigation, and food-grade nutritional supplementation, the patients can often see major changes in laboratory profiles in very short duration, and improvement in many conditions over time. It is important to consider any therapy that has potential merit, and to not allow any doctor to discourage you from trying it.

BW: What forms of IV therapy does your practice provide?

REC: Holistic Medical Clinic of the Carolinas is one of the oldest integrative health-care practices in the southeastern United States. What makes a practice like ours unique is that we include all forms of integrative practitioners in one clinic to provide the most benefit and the most varied services to the patients. Our clinic has medical, chiropractic, and naturopathic physicians on staff who all work together to evaluate and treat each patient. We include all of these medical philosophies and use them interactively with IV nutrition, chelation, massage therapy, acupuncture, homeopathy, colonic irrigation, and many other therapies.

The majority of the patients seen in an integrative clinic like ours have complex physical problems that other practitioners have been unable to treat. Many of our patients have been diagnosed with irritable bowel syndrome, celiac disease, cardiovascular disease, diabetes, or chronic thyroid problems. We also see a large percentage of patients with fibromyalgia, chronic fatigue, Lyme disease, and many metabolic diseases that have failed with conventional therapies. Most integrative clinics do not see

We use chelation for many of these chronic metabolic problems, not only to treat the patient but to help find out why these conditions may have occurred. Most disease is brought on by the environment in which we live. There are two expressions integrative practitioners often use: 1) "You are what you eat" and 2) "Above, down, inside, and out." What I mean by this is, everything that is put into the body will affect you

"We have found that patients with chronic metabolic diseases, including cancer, will greatly improve if they alter their lifestyle and determine the true cause of their underlying problem."

cancer patients, but with more than 35 years of clinical experience treating nutritional diseases, we are one of the few that does. We have found that patients with chronic metabolic diseases, including cancer, will greatly improve if they alter their lifestyle and determine the true cause of their underlying problem.

and your health. Everything goes in from above (the mouth or respiratory tract), then travels through the body downward from the inside to the tissues and then out. We therefore use chelation to help evaluate patients for toxicities such as lead, mercury, arsenic, aluminum, cadmium, or other toxic metals (which are known as potential carcinogens). The test results will often find high levels of these toxins and help guide us to provide treatment for toxin removal. Together with moderate dietary changes, proper supplementation, and detoxification, we see many patients each year who continue to live healthy and productive lives, even after being told they might not.

BW: How would a patient find a doctor in their area who is experienced in using chelation and other IV therapies in the treatment of cardiovascular or other diseases?

greater distances. I often recommend that patients find the best clinical practitioner and make the effort to travel to see him or her. There are integrative and holistic professional associations in the medical, chiropractic, and naturopathic professions accessible through the Internet. Doctors certified in chelation therapy are usually members of the American College for Advancement in Medicine (www.acam.org). ACAM certifies doctors who meet the educational and clinical expertise requirements and who utilize chelation therapies in their practices. I always

"While it can be helpful to read about doctors on chat rooms or similar sites, it does not always reflect an accurate description of the practitioner; often it is the loud response of a minority of disgruntled patients."

REC: The Internet is a good source for finding names of practitioners in a patient's geographic area. However, many of the experienced integrative practitioners can only be found at

advocate that a patient get recommendations from friends or relatives who have had experience with integrative practitioners to see if that practitioner is a proper fit for them.

BW: What are the right questions to ask when seeking an integrative practitioner?

REC: If a doctor has been recommended to you by friends or family, you want to make sure that what they have told you is correct. If you can, check out the practitioner's website to determine if the services offered are what you are looking for. While it can be helpful to read about doctors on chat rooms or similar sites, it does not always reflect an accurate description of the practitioner; often it is the response of a minority of disgruntled patients. If that practitioner has been in practice for many years and you have heard positive feedback about him or her, that is typically a good indication that your experience will be positive.

Ask the doctor's staff some specific questions when you call. Find out if he or she is available to e-mail or call you later that day to answer a few questions about what you are looking for. Another option is to make an appointment to meet the doctor for a few minutes to see if you both connect (remember this will not be a complete consultation). Once you feel this office may be right for you, make an appointment and bring with you the most important questions and information (labs, CT, MRI, biopsy, and reports) you want the doctor to know about you as a new patient.

If the office is busy when you arrive, this is usually a good sign that many people are seeking the care of this doctor. Feel free to ask some general questions of others in the waiting room, such as 1) does the doctor listen to your concerns, 2) does he or she make recommendations that have been helpful, and 3) does the doctor have enough time to work with you, or is he or she too busy?

Remember to fill out the entire form(s) that are provided to you, being sure to include personal information. While you may not think some of the information is important, it is. Doctors need to gather a lot of information from which to base their diagnosis and recommendations. They are trained to organize little bits of information into groups that represent potential diagnoses, and from which they determine the most probable cause of your condition. In addition to signs and symptoms, they must know family history and personal information. This is part of working with your doctor.

Expect, as a new patient, that while your appointment may be at 2:00 in the afternoon you may not see the doctor until 30 to 45 minutes after that time. This time is allowed for new patients to complete the entrance data and forms and still have time to be seen. Next, you will speak to the doctor in private. Most integrative practitioners will spend more time here because they have learned in school that the majority of all diagnoses are made during the patient's history. That is correct—most diagnoses are made when the doctor speaks with you! The most valuable aspect of the doctor-patient relationship is the time a doctor takes to sit with you as a patient to discuss what you feel is wrong. Functional testing helps to augment the information gathered during these times, but it cannot substitute for this interaction.

BW: What should people know if they have already been diagnosed with a health condition?

REC: You need to take time to research your condition. Know the standard options, along with the alternatives, that are available to you. Remain open to all information that you find might be of help, even if it is not familiar to you. Then return to your doctor (each doctor if you have more than one) and sit down to discuss all of these options. If the doctor seems too busy, he or she is not the right doctor. If the doctor belittles you for seeking alternatives to what he or she has recommended, the doctor's approach may be too conventional. By dismissing your alternatives, you may miss opportunities that could benefit your health. Conversely, if the doctor speaks terribly about all conventional therapies and only recommends his or her own procedures, be concerned that you are being swayed in only one direction.

If you have found alternative or natural therapies, ask the doctor if he or she has any experience with these, or if you can be referred to someone who does. Write down all you have learned in your search and find someone who is knowledgeable and open to everything you have investigated. You need someone who

"You also want to learn as much as you can about any test results obtained, and what they mean. Ask that each test be explained to you and make sure you understand them. When dealing with common conditions such as constipation, diarrhea, weight gain or weight loss, swelling, loss of breath, fatigue, or other issues, the laboratory testing can tell a lot about why you are not feeling well."

is better educated than yourself to guide you down this path so you will feel comfortable in your final decisions.

You also want to learn as much as you can about any test results obtained, and what they mean. Ask that each test be explained to you and make sure you understand them. When dealing with common conditions such as constipation, diarrhea, weight gain or weight loss, swelling, loss of breath, fatigue, or other issues, the laboratory testing can tell a lot about why you are not feeling well. If a doctor simply tells you "everything looks OK," and does not review the results with you, ask for a copy of your tests, and ask that he or she review it with you anyway. Determine if your test results are on the outside edge of normal ranges or if they are more in line with the healthiest individuals. Ask what you can do to move toward the healthiest test result ranges.

Normally an integrative and preventative medicine physician will take the information from this testing, your examinations, and history, and sit down to review the findings with you. Take for example a history of constipation or alternating constipation and loose bowels. During this consultation with the doctor it would be important to discuss your bowel habits. If you only have one bowel movement a week, three times a week, or just one small movement each day, it may be determined that magnesium deficiency (below 2.1 mg/dL) could be a cause, as could a history of taking antibiotics, during which the good intestinal bacteria is depleted. A lack of fresh raw foods in your diet (and thus a lack of dietary fiber necessary to clean your intestine) may also be part of the problem. Further, medication, such as narcotic pain medicines, could also cause constipation. This is why it is so important to completely fill out your initial history form and to discuss these issues with the doctor.

Combining the knowledge obtained from these exams, the doctor should be able to recommend cleansing of the bowel with either colonic irrigation or gentle herbal cleansers, followed by re-establishment of the missing probiotics. If there is a history of irritation causing poor nutrient absorption, the addition of L-glutamine might be necessary to nourish the tiny villi that line the intestine. Removal of poor-quality foods and replacement with fresh, whole foods including plenty of raw vegetables and fruit will help support the restoration of health. Over time you will notice that your malaise, body odor, fatigue, and flatulence decrease. Soon the color of your skin (the largest excretory organ of your body) will clear and brighten up. The whites of your eyes may brighten and many of the everyday aches and pains disappear—all of this without the addition of any medications.

BW: Thank you, Dr. Cohn, for the information you've shared with us. So many people become frustrated while trying to manage their health care. The suggestions you have provided will help many people take back control of their health, and their health care, while establishing a beneficial doctor-patient relationship.

section two

LOVE YOUR HEART

Love Your Heart: A Guide for Taking Control of Your Health

Up until now, you have learned about many contributors to heart disease, some of which you probably were not aware of previously. You learned that high cholesterol, and even high LDL cholesterol, is not necessarily bad. Rather, it's the state in which the cholesterol is found that truly determines heart health. You learned to monitor your blood pressure because it can be a silent killer. You learned the importance of maintaining healthy blood sugar levels, and how this goes a long way toward preventing metabolic syndrome, type 2 diabetes, and cardiovascular disease.

You learned about silent inflammation, which underlies all of these heart disease risk factors and is intimately involved in the development and worsening of heart disease itself. You learned about different sources of inflammation, the gut being a primary source. You learned about how healthy digestive function is the foundation upon which total-body health is built. You learned that to heal your heart, you must begin by healing your gut. You also learned about how stress and toxins can take their toll, triggering inflammation and contributing to heart disease.

You are now armed with so much information. Educating yourself is an important part of becoming your own health advocate. It is why I have written so many books, why I do so many PBS shows, and why I continue to focus so much of my time and energy on spreading the word about healing your gut to heal your body. When it comes to our own health, we often come to rely completely on the advice of one or a few doctors without fully understanding the extent of our options. I encourage you to seek out all possible options for achieving health, and to then make your decisions based on what you feel is the best option for you.

Now that you have learned so much about heart health, it's time to put your knowledge into action. I've passed you the ball. Now run with it. The rest of this book will give you the tools you need to create a new lifestyle—a lifestyle in which you choose health as a natural way of being. You will learn the truth about what we have been led to believe is a healthy diet, and you will be given the tools to implement a truly heart-healthy diet and lifestyle. I wish you all the best on your journey.

From my heart to yours,

Brenda Watson

"The part can never be well unless the whole is well."

—Plato

Chapter 12

Love Your Heart: The History of Diet

Modern humans do not differ much, genetically, from our ancient Paleolithic ancestors.[1] Since Paleolithic times between 50,000 and 10,000 years ago, our genes have remained essentially unchanged. Our genes have not yet adapted to the world in which we currently find ourselves. This means our bodies are not adapted to modern diets, comprised of agriculturally and industrially produced foods, which is thought to be one main reason for the increase in chronic, diet-related diseases of modern times. Bluntly put, our bodies are not made for the junk we are feeding them.

The diet of our hunter-gatherer ancestors consisted of about 35 percent fats (though this varied by region), 35 percent carbohydrates, and 30 percent protein.[2] Carbohydrates came from fruits and vegetables, with honey only comprising 2 to 3 percent of total food intake. Saturated fats made up about 7.5 percent, trans fats were barely detectible, and polyunsaturated fats were high, with an omega-6/omega-3 ratio of about 1:1. Dietary cholesterol accounted for about 480 milligrams per day. Fiber consumption was very high, at about 100 grams daily, and so was vitamin and mineral intake. The hunter-gather diet was an alkaline-producing diet, which is associated with a number of protective health effects.

Compare this to the Standard American Diet (SAD—an apt acronym): Fat makes up 32.8 percent, carbohydrates 51.8 percent, and protein 15.4 percent.[3] Cereal grains (85 percent refined and 15 percent whole) are the main source of carbohydrates, with only 23 percent of total carbs coming from fruits and vegetables and 15 percent coming from added sugar.[4] Saturated fats make up 11 to 12 percent of the SAD diet, and trans fats make up about 2 percent. Total polyunsaturated fatty acid intake is thought to be half as much as that of our hunter-gatherer ancestors, and has an omega-6/omega-3 ratio of about 10:1.[5] Current dietary cholesterol intake is about 260 milligrams per day.[6] Fiber intake is only about 12 to 15 grams daily, and vitamin and mineral intake is less than that of our Paleolithic ancestors (with the exception of sodium, which is higher). The SAD contains many acid-producing foods, which creates a chronic, low-grade metabolic acidosis.[7]

Our bodies are not made for the junk we are feeding them.

Nutrient Comparison of Standard American Diet (SAD) to Hunter-Gatherer Ancestors' Diet

	Hunter-Gatherer Diet	Standard American Diet (SAD)
CARBOHYDRATE %	35%	51.8%
added sugar	2-3% (from honey)	at least 15%
fiber	100 g/day	12-15 g/day
FAT %	35%	32.8%
saturated fats	7.5%	11-12%
trans fats	Negligible	2%
omega-6:3 ratio	1:1	10:1
Cholesterol*	480 mg/day	265 mg/day
PROTEIN %	30%	15.4%
ACID/BASE BALANCE	alkaline-producing	acid-producing

*See the end of the chapter for an explanation of the higher cholesterol levels seen in hunter-gatherer diet.

Vitamin/Mineral Content of Standard American Diet (SAD) to Hunter-Gatherer Ancestors' Diet

	Hunter-Gatherer Diet	Standard American Diet (SAD)
Riboflavin (B2)	6.49 mg	2 mg
Folate (B12)	357 mg	361 mg
Thiamin (B1)	3.91 mg	1.6 mg
Vitamin C	604 mg	77 mg
Vitamin A	2870 mg	983 mg
Vitamin E	32.8 mg	8.8 mg
Iron	87.4 mg	15.2 mg
Zinc	43.4 mg	11.4 mg
Calcium	1956 mg	863 mg
Sodium	768 mg	3375 mg
Potassium	10,500 mg	2628 mg

Where Did We Go Wrong?

Over time, diets have shifted from being high in vegetables and fruits (and thus, fiber), lean meats, and seafood (and thus, omega-3 fatty acids) to a diet low in all these foods yet high in processed, refined, chemical-laden non-foods, grain-fed fatty meats, carbohydrates, and sugar. Grains, refined sugars, dairy products, and refined oils became major components, together comprising more than 70 percent of the modern SAD diet, usually in processed form.[8]

With the advent of agriculture and animal husbandry, the characteristics of diet began to change. The most notable change was the addition of grains to the diet. Humans went from eating no grains to eating grains as the main staple. The cultivation of early wheat—emmer and einkorn—about 10,000 to 11,000 years ago marked the beginning of what was to become a long-term experiment in alteration of a food until it no longer resembles its original form. See the interview with Dr. Davis on page 76 for more information on the negative health effects of modern wheat.

Paleolithic Diet

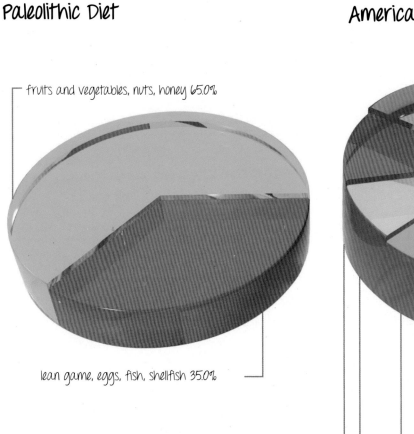

fruits and vegetables, nuts, honey 65.0%

lean game, eggs, fish, shellfish 35.0%

American Diet

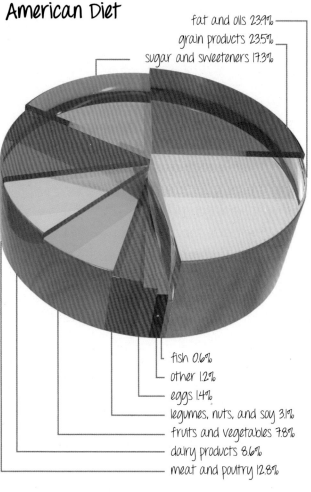

fat and oils 23.9%
grain products 23.5%
sugar and sweeteners 17.3%

fish 0.6%
other 1.2%
eggs 1.4%
legumes, nuts, and soy 3.1%
fruits and vegetables 7.8%
dairy products 8.6%
meat and poultry 12.8%

Myth:

A low-fat diet is a heart-healthy diet.

The Industrial Revolution: It's All Downhill From Here

From Paleolithic times all the way until the Industrial Revolution in the 1700s and 1800s, dietary changes came slowly. With the advent of the Industrial Revolution came food processing, which completely changed food as we knew it, heralding the biggest dietary changes in human history.[10] Mechanized milling took an already foreign-to-the-body food (wheat) and stripped it of its beneficial components, the germ and bran—where all the fiber and vitamins are found. With food processing, nutrient-dense foods were replaced with nutrient-poor, high-carbohydrate foods. The result of these changes has been an epidemic of obesity and diabetes (also called diabesity), along with heart disease death rates topping the charts.

In the 1950s began the idea—generated by the observations of one man (Ancel Keys), and fueled by his connections to the American Heart Association and the government—that a low-fat diet is a heart-healthy diet. This observation drew on findings in animal studies that showed one form of fat—saturated fat—raises total cholesterol levels,[11] and that decreased dietary saturated fat intake was associated with heart disease protection.[12]

For many years the idea that a low-fat diet is protective against heart disease was perpetuated, based on little evidence.[13] In 1961 the Framingham Heart Study linked cholesterol levels to heart disease, and Ancel Keys published a famous article in *Time* magazine claiming that a low-fat diet would lower cholesterol levels. Thus continued the idea that a low-fat diet is a heart-healthy diet.

The 1977 *Report on Dietary Goals for the United States*, strikingly similar to the current 2010 *Dietary Guidelines for Americans*, further

Fact:

A low-fat diet is often a high-carbohydrate diet, which lowers HDL cholesterol and raises triglycerides, blood sugar, and insulin levels, all contributors to heart disease risk.

---

pushed the recommendation of a low-fat, high-carbohydrate diet. The American Medical Association did not support these guidelines, however: "We believe that it would be inappropriate at this time to adopt proposed national dietary guidelines as set forth in the *Report on Dietary Goals for the United States*. The evidence for assuming that benefits to be derived from such universal dietary goals as set forth in the *Report* is not conclusive and there is potential for harmful effects from a radial long-term dietary change as would occur through adoption of the proposed national goal." Boy, were they right about that!

In the 1980s the National Institutes of Health (NIH) sponsored a study that demonstrated that the use of a drug, cholestyramine, reduced total cholesterol levels and was associated with a reduction in overall death rates.[14] Studies using statin drugs further validated the association

between heart disease protection and lower cholesterol levels. So what does all this have to do with diet?

Here is where it gets shady. The NIH, the National Cholesterol Education Program, and the American Heart Association came to a conclusion:[15] If lowering cholesterol levels with medication was effective for prevention and management of heart disease, then reducing dietary fat intake—all dietary fat, not just saturated fat—would also lower cholesterol levels and have the same result.

Thus began, according to one scientific review, "one of America's most extensive public relations campaigns: convincing the profession as well as the public that avoiding dietary fat was a key element in the prevention and treatment of atherosclerotic coronary heart disease."[16] As you can see, this idea is not based on scientific findings but rather exemplifies a leap of faith.

What seems to be missing from dietary recommendations for heart disease protection is a closer look at the contribution of carbohydrates to the development of heart disease.

The Not-So-Healthy Low-Fat Diet

The widely believed—even today—idea that low-fat foods are heart healthy is fatally flawed. In fact, many studies have demonstrated that it's not the amount of fat, but the type of fat that is important to heart health.[17] In general, it is thought that replacing saturated and trans fats with healthy polyunsaturated and monounsaturated fatty acids (such as canola oil or olive oil) is more heart healthy than lowering intake of all dietary fats.

The idea that even saturated fats are unhealthy for the heart is debated, however.[18] An analysis of 24 studies found that there is not enough evidence to conclude that dietary saturated fat is associated with an increased risk of heart disease or stroke.[19] What is known is that monounsaturated and polyunsaturated fats are heart healthy, especially those high in omega-3 fatty acids. Increasing consumption of these fats is a good idea. Limiting saturated fats to moderate consumption is probably a good idea until more studies are done.

What seems to be missing from dietary recommendations for heart disease protection is a closer look at the contribution of carbohydrates to the development of heart disease. The low-fat diet craze saw a proliferation of low-fat processed foods. It quickly became obvious, however, that when fat is removed from food, taste is compromised. To remedy this, food manufacturers began to add sugar and carbohydrates to low-fat and non-fat foods to improve taste and texture. People believed—and they still do—that low-fat foods are healthy.

To the contrary, a low-fat, high-carbohydrate diet lowers HDL cholesterol particles (remember these are the heart-healthy "pickup trucks" carrying cholesterol back to the liver) and raises triglyceride levels,[20] both of which are independent risk factors for heart disease.[21] Further, this diet increases the amount of small, dense LDL particles.[22] (Remember from chapter 2 that these are the artery-damaging LDL particles.) A high-carbohydrate diet also raises blood sugar and insulin levels, both leading to the development of metabolic syndrome and diabetes. Because the low-fat diet became a low-fat, high-carbohydrate diet,[23] the belief took hold that carbohydrates are heart healthy. The result has been, quite plainly, epidemic increases in obesity and diabetes,[24] both of which can lead to heart disease, the number one killer of Americans.

The Sweetening of America

In 1981, around the time when obesity rates began to rise, the glycemic index was developed as a way to compare the blood glucose–raising potential of various foods, as compared by carbohydrate, gram for gram.[25] In 1997 the glycemic load was introduced as a way to assess the blood sugar–raising potential of foods based on how many carbs are consumed in a portion of food.[26] Thus, glycemic load gives a more accurate picture of how much a portion of food will raise blood sugar levels.

Increased consumption of refined sugar is another contributing factor to blame for the 60 percent overweight/obesity rate currently plaguing the United States. In 1815 annual sugar consumption in England averaged 15 pounds per person,[27] with U.S. consumption thought to be similar. By 1970 in the United States it had risen to 120 pounds. And it doesn't stop there— from 1970 to 2000 annual sugar consumption rose to 152 pounds![28]

Soft drinks and sweetened beverages are the main source of added sugars in the SAD diet. Sugars, candy, cakes, cookies, pies, dairy desserts, milk products, and sweetened grain products make up most other sources of added sugar. In the 1970s the mass-quantity manufacture of high-fructose corn syrup began.[29] HFCS is a sweetener made from corn syrup, chemically altered by an enzymatic process that increases the amount of fructose in the sweetener. HFCS became the preferred sweetener in processed food due to its lower cost. Since the 1970s, the consumption of HFCS has risen dramatically. HFCS is quickly becoming the most consumed added sugar in the United States, largely due to its presence in soft drinks and sweetened beverages.

The American Heart Association, along with many other organizations and doctors, recommends lowering added sugar consumption to less than six teaspoons for women, and less than nine teaspoons for men. You know what I say? Eliminate added sugar completely. Added sugar adds nothing to the diet but chronic disease risk. Most holistic-minded health practitioners and doctors give the same advice. And don't be fooled by fancy names. Whether it's sugar, brown sugar, HFCS, fructose, cane sugar, agave nectar, molasses, corn sweetener, dextrose, evaporated cane juice, fruit juice concentrates, glucose, honey, lactose, maltose, malt syrup, or syrup (see how sneaky the processed food industry is?), it's added sugar.

Dietary Cholesterol Revisited

You may have noticed at the beginning of the chapter the high amount of dietary cholesterol found in the diet of hunter-gatherers compared to the Standard American Diet—480 milligrams daily compared to 265 milligrams daily in the SAD diet. Despite high dietary cholesterol intake, average total cholesterol levels of modern-day hunter-gatherers are substantially lower than those of today's average American.[30] Dietary cholesterol does not have as big an effect on blood cholesterol levels as we are led to believe.[31] The hunter-gatherer diet displays close to ideal nutrient components. For modern-day humans, however, the many restrictions of this diet make it difficult to adhere to. See the Love Your Heart Eating Plan for a practical way of eating that is much closer to what our bodies are adapted for than the SAD diet.

HISTORY OF DIET TIMELINE

48,000-8,000 BC	Hunter-gatherer diet based on foods that could be obtained from the wild
8,000 BC	Food cultivation & livestock farming begins -> Grains become a dietary staple
4,000-3500 BC	Dairy foods (other than breast milk) enter diet
1700-1800s	Industrial Revolution -> Mechanized agriculture, food processing, manufacturing, widespread transportation
1815	Annual sugar consumption: 15 lbs. per person
1897	Hydrogenation of oils creates trans fats
1900	Heart disease becomes leading cause of death in the United States
1909	Use of refined vegetable oils increases -> Omega-6/Omega-3 fatty acid ratio becomes imbalanced
1910	Lifetime risk of diabetes: 1 in 30
1970	Annual sugar consumption: 120 lbs. per person
1970's	High-fructose corn syrup developed
1977-1980	Low-fat diet goes mainstream-> Carbohydrate intake increases as fat decreases
1980	Obesity rate begins to increase
1992	Food Guide Pyramid recommends 6-11 daily servings of bread/cereals/rice pasta
1995	Average sugar consumption: 150 lbs per person
2000	Average sugar consumption: 152 lbs per person
2004	Obesity rate over 30% of Americans
2010	Lifetime risk of diabetes: 1 in 3
2012	Heart disease continues to be the number one cause of death in United States

"No disease that can be treated by diet should be treated with any other means."

—*Maimonides*

Chapter 13

Love Your Heart: The Whole Story

In the last chapter you learned that the Standard American Diet is unhealthy (big surprise!). You also learned that the supposed heart-healthy low-fat diet is actually unhealthy despite decades of unsubstantiated propaganda to convince you otherwise. What do these two unhealthy diets have in common? They are both high-carbohydrate diets. We also learned that a high-carbohydrate diet is a relatively recent introduction to humans, evolutionarily, and that our bodies have not yet genetically adapted to this diet.

Yet mainstream medical, governmental, and nutritional institutions promote a diet high in carbohydrates.[1] Since the *Report on Dietary Goals for the United States* was released in 1977, a low-fat, high-carbohydrate diet has been widely pushed, based on little evidence. The current 2010 *Dietary Guidelines for Americans* are strikingly similar to the 1977 goals. The U.S. Department of Agriculture (USDA) and the U.S. Department of Health and Human Services are responsible for putting out these reports, but there is concern that the USDA's ties to the food industry influence the guidelines.[2]

I have no doubt about this. The food industry and the pharmaceutical industry are both in bed with policy makers. The *Dietary Guidelines* report is no exception.

The idea that a high-carbohydrate diet is healthy, and even that whole grains are healthy, does not tell the whole story.

Recommendations have been made by major medical associations for reduction of cardiovascular disease risk by restricting fat intake to 30 percent, raising carbohydrates to 55 to 60 percent, and keeping protein at 15 percent.[3] These recommendations are fatally flawed, however. I'm going to explain why.

The idea that a high-carbohydrate diet is healthy, and even that whole grains are healthy, does not tell the whole story. The increase in calories that has occurred over the last 30 years has come almost entirely from carbohydrates.[4] In fact, since 1970 the average daily calories from flour and cereal products have increased by 10 times.

The epidemic increase in diabetes and obesity rates has coincided with this increase in carbohydrate consumption. Obviously, a closer look at carbohydrates, particularly from grain sources, is needed. To cite the *Dietary Guidelines* 2010: "Studies of carbohydrates and health outcomes on a macronutrient level are often inconsistent." This basically means that the science behind carbohydrates and health is inconclusive. Yet they claim, "Healthy diets are high in carbohydrates."[5]

Type 2 diabetes, a major health concern of modern times and a risk factor for heart disease, involves an impairment of blood sugar control as the result of an increased intake of digestible carbohydrates.[6] Yet the focus of most dietary recommendations for diabetes minimizes the effects of total carbohydrate intake. Focus is placed only on added sugars, and the recommendation for "healthy whole grains" abounds. Yet the definition of a healthy whole grain has not even been established. For example, the addition of "more whole grains" to General Mills Lucky Charms, Cinnamon Toast Crunch, and similar cereals certainly should not be promoted as healthy, but it is. Processed whole grain foods can be just as unhealthy as refined sugar products, as Dr. William Davis has

highlighted in his book *Wheat Belly*: 2 slices of whole grain bread raise blood sugar more than 2 tablespoons of sugar. See the interview with Dr. Davis on page 76 for more information.

Carbs Turn to Sugar

It is well known that added sugar is not a heart-healthy food.[7] High-sugar diets lower HDL cholesterol particles[8] and raise triglyceride levels.[9,10] Sugar-sweetened beverages are particularly to blame for their negative effects on heart health. There is really no place for added sugar in a heart-healthy diet.

Now consider this: Carbohydrates break down into sugar in the body. In fact, sugar itself is a carbohydrate—a simple carbohydrate. Sugars are called simple carbohydrates because they are simple molecules—monosaccharides or disaccharides. Complex carbohydrates, or polysaccharides, are actually long chains of sugar molecules, or saccharides. "Poly"-saccharide means "many" sugars.

There are three types of polysaccharides: starch, glycogen, and dietary fiber. Starch is the major storage carbohydrate in plants, made of amylose and amylopectin. Glycogen is the storage unit of carbohydrates in the body (just like triglycerides are the storage unit of fat in the body). And dietary fiber is a nondigestible form of carbohydrate. This is why dietary fiber passes through the digestive tract undigested, until it reaches the colon, where gut bacteria ferment it, essentially breaking it down.

Carbohydrate foods high in fiber will break

down more slowly in the digestive tract, resulting in a more even release of sugar molecules for absorption into systemic circulation. Thus, a high-fiber diet helps to regulate blood sugar levels.[11] High-fiber diets are also associated with lower insulin levels, less weight gain, and improvements in other heart disease risk factors.[12]

TIP:

The high-fiber carbohydrate foods I recommend for heart health are non-starchy vegetables and low-sugar fruits.

Processed carbohydrate foods, like those made from refined flours, break down into sugar quickly in the digestive tract. Even processed "whole grain" bread products break down quickly into sugar—perhaps not as quickly as their white-bread counterparts, but they still convert rapidly to sugar.

The best place to find fiber from carbohydrates is in non-starchy vegetables and low-sugar fruits. Vegetables and fruits contain fiber intact, so it takes the digestive system more time to break them down. In the process, many beneficial phytonutrients are released. Compare that to the empty calories of bread. Not many nutrients are gained from those carbs. The carbs you should be eating need to come from plenty of vegetables and some fruits. These are truly healthy carbs.

What About Whole Grains?

The idea that whole grains are healthy is being spread far and wide. We have made the case here that processed whole grains, as are found in whole wheat bread/cereal/cakes and so on, can be just as detrimental as sugar itself because they quickly break down into sugar in the body. But you might be wondering about whole grains that aren't processed, such as quinoa, oats, and rice.

Well, if the whole grains contain gluten (wheat, rye, barley, or oats) it is very possible they are triggering a food sensitivity that you are not even aware of. Trying a gluten-free diet, or doing the gluten sensitivity test from EnteroLab, is usually the first advice I give most people coming to me with health issues. So many people have found relief from a wide array of health problems by cutting gluten out of the diet. Further, gluten produces exorphins in the gut, which are opiate-like peptides known to have addictive effects, explaining the strong carb cravings (and sometimes withdrawal) many people experience. See the interview with Dr. Davis on page 76 for more information about the addictive qualities of wheat.

So what about the non-gluten whole grains? All grains contain a high amount of carbohydrates. These foods break down into sugar in the body. Whole grains (not processed whole grains) may take slower to break down into sugar, but they still break down. For someone with heart disease risk factors, all grains have got to go. What's more, grains are particularly abundant in antinutrients known as lectins.[13] The lectins in grains, like the agglutinin of wheat, are known to damage the intestinal lining[14] and trigger an immune response leading to autoimmunity.[15]

All this is in line with the idea that our bodies are not genetically adapted to eat grains. If you are dealing with health issues that you can't get to the bottom of, eliminating grains may just be the missing piece to your health puzzle.

Will the Real Heart-Healthy Diet Please Stand Up?

We have established the health detriments of a high-carbohydrate diet. What about the health benefits of a low-carbohydrate diet? Because low-carbohydrate diets are, by nature, higher in fat and protein (you have to replace the carbs with something), it has been thought that they might have potentially negative effects on blood lipids and cardiovascular risk.[16]

With such widespread promotion of a low-fat, high-carbohydrate diet, and the accompanying bad-mouthing of low-carb diets, you would think the science behind low-carb diets is scant. To the contrary, there are many studies demonstrating the health benefits of reducing carbohydrate consumption. I was shocked—delightedly shocked. You see, I had already seen this diet work wonders on my husband, Stan, and my sister, Sandee.

My own diet had essentially been a low-carbohydrate diet because I was eating gluten free—the kind of gluten free that isn't chock full of processed gluten-free breads, pastas, and so on. When I saw how well Sandee and Stan did on the Love Your Heart Eating Plan, and when I learned about how much science there is behind this diet—and how much industry-supported propaganda is behind the so-called healthy low-fat, high-carbohydrate diet—it was easy for me to fully implement the diet as my way of eating. In fact, I don't even think of it as a diet. This is simply how I eat.

Gluten produces exorphins in the gut...

...which are opiate-like peptides known to have addictive effects.

TIP:

The Love Your Heart Eating Plan is so easy. I don't even think of it as a diet.

This is simply how I eat.

Many studies have found the low-carbohydrate diet to be more effective for weight loss, increase in HDL cholesterol, reduction of triglycerides, and lowering of blood pressure when compared to—you guessed it—a low-fat, high carbohydrate diet.[17,18] Not to mention, people stick with low-carbohydrate diets better than the conventional low-fat, high carbohydrate diets.[19] Carbohydrate-restricted diets have been found to lower blood sugar and insulin, improve triglycerides, HDL cholesterol levels, and LDL particle distribution (decreased small, dense LDL particles and increased large, fluffy LDL), and increased weight loss when compared to a conventional low-fat, high-carbohydrate diet.[20]

Some studies have found an increase in LDL cholesterol with a low-carbohydrate diet,[21] but this is likely due to the switch from the atherogenic small, dense LDL particle size to large, buoyant (less atherogenic) LDL particles, which ends up increasing total amount of LDL cholesterol, making it look bad when it's really not. If you remember from chapter 2, the condition in which the LDL cholesterol particle is found is what really determines its potential to trigger atherosclerosis. A low-carbohydrate diet favorably improves the condition of LDL cholesterol particles.

The Paleo diet, which mimics the diet of our hunter-gatherer ancestors, is one form of low-carb diet that is thought to be more in line with what our bodies are designed to eat. The current high rate of cardiovascular disease is thought to be the result of the mismatch of our current genes (still adapted to a Paleolithic-era diet) with the current Standard American Diet (SAD).[22] Thus, the Paleo diet is thought to be a heart-healthy diet.

Indeed, studies have been done to support the heart-health benefits of a Paleo diet. In one study, patients with ischemic heart disease and either glucose intolerance (basically prediabetes) or type 2 diabetes showed a 26 percent reduction in blood sugar levels compared to people on a whole grain, low-fat diet.[23] Another study found the Paleolithic diet produced lower average levels of A1c blood sugar (a measure of long-term blood sugar control) and lower levels of: triglycerides, diastolic blood pressure, weight, body mass index, and waist circumference when compared to the standard diabetes diet recommended by the American Diabetes Association (low-fat, high-carbohydrate diet).[24]

Low-carb diets, and the Paleo diet specifically, are both low in carbohydrates because they eliminate grains. Grain-based foods—whether refined grains or the so-called healthy whole grains—in addition to added sugar and starches, are contributing to the obesity and diabetes epidemic, the carbohydrate cravings driving these epidemics, and the ultimate development of heart disease to which all of these factors lead.

The Downside of Low-Carb and Paleo Diets

Both the low-carbohydrate diet and the Paleo diet have many positive attributes and heart-health benefits. What about the drawbacks of these diets?

Many low-carbohydrate diets are also low-fiber diets, for two reasons: not enough vegetable and fruit intake and removal of whole grain foods. Fiber is an important component of the diet. I recommend at least 35 grams of fiber daily. (See the chapter 15 section for more information about fiber.) If you follow a standard low-carbohydrate diet (there are many to choose from), you likely won't be getting the important benefits of high intake of dietary fiber.

TIP:

Due to the methylmercury contamination of many fish, purified fish oil supplements are the best way to get your daily omega-3s.

Another downfall of low-carb diets is the initial stage of the diet, which involves severe carbohydrate restriction of under 20 grams daily. This intense restriction rapidly puts the body into a state of ketosis, whereby fat is burned for energy in the absence of available glycogen (the storage form of glucose, or sugar, in the body). This kind of strict carbohydrate restriction requires monitoring of ketone bodies in the urine (a dipstick test that can be done daily) to be sure that ketones do not become excessive to the point of triggering ketoacidosis, a dangerous condition common in undiagnosed diabetics. Ketosis is induced by a very-low-carbohydrate diet containing less than 30 grams of carbohydrates daily. Ketosis (not to be confused with ketoacidosis) is thought to be a beneficial, natural process, but it must be monitored by measuring ketones.

Further, some low-carb diets put no limit to the amount of saturated fat you can eat. Although I am not completely convinced that saturated fat needs to be greatly limited, I'm also not convinced that eating excessive amounts of saturated fat is safe. I say eat saturated fat in moderation. Don't forgo that pat of butter because you think it will go straight to you heart, but do refrain from eating bacon for breakfast, lunch, and dinner. Practice moderation here, folks.

Now let's look at the modern Paleo diet. While higher in fiber (due to the emphasis on eating plenty of vegetables and fruits), this diet tends to contain insufficient amounts of calcium and vitamin D.[25] Hunter-gatherers lived outdoors with plenty of sun exposure, and so were not at risk of vitamin D deficiency. The absence of dairy foods in the Paleo diet, and the low sun exposure of modern people both contribute to low calcium and vitamin D levels when following the Paleo diet.

Further, the omega-3 content of modern meats is not what it was in Paleolithic times, so to obtain enough omega-3s, high amounts of cold-water fatty fish are recommended. However, due to the methylmercury contamination of many of these fish,[26] high fish consumption may not be safe.

The Paleo diet does not limit fruits or starchy vegetables such as potatoes. Fruits contain high amounts of fructose, which does not raise blood glucose levels but can have many detrimental effects. Fructose is processed in the liver and contributes to increases in LDL cholesterol, triglycerides, and apolipoprotein-B (a protein that can lead to plaques and heart disease).[27] Starchy vegetables, on the other hand, which rapidly break down into sugar, do contribute to increases in blood sugar levels.

The Love Your Heart Solution

The Love Your Heart Eating Plan, outlined in the next section, is essentially a hybrid between a low-carbohydrate diet and the Paleo diet, taking from each the positive attributes while removing the negative attributes, creating a heart-healthy diet rich in nutrients, full of flavor, and without the characteristic hunger pangs and carb and sugar cravings of the conventional low-fat, high-carbohydrate diet.

"Sorry, there's no magic bullet. You gotta eat healthy and live healthy to be healthy and look healthy. End of story."

—Morgan Spurlock

Chapter 14

Love Your Heart: Eating Plan

The Love Your Heart Eating Plan is a simple way to eat healthfully without having to spend your day counting calories and grams of this or that nutrient. It makes eating healthy a cinch. You've already learned about how high-sugar, high-carbohydrate foods contribute to the many factors involved in heart disease, so you won't be surprised to find out that these foods are not part of the Love Your Heart Eating Plan.

Instead of relying on the usual comfort foods—breads, pastas, cereals, and sweets—the focus is placed on filling your plate with lean proteins and vegetables. You will enjoy a filling, delicious breakfast, a mid-morning snack, a nutritious lunch, another snack in the afternoon, and a dinner of foods that you enjoy. This healthy eating plan will not leave you hungry or craving carbohydrates.

What's more, you'll learn how to make the right choices when it comes to food. This empowerment, along with how great you feel from eating such healthy foods, will be the driving force that helps you make these changes to your diet a way of life. This is not a fad diet. This is not a quick fix. This is you taking control of your health because you deserve it.

TIP:
The Love Your Heart Eating Plan provides you 3 simple rules.

The Love Your Heart Eating Plan gives you three Eating Plan rules. Once you learn these three rules, you can begin to apply them. A one-week Menu Planner including simple, delicious recipes is provided to give you meal and snack ideas to plan your week. Use the Menu Planner as a guide, and feel free to add your own favorites as long as they follow the three

3 [Simple] Rules

1. Track teaspoons of sugar

2. Eat between 6 to 8 teaspoons of sugar daily

3. Eat 12 portions of lean protein daily

Rule 1: Track teaspoons of sugar

That's right—it all comes down to how much sugar is contained in your food. And I don't just mean the added sugar or the sugar found naturally in foods. I also mean the sugar produced by the breakdown of carbohydrates, including fruits and vegetables, in your body. As I said before, carbohydrates break down into sugar in your digestive tract. The only exception is fiber. Remember that fiber is a carbohydrate that resists digestion. That means fiber is your friend because it doesn't break down into sugar.

Rule 2: Eat between 6 to 8 teaspoons of sugar daily

If you are overweight or obese, have a high BMI, waist circumference, or waist-to-hip ratio (see chapter 5 to figure out if this is you), you will eat between 6 and 8 teaspoons of sugar—from all sources—daily. You will eat this way until your weight is under control. When you reach normal weight, or if you are beginning at normal weight, BMI, etc., but with other heart disease risk factors, you will begin in the Maintenance Phase, discussed later.

Please keep in mind that the 6 to 8 teaspoons of sugar are those coming from the calculation from Rule Number 1: total carbohydrates – dietary fiber ÷ 5. Do not use grams of sugar as found on Nutrition Facts panels on food packaging, which only accounts for the added sugar and the sugars found naturally in foods, not the sugars that come from the breakdown of carbohydrates.

Rule 3: Eat 12 portions of lean protein daily

Protein is an important part of the Love Your Heart Eating Plan. You will eat 12 portions of lean protein throughout the day. Choose lean poultry, meat, seafood, low-fat cheese and yogurt, eggs, tofu, tempeh, or nuts for your protein foods.

Eating protein at each meal and snack will help keep your appetite satisfied. At breakfast, eat 2 portions of protein, at lunch and dinner eat 3 to 4, and eat 1 to 2 at snack times, for a total of 12 portions throughout the day. Three to four portions of protein make up a standard serving. For example, a standard grilled chicken fillet added to a salad is 3 to 4 ounces, or 3 to 4 portions in the Love Your Heart Eating Plan.

Studies have found that a high-protein breakfast makes you feel full longer. Eating protein at breakfast is essential to help you avoid carb cravings later. Most people are used to starting their day with cereal, oatmeal, a muffin, or a donut, and wonder why they crave more carbs mid-morning. Instead, begin your day with protein and low-sugar fruit or vegetables.

To track teaspoons of sugar contained in the foods you eat, you have only to use the following:

$$\text{teaspoons of sugar} = (\text{total carbohydrates} - \text{dietary fiber}) \div 5$$

It all comes down to the choices you make. On the Love Your Heart Eating Plan, you will learn what foods you can eat by simply tracking teaspoons of sugar. You will find that your plate fills with lean proteins and healthy vegetable options. Experiment with new foods. Fall in love with vegetables— the diverse flavors available in phytonutrient-rich vegetables have simply been taken for granted in the Standard American Diet.

Portion sizes are as follows:

Protein	Portion
Poultry, meat, seafood, cheese	1 ounce
Eggs	1 egg or 2 egg whites
Tofu	3 ounces
Tempeh	1 ounce
Nuts	1 ounce (handful)
Nut butters	2 tablespoons
Low-fat Greek yogurt	3 ounces

Portions per meal:

Protein	Portion
Breakfast:	2+
Snack:	1–2
Lunch:	3–4
Snack:	1–2
Dinner:	3–4
Total	12

To make protein portions easy, incorporate protein snacks into your day. I recommend preparing some protein snacks ahead of time and storing them in containers for easy-to-grab snacks whenever you need them. Take these containers with you on the go.

Easy as 1-2-3

On the Love Your Heart Eating Plan you'll quickly and easily be on your way to creating a heart-healthy way of eating. By following the three basic rules, you will naturally exclude sugars, grains, and all the processed foods that contribute to heart disease. Your plate will be filled with lush vegetables, lean proteins, low-sugar fruits, and healthy dairy products. The three basic steps will naturally help get you moving in the right direction—a heart-healthy direction. It's as easy as 1-2-3.

The Love Your Heart Eating Plan allows you look at food in a new way. You will begin to see food in terms of how it nurtures your body rather than fulfills your cravings. Try new recipes and new ways to cook old favorites and new delights. You will be surprised at the selection available to you when you look for it.

Maintenance Phase

When you reach your health goal, whether it's healthy weight, normal BMI, or optimal waist circumference or waist-to-hip ratio, you may begin to gradually add more teaspoons of sugar and portions of protein. Begin by adding 1 to 2 teaspoons of sugar and 2 to 4 portions of protein during a 6-week transition period to find the right amounts that keep you at a steady weight. If you are already normal weight, BMI, etc., but you have other heart disease risk factors you want to control, begin with 8 to 10 teaspoons of sugar and 12 to 14 portions of protein daily. The total teaspoons of sugar and portions of protein will vary somewhat depending on many factors, so you will have to do some fine-tuning during this transition. Monitor your heart disease risk factors to help determine the optimal amounts of sugar and protein for you.

After you determine your optimal teaspoons of sugar and portions of protein, I hope you also realize that this is a heart-healthy eating plan for life. This is not meant to be a fad diet for you to follow until you look and feel great, only to turn back to sugars and carbohydrates once you're there. That is likely how you've dieted in the past. The Love Your Heart Eating Plan is different. In this book I have taken you deep into the depths of your body to help you understand how heart disease develops. I did this so that you would understand how imperative it is to make the fundamental changes to your diet and lifestyle so that you can truly have a healthy heart. You have the information in your hands. Now it's up to you to carry out this change as a new way of life.

FAQs In the following section I answer some of the most frequently asked questions I hear about the eating plan. I designed the eating plan as a simple guide to help you develop a way of eating that easily incorporates whole, healthy foods.

Q: What if I am already a healthy weight and don't have any other risk factors for heart disease?

A: This diet was designed specifically for people dealing with the issues outlined in this book. If you are currently enjoying optimal health—your blood cholesterol levels are healthy (not just the standard lipid panel, but also the additional tests that assess the condition of the LDL particle), blood sugar, and insulin levels are normal, you do not have excess abdominal fat, blood pressure is normal, your digestion is optimal, diet includes plenty of non-starchy vegetables, and your exposure to toxins is minimal—then I say keep doing what you're doing. Just don't make the mistake of thinking you are healthy because you feel good, eat "healthy," and your cholesterol levels are healthy based on the standard lipid profile alone. It is best to rule out the underlying causes of poor health that are not always obvious.

You can certainly follow the Maintenance Phase,

experimenting with your own optimal teaspoons of sugar and portions of protein. You may also be able to eat whole grains with no problems, but I do still recommend gluten-free whole grains—non-processed whole grains, that is.

Q: What if I am vegetarian? This diet calls for a lot of animal products.

A: You're right. This diet emphasizes lean proteins, many in the form of animal products. If you are lacto-vegetarian, or lacto-ovo-vegetarian, you will be able to eat dairy and eggs to obtain enough protein. For vegans, however, it will be difficult to eat a diet low in teaspoons of sugar. Beans, though high in protein and fiber, tend to also be very high in carbohydrates, so you are likely to not obtain enough protein when trying to eat this way as a vegan. However, you will likely still benefit if you focus on obtaining your carbohydrates from vegetables and fruits (rather than grains and processed foods), while being sure to eat enough protein daily.

Q: I have been on the Love Your Heart Eating Plan for a while, but I am experiencing a lot of fatigue. Why is that?

A: For some people, it is helpful to begin the eating plan gradually. For the first week, begin by eating a breakfast low in teaspoons of sugar. The next week, eat both breakfast and lunch low in teaspoons of sugar. The third week, add dinner. This may help your body adjust more gradually to the change.

Another contributor to low energy could be low thyroid function, a condition known as hypothyroidism. The thyroid gland produces hormones that are involved with metabolism. When thyroid function is low, these hormones are not produced efficiently, and symptoms of fatigue, sensitivity to cold, and even weight gain are common. A thorough assessment of thyroid function, looking at more than the standard TSH (thyroid stimulating hormone) and T4 (thyroxine) hormones, is recommended. Find an integrative or functional medicine physician who can help you get to the bottom of thyroid imbalance.

Q: You talk about the poor health that results from a low-fat diet, and then you recommend low-fat dairy. This seems contradictory. Could you explain?

A: The low-fat diet is unhealthy for two main reasons: One, when fat is reduced, it is replaced with carbohydrates, usually in the form of sugar and refined flours; and two, by cutting total fat you miss out on an essential nutrient. What is important is the type of fat you eat. Reducing omega-6 fats found in soybean, cottonseed, sunflower oil, and similar oils, and increasing omega-3 fats found in fish, flax, and canola oil is important. Saturated fat should be eaten in moderation. As I mentioned, some studies are finding that saturated fat is not the villain it is made out to be, but because other studies show harmful effects, I think it's best to eat it in moderation for now, until we know more. This is why I recommend low-fat dairy—dairy is high in saturated fat. Use your judgment here.

Q: This is a relatively low-carbohydrate diet; what about ketoacidosis?

A: Low-carbohydrate diets restricting carbs to fewer than 20 or 30 grams of carbohydrates a day produce ketosis, or the burning of fat instead of glycogen for energy. Ketosis needs to be monitored so that ketone bodies are not produced in excess, which could trigger ketoacidosis in certain individuals, especially those with undiagnosed type 2 diabetes. The Love Your Heart Eating Plan delivers between 30 and 45 grams of carbohydrates daily, so you do not need to monitor ketones.

Q: What if I am diabetic?

A: If you are diabetic, it is recommended that you consult with your doctor before beginning the Love Your Heart Eating Plan. Because the Love Your Heart Eating Plan can have positive effects on blood sugar levels, it is important to work with your doctor to monitor blood sugar.

"If we are creating ourselves all the time, then it is never too late to begin creating the bodies we want instead of the ones we mistakenly assume we are stuck with."

—Deepak Chopra

Chapter 15

Love Your Heart: The HOPE Solution

HOPE = High Fiber

In addition to diet, there are four main supplements that should be incorporated into your daily heart-health maintenance: High fiber, Omega-3s, Probiotics and Enzymes. I call this the HOPE Formula, a daily digestive health maintenance formula that supports digestive and total-body health. The first supplement to incorporate into your daily heart-health maintenance is a high amount fiber. Dietary fiber is found only in plant foods such as fruits, vegetables, nuts, legumes, and grains. Fiber makes up the nondigestible part of plants. The average American eats only between 12 and 15 grams of fiber daily. I recommend 35 grams of dietary fiber daily for optimal digestive and heart health. Achieving the goal of consuming 35 grams of dietary fiber each day requires major dietary changes for most people.

Increasing the consumption of fruits and vegetables is the best way to reach 35 grams of fiber each day. But even with an increase of fruit and vegetable intake, it can be difficult to eat this much fiber from food alone. For this reason, a fiber supplement is recommended as an easy way to increase daily fiber intake.

Soluble and Insoluble Fiber

There are two types of fiber: soluble and insoluble. All plant-based foods contain both soluble and insoluble fiber. The natural ratio of a healthy diet is 65 to 75 percent insoluble fiber to 25 to 35 percent soluble fiber. Soluble fiber slows the passage of food through the digestive tract, helping to control appetite and blood sugar elevations. Soluble fiber also helps to bind toxins and other gut contents such as cholesterol; hence soluble fiber's cholesterol-lowering effect. Some soluble fibers also act as prebiotics, or food for the friendly gut bacteria, helping to increase the amount of good bacteria in the gut, a process that produces the short-chain fatty acids butyrate, acetate, lactate, and propionate, some of which provide fuel for the cells that line the colon.[1] Insoluble fiber increases the bulk of stool, helping to move waste through the intestines. Insoluble fiber does not break down in the digestive tract, and helps improve the consistency of stool.

Think of fiber like a two-sided sponge. Soluble fiber is like the yellow side, soaking up unwanted toxins as it moves through the digestive tract. Insoluble fiber is like the green part of the sponge, helping to scrub the colon free of debris. Soluble fiber dissolves in water and leaves the stomach slowly. Insoluble fiber does not dissolve in water and travels though the intestine in much the same form as it was consumed. Foods high in soluble fiber are primarily fruits and vegetables. Foods high in insoluble fiber tend to be cereal grains. All plant-based foods contain both types, however.

Fiber and Heart Health

A high-fiber diet is the hallmark of heart health. High-fiber diets have been associated with:[2]

- Lower LDL-cholesterol levels
- Lower blood sugar levels in people with diabetes
- Lower blood pressure in people with high blood pressure
- Lower risk of heart disease
- Lower risk of diabetes
- Healthier weights and lower rates of obesity

Many studies have found a relationship between increased dietary fiber consumption and decreased risk of heart disease. The greater the dietary fiber intake, the lower the risk of developing heart disease. This has been found true of fiber from fruits and vegetables, as well as fiber from cereal grains. Interestingly, some studies have found that fiber from vegetables does not have as protective an effect, but this is thought to be due to the inclusion of starchy vegetables such as potatoes, corn, and peas (all high-carbohydrate vegetables) when considering total vegetable consumption.[3]

LDL Cholesterol

Soluble and Insoluble Fiber

Inside the digestive tract, soluble fiber absorbs LDL cholesterol and toxins and begins to dissolve into digestive contents, resulting in slower release of sugars from food. Insoluble fiber remains intact, and helps to sweep, or scrub, the intestinal wall, bulk the stool, and improve gut motility.

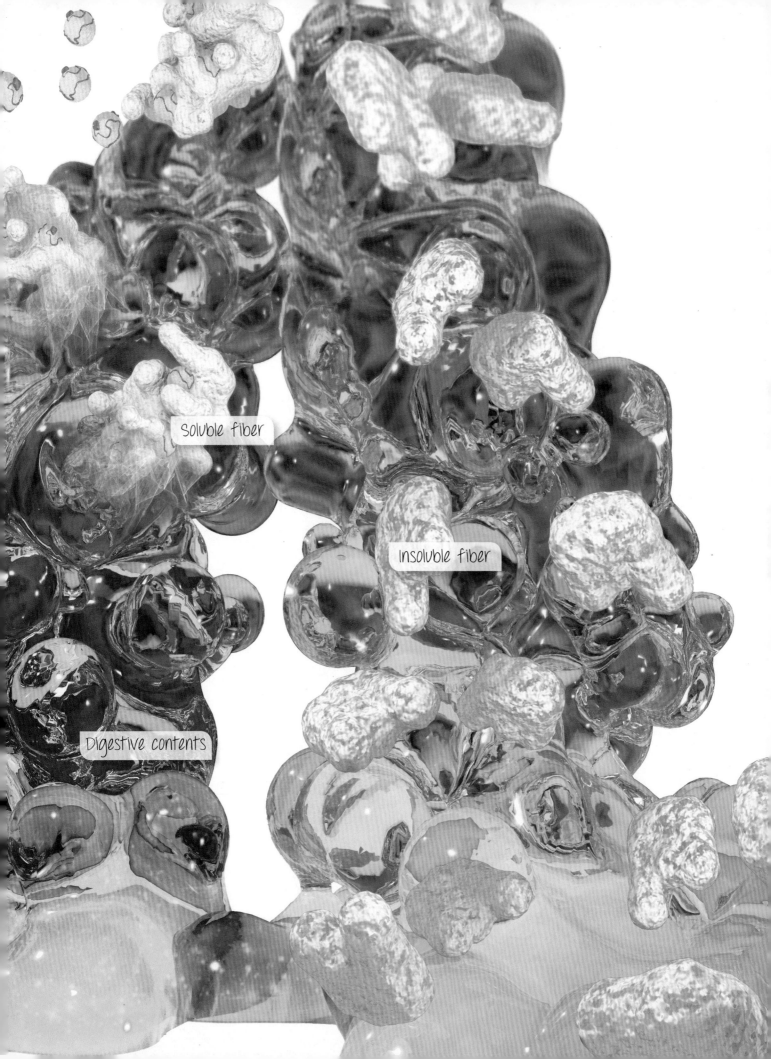

Fiber from low-sugar fruits and non-starchy vegetables is particularly heart healthy. In one study, consumption of green leafy vegetables and vitamin C–rich fruits and vegetables was found to have a protective effect against heart disease.[4] People who ate eight or more servings of fruits and vegetables per day experienced the greatest heart disease protection. A diet high in fruits and vegetables has also been found to protect against stroke.[5]

The heart-health benefits of eating a diet high in low-sugar fruits and non-starchy vegetables are multiple. Antioxidants, folate, fiber, minerals, and a wide array of phytochemicals likely all play a role in the protective effects of these foods. Soluble fiber has been found to be particularly protective against the development of heart disease.[6] Soluble fiber is high in fruits and vegetables, as well as in oat, flaxseed, and acacia fiber.

The American Heart Association and other organizations recommend a diet that includes five or more servings of fruits and vegetables daily, yet it has been estimated that the average American eats less than one serving of vegetables and less than one serving of fruits daily.[7]

People who eat diets low in fiber tend to gain excess weight and belly fat, and have high blood pressure and triglycerides, low HDL-cholesterol, and high LDL-cholesterol.[9] Dietary fiber also plays an important role in regulating blood sugar, and therefore insulin response. As you can see, fiber works in many ways to help reduce the overall risk of cardiovascular disease.

Fiber in the Love Your Heart Eating Plan

Foods high in fiber, especially non-starchy vegetables, are encouraged in the Love Your Heart Eating Plan because fiber is a type of carbohydrate that is not digested by enzymes in the digestive tract. High-fiber foods decrease the absorption of carbohydrates after a meal, and thus help control blood sugar and insulin response to carbohydrates.[10] I recommend 35 grams of fiber daily. Non-starchy vegetables and low-sugar fruits are recommended to be eaten in high amounts, and the addition of a fiber supplement is a great way to ensure that 35 grams are consumed daily.

What to Look for in a Fiber Supplement

Even if you eat plenty of vegetables and fruits, and strive to maximize your dietary fiber intake, it can be difficult to reach 35 grams daily. The addition of a daily fiber supplement is recommended to help you achieve your goal.

- Made with natural and organically-grown ingredients
- Made with lignin-rich flax fiber, soluble acacia fiber, or natural chia seed
- Psyllium-free to prevent cramping, gas, or bloating

H O P E = OMEGA 3s

In addition to diet, there are four main supplements that should be incorporated into your daily heart-health maintenance: The second supplement to incorporate into your daily heart-health maintenance is omega-3s. The first of these three is the omega-3s. Omega-3 fatty acids found in fish are probably the most well-known—and well-studied—natural supplements for heart health.

Fats 101

To understand omega-3 fatty acids, it helps to know how fats are categorized. There are two main types of fats: saturated fats and unsaturated fats. Saturated fats mostly come from animals, but can also be found in coconut oil, cottonseed oil, and palm kernel oil. Unsaturated fats are further categorized as either monounsaturated or polyunsaturated fats. Monounsaturated fats are most commonly represented by omega-9 oils found in

Omega-3s are the most well-known and well-studied natural supplements for heart health.

olive oil, avocados, peanuts, and almonds. Polyunsaturated fats are made up of two groups: omega-6 and omega-3 fatty acids. Oils that contain omega-6 fatty acids include corn oil, safflower oil, sunflower oil, soybean oil, and cottonseed oil. Omega-3 fatty acids are further comprised of ALA (alpha linolenic acid), found in flaxseed, canola oil, and walnuts, and EPA (eicosapentaenoic acid) and DHA (docosahexaenoic acid), both found in fish. In the body, ALA is converted into EPA, and EPA is converted into DHA. Only a small percentage of ALA is converted to EPA,[1] however, and the final conversion to DHA is even less.[2] For this reason, it is important to obtain EPA and DHA from fish or fish oil supplements.

Omega-3/Omega-6 Balance

The diet humans evolved on (the hunter-gatherer diet) had an omega-6/omega-3 ratio of 1:1 to 2:1. That is, hunter-gatherers ate an almost equal portion each of omega-3 and omega-6 fatty acids in their diets. The omega-6/omega-3 ratio of the Standard American Diet (SAD) has been estimated to be from 10:1 to 25:1.[3,4] This means we are eating a lot more omega-6 and a lot less omega-3 than our ancestors, a pattern that promotes the development of many diseases, including heart disease.[5] Both omega-6 and omega-3 fatty acids are considered essential, meaning they must be obtained through the diet. The SAD diet is plentiful in omega-6 owing to the widespread use of vegetable oils in cooking, and is considered deficient in omega-3 because of the lack of omega-3-rich foods in the diet.

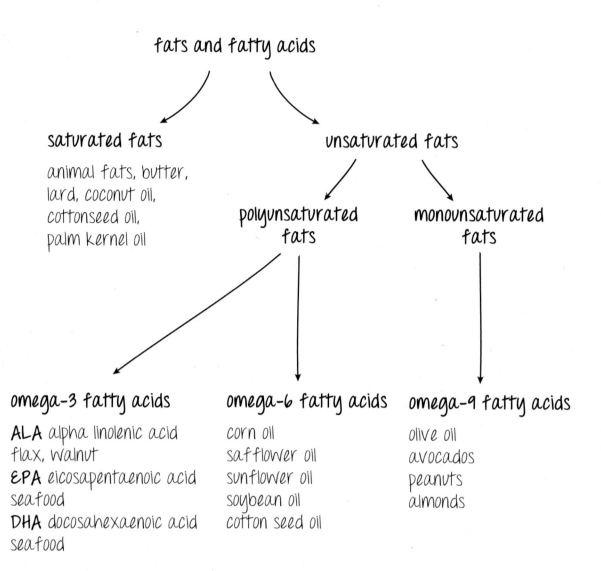

fats and fatty acids

saturated fats

animal fats, butter,
lard, coconut oil,
cottonseed oil,
palm kernel oil

unsaturated fats

polyunsaturated fats

monounsaturated fats

omega-3 fatty acids

ALA alpha linolenic acid
flax, walnut
EPA eicosapentaenoic acid
seafood
DHA docosahexaenoic acid
seafood

omega-6 fatty acids

corn oil
safflower oil
sunflower oil
soybean oil
cotton seed oil

omega-9 fatty acids

olive oil
avocados
peanuts
almonds

Omega-3s and Heart Health

The discovery that omega-3 fatty acids have heart-health benefits began with anecdotal reports of a low prevalence of heart disease among Greenland Eskimos (Inuits), inspiring expeditions to Greenland by the researchers Hans Olaf Bang and Jorn Dyerberg beginning in the late 1960s.[6] These researchers found very low heart attack rates, healthy blood lipid patterns, and reduced platelet reactivity in the Greenland Eskimos when compared to healthy people in Denmark. Hans Olaf Bang and Jorn Dyerberg later found high levels of the omega-3 fatty acid EPA (eicosapentaenoic acid) and low levels of the omega-6 fatty acid AA (arachidonic acid) in the Eskimos, suggesting that the high levels of EPA were responsible for the heart-protective effects in this population.[7]

Since those first investigations, interest in the heart-health benefits of omega-3s, specifically the marine-derived omega-3s EPA and DHA, increased. Today, thousands of studies can be found that exploring the effects of EPA and DHA on heart health. One review of 25 clinical trials evaluating levels of omega-3 and omega-6 in the body found that the people with the lowest levels of EPA and DHA are more likely to experience a cardiovascular event such as a heart attack.[8] Further studies have found that men who eat at least some fish weekly have lower death risk from heart disease than men who eat no fish. This is also true in women—women from the Nurses' Health Study who consumed more fish and omega-3 fatty acids were at lower risk for heart disease death.[9]

Four large randomized, controlled clinical trials have demonstrated the heart disease prevention effects of the omega-3s. In the first, the Diet and Reinfarction Trial (DART), involving 2,033 male heart attack survivors, the group consuming oily fish (providing the equivalent of an additional 500 to 800 milligrams of omega-3s daily) experienced a 29 percent reduction in the rate of death from any cause over two years.[10]

In the second trial, the Gruppo Italiano per lo Studio della Sopravvivenza nell'Infarto Miocardico (GISSI)-Prevenzione trial, involving 11,324 heart attack survivors, the group receiving 1 gram daily of omega-3s (with 850 to 882 milligrams EPA and DHA) experienced a 15 percent reduction in death, heart attack, or nonfatal stroke, along with a 20 percent reduction in death from any cause.[11] The rate of sudden death was lowered even further, by 45 percent. In the fourth clinical

trial, a follow-up study to this trial, the GISSI Heart Failure Study, patients with chronic heart failure receiving standard treatment and given 1 gram of omega-3 fish oil daily experienced a small reduction in death rate.[12]

In the fourth trial, the Japan Eicosapentaenoic Acid (EPA) Lipid Intervention Study (JELIS), involving 16,645 patients with high cholesterol given either a statin drug, or a statin drug plus 1800 milligrams EPA, those patients receiving the statin drug plus EPA experienced a 19 percent reduction in major coronary events.[13]

In addition to these trials evaluating the effects of omega-3s on heart disease prevention, numerous studies have identified an array of heart-health benefits of the omega-3s.

Heart Health Benefits of Omega-3s[14,15,16,17,18]

- Decrease free radicals
- Decrease inflammation
- Decrease C-reactive protein (CRP)
- Increase sensitivity to insulin
- Decrease triglycerides
- Increase HDL cholesterol
- Lower blood pressure
- Improve endothelial dysfunction
- Reduce inflammatory atherosclerotic plaque
- Improve heart rate variability
- Lower homocysteine levels

As a result of such robust science behind the heart-health benefits of omega-3s from fish, the American Heart Association makes the following recommendations:[19]

All adults should eat fish (particularly fatty fish like salmon and sardines) at least two times a week. This is the equivalent of about 500 to 800 milligrams of EPA+DHA per day.

Patients with coronary heart disease should consume about 1 gram (1000 milligrams) of EPA+DHA per day from fatty fish or fish oil capsules. Patients who need to lower triglycerides should take 2 to 4 grams of EPA+DHA per day from fish oil capsules.

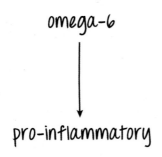

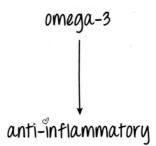

Omega-3s and Inflammation

Anti-inflammatory properties were attributed to omega-3s in the 1970s with the observation of an absence of many autoimmune and inflammatory conditions among the Greenland Eskimos when compared with groups in Denmark.[20] Over the decades since, a number of anti-inflammatory properties have been attributed to the omega-3s.[21]

The SAD high in omega-6 and low in omega-3, creates a pro-inflammatory state in the body that is said to contribute to the development of cardiovascular disease and other inflammatory disorders.[22] In general, omega-6 fatty acids promote inflammatory processes in the body, and omega-3s promote anti-inflammatory processes. Omega-6 fatty acids are converted into the omega-6 eicosanoid PGE2, a pro-inflammatory compound. The omega-3 fatty acid EPA directly competes with omega-6, displacing the pro-inflammatory omega-6 PGE2 with the anti-inflammatory omega-3 eicosanoids PGE1 and PGE3.[23]

Reversing this imbalance by increasing consumption of omega-3s, especially those found in fish oil, reduces the burden of inflammation in the body.[24] Chronic, low-grade inflammation is an underlying feature of most, if not all, chronic disease, especially heart disease. The anti-inflammatory properties of omega-3 EPA and DHA are one means by which these beneficial oils work to help prevent heart disease.

Omega-3 fatty acids become incorporated into the cell membrane (outer coating) of cells throughout the body. The cell membrane plays a particularly important role in cell-to-cell communication. Higher amounts of omega-3 incorporated into the cell membrane increase the flexibility (also known as fluidity) of the cell membrane, improving its ability to send and receive a variety of chemical messages—all vital to the functionality of the cell. The anti-inflammatory properties of omega-3s are particularly important at the cell's surface—again, acting as a method of communication. Think of omega-3s as the ambassadors of the cell—keeping the lines of peaceful, productive communication open between cells and tissues of the body.

One particularly interesting finding with regard to the anti-inflammatory properties of omega-3s has been the concept of inflammation resolution. As discussed in chapter 6, inflammation is a necessary process in the body. But its occurrence should be limited, resolving in due time. Compounds called resolvins, derived from the omega-3s EPA and DHA, do just that—they allow inflammation to run its natural course, and then resolve the inflammation at the appropriate time.[25] This is an important immune-balancing feature of the omega-3s, for the immune system regulates inflammation.

Fish Contaminants

Some types of fish contain high amounts of methylmercury (a particularly toxic form of mercury), polychlorinated biphenyls (PCBs), dioxins, and other contaminants.[26] These contaminants are present in fresh waters and oceans, and concentrate up the food chain: Medium-sized fish eat small fish, accumulating the toxins from the small fish (especially in fat cells); large fish eat medium fish, accumulating yet more toxins up the food chain. This is why older, larger, fatty fish tend to be the most toxic. In humans, these toxins, especially PCBs and methylmercury, accumulate in the body. Indeed, increased mercury levels in adults have been found to be directly associated with heart attack risk, while increased levels of omega-3 DHA in these adults are associated with decreased heart attack risk.[27]

Because of the health risk posed by the mercury content of fish, the Environmental Protection Agency recommends that children and pregnant or nursing women limit their intake of fish.[28] Pregnant or nursing women are advised to limit their consumption of fish to one 6-ounce portion per week, and young children are advised to eat 2 or less ounces of fish weekly. The FDA takes these recommendations further by suggesting that women and children eliminate shark, swordfish, king mackerel, and tilefish from their diets completely, and limit other fish to 12 ounces per week.[29] For men, and women after menopause, these agencies consider the benefit of fish consumption to outweigh the health risk of methylmercury intake. They may be underestimating the risk from mercury, however.

Purified Fish Oil

The best way to obtain the benefits of omega-3s from fish while avoiding the toxic contaminants they may contain is to consume a purified fish oil supplement. Not all fish oil supplements are without toxins, however, so be sure to read the label. Look for the International Fish Oil Standards (IFOS) icon on the bottle to be sure you are getting a purified, high-quality fish oil.

ALA or EPA/DHA?

Although not all studies agree, alpha-linolenic acid (ALA), sometimes called the parent omega-3 because of its conversion to EPA and DHA (although in limited amounts), has also been found to have beneficial heart-health effects. Some trials have found a beneficial effect from ALA,[30,31] and some have not.[32,33]

These benefits are often attributed to the conversion of ALA into EPA and DHA in the body. Both EPA and DHA are considered more biologically potent than ALA.[34] Due to the low conversion rate, however, in addition to the large volume of research supporting EPA+DHA, most experts recommend that omega-3 come from EPA+DHA for heart health protection.

EPA, DHA, or Both?

The beneficial effects of fish oil were originally attributed to EPA even though more DHA accumulates in all tissues of the body, and DHA has many similar effects as EPA.[35] Although one large trial (the JELIS trial) administered only EPA, most studies have used a mixture of both EPA and DHA, or have evaluated fish intake (which contains both EPA and DHA). Because of this, both EPA and DHA together are recommended for optimal heart health.[36,37,38]

TIP:

To obtain the same amount of omega-3s from a standard non-concentrated fish oil, you would have to take almost three times the amount of softgels as one concentrated fish oil softgel.

Omega-3 Index

The Omega-3 Index is a blood test that detects omega-3 levels. Although not a standard blood test—yet—the Omega-3 Index is an easy finger prick test that determines the levels of omega-3 EPA+DHA in red blood cell membranes. Detecting EPA and DHA in red blood cell membranes is thought to more accurately reflect heart tissue levels of EPA and DHA.

A high Omega-3 Index has been associated with lower risk of death from heart disease.[39] An index of ≥8 percent offered the greatest protection, and an index ≤4 percent was associated with the least protection. In one study, coronary heart disease patients taking omega-3 fish oil supplementation (3 grams EPA+DHA daily for 3 months followed by 1.5 grams daily for 18 months) experienced a slower rate of heart disease progression in association with a raise in their Omega-3 Index from 3.4 percent to 8.3 percent.[40]

The Omega-3 Index test can be purchased by mail order and done from home, or can be requested from a doctor. LabTestingTirect.com offers the Omega-3 Index test by OmegaQuant.

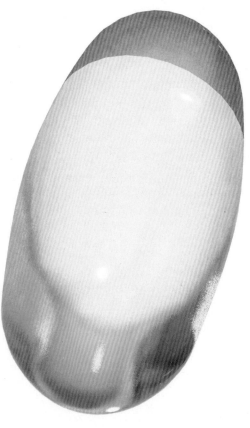

omega-3 Fish Oil

concentrated softgel

Omega-3s and Gut Health

Not only do omega-3s have a beneficial effect on the heart, but they also play a big role in gut health. The anti-inflammatory and immune effects of omega-3s play an important role in the gut,[41] especially since up to 80 percent of the immune system resides in the gut. Omega-3s have been found to decrease oxidative stress in people with ulcerative colitis[42] and maintain remission of Crohn's disease[43] (both inflammatory bowel diseases).

Gut inflammation is a hallmark feature of most digestive conditions. The anti-inflammatory effects of omega-3s help

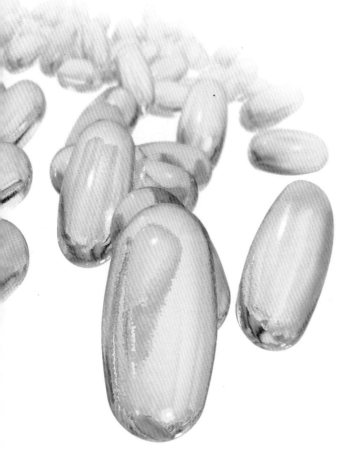

Non-concentrated softgel

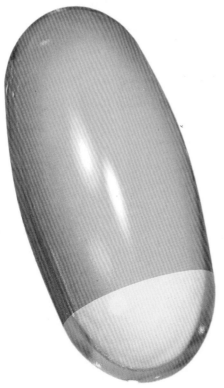

Total omega-3

Saturated and monounsaturated fat

to soothe this inflammation, which is an important part of keeping the inflammation under control and out of systemic circulation, where it can trigger yet more inflammation throughout the body.

Gut inflammation is a major contributor to the development of leaky gut, or intestinal permeability, a condition responsible for the spread of gut inflammation into systemic circulation. Omega-3 fish oils have been found to improve inflammation-induced leaky gut[44,45] and support the integrity of the intestinal lining.[46]

What to Look for in a Fish Oil Supplement

Fish oil supplements provide the heart-healthy omega-3s EPA and DHA in an easy delivery method for obtaining the amounts recommended by the American Heart Association and other omega-3 experts worldwide. Not all fish oil supplements are created equal, however. There are some important factors to consider when purchasing an omega-3 fish oil supplement.

Potency   Most people do not realize how many softgels are needed to obtain 1 gram of omega-3s daily. On this page is an illustration of two fish oil softgels.

- The one on the right is a standard fish oil softgel. It only contains one-third omega-3s. The rest of the oil in the softgel is made up of saturated fat and other fatty acids.

- The one on the left is a concentrated fish oil, which contains a much higher percentage of omega-3 oils—anywhere from 60 to 95 percent. Taking a concentrated fish oil supplement will require fewer softgels to get the recommended amounts of healthy omega-3s.

How do you know your fish oil is concentrated? Look at the total amount of omega-3s per softgel—don't be fooled if there are 2 softgels per serving. A standard fish oil softgel (which tends to be on the large side) should contain at least 800 to 1000 milligrams omega-3s.

Purity As mentioned previously in this chapter, fish contain varying amounts of contaminants. To obtain the recommended amounts of omega-3s by eating fish alone, the accumulation of these harmful contaminants is a risk, so much so that pregnant or nursing women and children are cautioned to limit the amount of fish consumed. To avoid potential accumulation of toxins, taking a purified fish oil supplement is the best option. Not all fish oil supplements are purified, however. Look for a product sourced from smaller, wild, cold-water fish that are naturally lower in environmental toxins such as mercury and dioxins.

Enteric-Coated, Dark-Colored Fish Gelatin Softgels Look for an enteric-coated fish oil supplement to ensure maximum absorption and minimum fish repeat (belching). Dark-colored softgels made of fish gelatin are the highest quality softgels, protecting the fish oil from light, which can induce oxidation.

Added Lipase Many people have difficulty completely digesting fats. For this reason, a fish oil with added plant lipase (a natural fat-splitting enzyme) helps the body digest and absorb the beneficial oils.

Recap: What to look for in an Omega-3 fish oil supplement:

- At least 1000 milligrams total omega-3 per one softgel as seen below in the Supplement Fact Panel.

- International purity standard (IFOS seal)

- Enteric-coated softgel

- Added lipase

Supplement Facts: Serving Size: 1 Fish Gel

	Amount per Fish Gel	%DV**
Vitamin D3 (cholecalciferol)	1,000 IU	250%
Total Omega 3•5•6•7•9•11	1,110 mg	
Omega-3	1,025 mg	***
EPA (Eicosapentaenoic Acid)	780 mg	***
DHA (Docosahexaenoic Acid)	120 mg	***
Omega-5	1 mg	***
Omega-6	56mg	***
Omega-7	1 mg	***
Omega-9	12mg	***
Omega-11	1 mg	***
Lipase (activity 50 FIP)	5 mg	***

** Percent Daily Values (DV) are based on a 2,000 calorie diet for 1 Fish Gel.
*** Daily Value not established

HOPE = PROBIOTICS

The third of the four main supplements to incorporate into your daily heart-health maintenance is a probiotic. Probiotics are the friendly gut bacteria that serve as your body's own Gut Protection System, or "GPS." The balance of bacteria in your gut determines the health of your digestive system and, in turn, the health of your entire body.

The entire digestive tract is colonized by bacteria. As a matter of fact, you have 10 times more bacteria cells in your gut than cells making up your entire body. There are more than 1,000 species of bacteria in your gut. Collectively, these gut bacteria weigh about four pounds—that's as heavy as a brick.

What's more, there are more than 100 times the genes present in your gut bacteria as there are in your own human genome.[1] This suggests that the genes of our gut bacteria may have more impact on our health than our own genes. In fact, the gut microbiota is considered by some experts to be an organ itself because its functions are essential for survival.[2]

There are three types of bacteria: beneficial, neutral, and harmful. The majority of bacteria in your gut should be beneficial, or friendly, bacteria—otherwise known as probiotics—and neutral, or commensal, bacteria. The friendly probiotic bacteria make up your GPS.

Your GPS works in three main ways:

1. It produces substances that neutralize harmful bacteria.

2. It protects the intestinal lining and improves the balance of good to bad bacteria in the gut by crowding out bad bacteria.

3. It influences the immune system so that it responds appropriately to invaders, such as harmful organisms, toxins, and even food.

The complex community of gut bacteria, also known as the gut flora or microbiota, is unique to each individual. Everyone has his or her own gut microbial fingerprint, which begins developing at birth. For example, major differences in gut bacteria are seen between infants born vaginally and those born by Cesarean. This is because the birth canal is also colonized by bacteria, inoculating the infant during birth. Infants born by C-section miss out on this colonization; they have lower numbers of the beneficial bifidobacteria and have been found to be more often colonized with the harmful bacteria *C. difficile* because they acquire bacteria from the hospital environment instead of from the mother.[3]

After birth, breastfed infants receive further advantage with improved gut bacteria as compared to exclusively formula-fed infants.[4] The establishment of gut flora is a progressive process, with increasing diversity important for overall health.[5] By age three, the major functions of the gut microbiota are established: nutrient absorption, immune stimulation, and protection against pathogens.

Throughout childhood, gut flora composition continues to develop until it reaches stability at the end of adolescence. In healthy adults, a diverse and stable gut flora (the GPS) will persist, contributing to digestive health as well as total body health. With age, however, modifications are seen in the gut microbial balance. Most notably, a decrease in beneficial bifidobacteria and an increase in potentially pathogenic bacteria occur.[6]

The GPS—What Can Go Wrong?

A careful balance of gut bacteria is what allows the Gut Protection System to function optimally. Although this balance is not yet completely understood, a balanced gut flora is generally accepted as a higher presence of good bacteria—such as lactobacilli and bifidobacteria (the Ls and the Bs)—along with a low presence of potentially pathogenic bacteria—such as clostridia or *E. coli*. A disruption in the balance of gut bacteria is known as dysbiosis, and can

lead to health consequences in the digestive tract and in other areas of the body seemingly unrelated to the gut. Many factors can lead to the development of dysbiosis. These include:

Age With age, levels of certain beneficial bacteria begin to decrease, especially bifidobacteria in the large intestine.

Poor Diet The Standard American Diet (SAD), high in sugar, processed foods, chemicals, and additives, and low in fresh vegetables and naturally fermented foods, can be disruptive to the balance of gut bacteria.

Environmental Toxins Toxins from the environment are known to destroy friendly bacteria in the gut. Since the middle of the twentieth century, more than 80,000 new chemicals have been introduced into the air, water, food supply, and into homes.

Antibiotics While antibiotics can be life-saving, overuse and misuse of antibiotics is a serious concern. The problem is that along with the bad bacteria, antibiotics also kill the good bacteria in the process. This

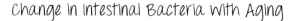

Change in Intestinal Bacteria with Aging

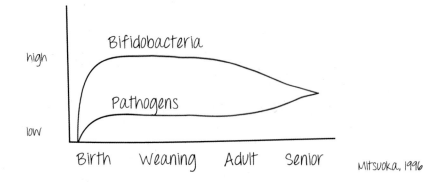

Mitsuoka, 1996

creates an imbalance that allows potential pathogens to quickly gain the upper hand, resulting in dysbiosis.

Acid-Suppressing Medications
These drugs reduce stomach acid, which is essential to the health of our GPS. Antacids work by changing the pH of the digestive tract, and in doing so create an environment favorable to the growth of harmful pathogenic bacteria.

Getting Your GPS Back on Track with Probiotics

Good bacteria have been part of the diet for thousands of years, largely in the form of fermented foods. One particular beneficial bacterium, *Bifidobacterium*, was isolated from breast-fed newborns in 1899, and was used to treat infants with diarrhea. The presence of *Bifidobacterium* in the digestive tract was, and still is, associated with good health.

In 1906 Elie Metchnikoff proposed the concept of the probiotic "Bulgarian bacillus," now known as *Lactobacillus bulgaricus*. Metchnikoff is known as the "Grandfather of Probiotics." His research and collaboration led to the modern interest in the ability of intestinal bacteria to benefit human health. He observed the long life spans of Bulgarians and attributed this to the fermented milk they drank. From this milk he isolated the *Lactobacillus* bacteria, and proposed that he could introduce this bacterium to the gut, producing a beneficial modification of the gut flora.

Metchnikoff's research pointed out the adverse effects of "autointoxication"—the production of toxic gut bacterial metabolites that reached the bloodstream, resulting in poor health. Though the idea of autointoxication was not completely accepted for some time, recent research is validating this concept, illustrating the harmful effects of an imbalanced GPS on other areas of the body seemingly unrelated to the gut.

Today probiotic research has greatly advanced. Probiotics are known to produce vitamins and enzymes and enhance nutrient absorption necessary to health; they are in close communication with the immune system—up to 80 percent of which resides in the gut—and help to balance immune response; and they help promote a healthy balance of bacteria in the gut, which protects against harmful bacteria and other pathogens.

Heart Health and Probiotics

The gut connection to heart disease is an indirect connection beginning with gut dysfunction and imbalance, all leading to inflammation. Gut inflammation increases intestinal permeability, creating a direct link from the gut to the cardiovascular system. Increased intestinal permeability, or leaky gut, allows toxins from bacteria and other sources and undigested food particles to enter circulation, triggering yet more inflammation that contributes to the chronic, low-grade inflammation characteristic of heart disease.

The hypothesis that bacterial infections are associated with atherosclerosis was first suggested more than 20 years ago.[7] Since then, bacterial toxins have been found to be an important factor in the development of atherosclerosis. Studies have found that patients with the highest levels of bacterial toxin, or endotoxin, are at increased risk of developing atherosclerosis.[8] The major source of bacterial toxins is the gut, highlighting an important link between gut health and heart health.[9]

Probiotics support digestive balance and digestive function in many ways. Probiotics help to protect the digestive lining against potential pathogens, help to reduce inflammation, and decrease leaky gut. A daily probiotic supplement is a foundational part of building gut health—and, thus, total-body health.

What to Look for in a Probiotic Supplement

Research on probiotics has increased dramatically over the past few decades. It is now recognized that individual probiotic strains have unique qualities. One strain may have specific immune-boosting properties, while another strain may have stronger ability to resist pathogens in the gut. For these reasons, and because of the wide diversity of bacteria that exists in the gut, a multistrain probiotic formula more resembles that diversity and may be more beneficial than a single-strain formula.[10]

Probiotics can be obtained through the diet by eating yogurt, kefir, and certain other fermented foods, but these products typically do not contain high amounts of probiotics. In fact, yogurt must be pasteurized, which involves high heat, so if live probiotic cultures are not re-added after pasteurization, the yogurt will not contain any beneficial bacteria.

Recently many new probiotic products have appeared on store shelves, in supplements, foods, beverages, and even in gum. With all the variety, it can be difficult to determine which products are of high quality. When shopping for an effective probiotic supplement, consumers should read labels carefully to ensure the following:

High Culture Count This refers to the total amount of bacteria per capsule. Look for a probiotic supplement with at least 15 billion (up to 100 billion) in a single capsule.

Number of Strains Your supplement should include at least 10 different strains of bacteria scientifically studied to benefit optimal health. Look for high amounts of *Bifidobacterium* to support the large intestine (colon) and *Lactobacillus* to support the small intestine and urogenital tract.

Delayed-Release Capsules Delayed-release capsules protect the probiotics from harsh stomach acid and deliver them directly to the intestines, where they are needed and utilized by the body.

Potency and Stability Guarantee The potency, or amount of active cultures, should be guaranteed through the product expiration date under recommended storage conditions.

HOPE = ENZYMES

Enzymes play an essential role in every function in the human body. In the digestive system, enzymes help break down foods by breaking apart the bonds that hold nutrients together. As a result, the body is able to use those nutrients for energy.

Although enzymes are typically present in raw, whole foods to assist with digestion, the majority of people do not obtain enough enzymes through diet alone. Today's diet of cooked and heavily processed foods depletes the natural enzymes from food and leads to poor digestion, because the body may not be able to completely break down food and obtain its valuable nutrients.

Several locations in the digestive system secrete enzymes: the mouth, stomach, pancreas, and cells of the small intestine. Proteins, fats, and carbohydrates are the three types of foods that the body breaks down and absorbs. The enzymes protease, lipase, and amylase, respectively, are made for this purpose. A healthy diet, exercise, and proper detoxification will help promote healthy enzyme production in the body. Additionally, there are several enzymes that the human body lacks, such as cellulase (the enzyme that breaks down cellulose) and phytase (the enzyme that helps break down phytates found in bran and seeds, such as nuts and beans).

Without the enzymes needed for proper digestion, the body may not completely break down foods to absorb nutrients. As a result, undigested food in the digestive tract can ferment, causing gas, bloating, and other digestive difficulties.

What to Look for in a Digestive Enzyme Supplement

When shopping for an effective digestive enzyme supplement, consumers should read labels carefully to ensure the following:

- High potency plant-based enzyme formula

- At least 100,000 HUT units of protease per serving for effective protein digestion

- Varied enzyme blend for full-spectrum digestion; look for an array of enzymes in addition to protease, amylase, and lipase

Low Stomach Acid

If you suspect you have low stomach acid, look for a formula that contains HCl. A quick test for stomach acid level involves taking a digestive enzyme capsule with HCl at the beginning of a meal. If a burning sensation is not felt, stomach acid levels are too low. The next day, take two of the HCl enzyme capsules at the beginning of a meal, increasing by one capsule each day until a burning sensation is felt. Once a burning sensation is experienced, you will know your dosage is one fewer capsule than that which caused the burning.

TIP:

Optimal heart health can be achieved with proper diet and nutritional supplementation that addresses underlying imbalances discovered by functional testing.

Support Supplements

In addition to the three main supplements to be implemented into your daily heart-health maintenance, there are a number of other heart-healthy supplements that may be beneficial. These include:

L-Glutamine The amino acid L-glutamine is the main fuel for the cells lining the small intestine. Glutamine is the most abundant amino acid in the bloodstream, but it can be depleted under a number of conditions, such as infection, injury, trauma, prolonged stress, starvation, or the use of steroid medications.[1] The intestinal tract is the primary user of L-glutamine. It increases the height of the intestinal villi, the fingerlike projections that make up the intestinal barrier and help maintain the integrity of the gut epithelial lining. L-glutamine also increases the secretion of the important anti-inflammatory mucosal antibody known as secretory IgA (sIgA).[2] In these two ways L-glutamine is important for the protection of the intestinal barrier, helping decrease leaky gut. Because leaky gut contributes to the silent inflammation characteristic of heart disease, maintaining the integrity of the intestinal lining with L-glutamine is important. Dosage: 5 to 10 grams daily.

Coenzyme Q_{10} (CoQ_{10}) CoQ_{10} is a powerful antioxidant found in almost every cell in the body. CoQ10 is naturally made in the body, but it decreases rapidly after age 40. CoQ_{10} has been found to help decrease oxidative stress in people with atherosclerosis,[3] improve blood pressure and blood sugar in people with diabetes,[4] and is recommended for people taking statin drugs because these drugs reduce the natural amount of CoQ10 in the body. Dosage: 100 milligrams daily.

Vitamin D Vitamin D deficiency is common

in the United States and worldwide.[5] Vitamin D is known as the sunshine vitamin because it is formed in the body by the sun's ultraviolet (UVB) rays on the skin. Vitamin D deficiency is associated with increased risk of heart disease, especially in people with high blood pressure.[6] Studies have found vitamin D supplementation to help reduce blood pressure and inflammation. Many experts recommend achieving vitamin D blood levels of at least 50 ng/mL. Dosage: 1000 to 5000 IU daily (an optimal blood level of vitamin D is 50 to 70 ng/mL).

Niacin (Vitamin B3) Niacin is a B vitamin effective at both lowering LDL cholesterol and raising HDL cholesterol. In fact, niacin is considered to be more effective than drugs at raising HDL cholesterol.[7] Some forms of niacin cause a skin-flushing reaction at high doses, so it is recommended that dosage be increased gradually. Dosage: 50 to 100 milligrams daily.

Vitamin C Because vitamin C status is connected to the very initiation of heart disease—endothelial dysfunction (see Dr. Levy's interview on page 184 for more information)—increasing intake of vitamin C is essential. Vitamin C is a powerful antioxidant. Low levels of vitamin C have been associated with atherosclerosis, high blood pressure, and stroke.[8] Dosage: 3000 to 9000 milligrams ascorbic acid daily in three divided doses (increase dosage gradually to determine bowel tolerance—if stool becomes loose, lower dosage).

Dark Chocolate Although not considered a supplement, dark chocolate has been found to have heart-protective effects by reducing inflammation[9] and blood pressure,[10] even when eaten in small amounts. Dark chocolate is high in flavonoid antioxidants, which help protect against oxidative stress, a main characteristic of atherosclerosis. Dosage: one square of dark chocolate daily (choose a dark chocolate that is low in sugar).

Functional Testing

Throughout this book a number of tests that can help you determine your heart disease risk have been mentioned. The following is a breakdown of those tests—all in one place—to give you an idea of what factors you can take a closer look at to assess your risk.

Some of these tests are available together, as a panel of tests, and others are available on their own. A good option is to work with an integrative doctor who can order the tests and help you to interpret the results. Alternately, most or all of these tests are available to order online through Lab Testing Direct (www.labtestingdirect.com), blood tests can be done through your local LabCorp, and some tests, like finger-prick tests or stool tests, can be done from your home and mailed in for analysis.

LIPID PROFILES

To assess your cholesterol and triglyceride status, most conventional doctors only order the standard lipid profile, which includes total cholesterol, triglycerides, HDL cholesterol, and LDL cholesterol. More comprehensive lipid panels, like the NMR LipoProfile, which includes the standard lipid profile in addition to lipoprotein particle number and particle size, will give a better picture of blood lipid status.

Total cholesterol The total amount of LDL cholesterol, HDL cholesterol, and other lipid components in the blood.

Triglycerides The form in which most fat exists in the body.

HDL cholesterol The total amount of cholesterol that is carried by the high-density lipoprotein carriers.

LDL cholesterol The amount of LDL is calculated based on the actual measures of total cholesterol, HDL cholesterol, and triglycerides. It represents an approximation of LDL cholesterol—not a measured value.

LDL/HDL ratio A high LDL/HDL ratio plus high triglycerides is associated with the highest heart disease risk. This ratio is calculated based on LDL and HDL levels, and is usually included in lipid panels.

LDL particle number The number of LDL particles is directly measured. LDL particle number can be high even if LDL cholesterol levels are low. This is possible because if the LDL particles have less cholesterol in each particle, the amount of actual cholesterol will be lower. But remember that it's not the cholesterol that is the problem—it's the carrier. A higher number of LDL particles means higher atherogenicity—likelihood of developing atherosclerosis.

LDL size (lipoprotein subfractions) The size of the LDL particle also determines its atherogenicity. Small, dense LDL particles are more likely to damage artery walls and get under the lining of the arteries. Large, buoyant LDL particles are more likely to bounce off of artery walls without damaging them. Size matters—the larger the better in the case of LDL particles. Small LDL particles carry less cholesterol, so LDL cholesterol numbers may be low yet still be in a form that damages the arteries.

Oxidized LDL Oxidated LDL particles are directly involved in the initiation and progression of atherosclerosis. Even if LDL cholesterol levels are normal, if the LDL is oxidized, it represents a substantial heart disease risk.

HDL particle number Not only does the number of LDL particles matter, so does the number of HDL particles. HDL particle number more closely correlates with HDL cholesterol levels than LDL particle number does with LDL levels, but HDL particle number is usually measured along with LDL particle number.

BLOOD GLUCOSE CONTROL TESTING

Fasting blood sugar Fasting blood glucose level testing is the most common test for first detecting high blood sugar levels. It detects blood glucose levels after at least eight hours of fasting.

Fasting insulin Insulin testing is often overlooked by conventional doctors, but because insulin is what regulates blood glucose, and insulin resistance plays a major role in the development of cardio-metabolic diseases, monitoring insulin levels along with blood glucose levels will give a better picture of blood glucose control.

Oral glucose tolerance test First, fasting blood sugar levels are taken, as with the fasting blood sugar test. Then the person receives a drink with 75 grams of glucose, after which blood is taken up to three more times—after 30 minutes, 1 hour, and/or 2 hours. This is the best way to determine how blood sugar levels change in response to food. The test gives the most accurate picture of blood glucose control.

Oral glucose and insulin tolerance test This test is essentially the oral glucose tolerance test with the addition of insulin testing. Both glucose and insulin are tested at fasting, and at 30 minutes, 1 hour, and/or 2 hours after eating. If insulin resistance is present, it can be determined by this test.[1] Because this test is not a standard profile but rather the combination of a few tests, you most likely will have to work with your doctor to obtain the test and interpret the results.

HbA1c (hemoglobin A1c test) Average blood sugar levels over the past two to three months are estimated by this blood test. This test gives a good idea of how well blood sugar is being controlled long term.

Blood glucose meter This finger-prick test is widely available and an easy method to regularly monitor blood glucose at home. Fasting, pre-meal, and post-meal blood sugar levels can be taken to determine blood sugar response to certain foods. Other factors that affect blood glucose levels, like exercise or illness, can also be tracked.

INFLAMMATION STATUS TESTING

hs-CRP (high-sensitivity C-reactive protein) C-reactive protein is a marker for systemic inflammation, and is an independent risk factor for heart disease. There are two CRP tests available, but the high-sensitivity test is the one to use, because, like the name suggests, it more accurately detects CRP levels than the standard CRP test.

Omega-3 Index This finger-prick test is an easy way to determine the status of 26 fatty acids, including omega-3, omega-6, saturated fatty acids, and trans fats, as well as omega ratios. The measure of omega-3 status is particularly associated with risk for heart disease death.

25(OH) vitamin D This test is the most accurate way to measure levels of vitamin D in the body. It is estimated that up to 90 percent of people[2] do not have sufficient vitamin D levels of around 50 ng/mL.[3] Low levels of vitamin D are associated with many aspects of heart disease.

Homocysteine Elevated homocysteine in the blood damages the artery wall, which leads to atherosclerosis.[4] Homocysteine levels can be reduced by taking vitamins B6, B12, and folic acid. (Active folate should be taken if you have the MTHFR polymorphism. See below.)

MTHFR polymorphism Up to 20 percent of people have the MTHFR mutation, which puts them at risk for having high levels of homocysteine.[5] Genetic testing to detect this mutation can be helpful to determine if supplementation is necessary.

GUT FUNCTION TESTING

Optimal gut function is at the heart of total-body health. Assessing gut function with the following tests can go a long way to help determine the underlying contributors to heart disease.

Lactulose-mannitol intestinal permeability test A drink of two sugars—lactulose (a disaccharide that normally is not absorbed unless the mucosal barrier is damaged) and mannitol (a monosaccharide that is readily absorbed though the gut lining)—is ingested, after which urinary levels of the sugars are measured to determine the extent of intestinal permeability, or leaky gut.

Gluten and food sensitivity test Underlying food sensitivities, especially to gluten and/or dairy, are much more common than most people realize. To determine if you have a food sensitivity, a stool test from EnteroLab (www.enterolab.com) is available. The test can be done from your home, with specimens sent via mail. If a food sensitivity is detected, eliminating that food from the diet often leads to improvement in an array of health problems.

Comprehensive stool analysis (CSA) with parasitology To detect imbalances in gut flora (dysbiosis), a comprehensive stool analysis is recommended. Gut imbalance increases inflammation and leaky gut, and can lead to food sensitivities. Healthy gut balance is the foundation upon which total body health is built. This test provides a great way to "look" at what is going on in your gut. It is available using either just one sample or three samples taken over the course of a few days. The three-sample option is recommended because of its greater ability to detect parasites that may not be present in a single sample.

Heidelberg pH Diagnostic Test To measure pH levels in the digestive tract, the Heidelberg pH Diagnostic System is recommended. The Heidelberg pH capsule is a technically advanced micro-electronic diagnostic tool that can accurately diagnose a patient who may have hypochlorhydria (low stomach acidity), hyperchlorhydria (high stomach acidity), achlorhydria (no stomach acidity), pyloric insufficiency, or heavy mucus. Unlike other pH tests, which require the use of an invasive nasal-gastric tube, or a standard endoscopic procedure, the Heidelberg pH Diagnostic Test is accurate and non-invasive, and very user- and patient-friendly. To find a doctor who can perform this test, visit www.phcapsule.com.

TIP:

If your physician is not aware of the tests described here, you may want to consider finding an integrative doctor who will be more educated in functional testing. One place to find a practitioner is through the Institute for Functional Medicine (check their website for a list of local practitioners).

section three

MEAL
PLANNER
& RECIPES

Love Your Heart: One-Week Meal Planner and Recipes

To attain good health, one of the most important factors to address is diet. Unfortunately, the word diet is often considered a four-letter word. But it doesn't have to be. Instead of taking the perspective that diet is a burden, or a chore that we relentingly give in to because we "should," why not begin by changing your mind right here and now? Decide that today is the day that you are going to take back control of your health by creating a new way of eating, of living, and even of being.

I don't call the Love Your Heart Eating Plan a diet because it's not just a six-week, or even six-month plan. It's a way of eating, period. So instead of saying, "I'm on a diet," choose to say, "I am changing the way I eat," or simply, "This is how I eat." By changing the way you feel about your eating habits, you will solidify those habits as a way of life. The choice is yours. It always has been. With the information you now hold, make the choice of health.

The following recipes, along with a one-week meal planner to help you organize your meals and snacks, offer a variety of foods low in teaspoons of sugar. The recipes are simple and delicious. My hope is that you will find these foods enticing and learn to find other similar foods that help make eating more enjoyable than ever. You will find that eating healthy is more about finding the right foods than avoiding the wrong ones. As it turns out, it's easy.

To help you plan your week, the one-week meal plan includes a variety of meals and snacks. Each day, your goal will be to eat between 6 to 8 teaspoons of sugar and 12 portions of protein. If you are on the Maintenance Phase, simply add more foods that increase your teaspoons of sugar and portions of protein to amounts that support your heart health, as determined by your weight or other risk factors. Use this meal plan as a guide to help you build your own meal plans according to your taste.

For each recipe, teaspoons of sugar (carbohydrates minus fiber, divided by five) have been calculated so that you can easily track your daily sugar intake. The one-week meal planner also includes teaspoon of sugar calculations along with protein portions. Feel free to mix and match the recipes and snacks in the one-week meal planner to find the perfect combinations for you.

From my kitchen to yours,

Brenda Watson

Love Your Heart: One-Week Meal Planner

18 new and delicious meals (shown in red) from my recipes on the following pages

	Breakfast	Snack	Lunch
Sunday	Mini Egg Frittatas	2 celery stalks with peanut butter	Eggplant Roulades with Basil Ricotta
Teaspoons Sugar	0.5	1	4.2
Portions Protein	2	1	4
Monday	2 eggs, any style, 2 slices turkey bacon, plus a handful of blueberries	Greek yogurt, plain, low-fat	Garlic-n-Lemon Shrimp
Teaspoons Sugar	2.4	1.2	1.4
Portions Protein	4	2	2
Tuesday	Greek yogurt (4 to 6 ounces), plain, low-fat, plus a handful of blackberries	Handful of nuts	Chicken Cobb Salad with Spicy Lime Drizzle
Teaspoons Sugar	1.6	0.4	2
Portions Protein	2	1	5
Wednesday	Turkey Sausage Patties	Veggies and guacamole (use 1 avocado, and add veggies such as celery, bell pepper, baby carrots)	Seafood Gumbo
Teaspoons Sugar	0.1	3.4	1.8
Portions Protein	6	1	3
Thursday	Veggie scramble (2 eggs plus low-starch veggies such as spinach, artichoke, bell pepper)	Turkey slices, 2 ounces	Sautéed Grouper over Southern Greens
Teaspoons Sugar	1.4	0.4	1.6
Portions Protein	3	2	4
Friday	Non-Oat Nutmeal	Baby carrots and hummus, 1/2 cup of each	Seared Sesame Tuna over Asian Slaw
Teaspoons Sugar	0.7	2	1
Portions Protein	3	1	2
Saturday	Veggie-Egg Patties	Shelled edamame, 1/2 cup	Athenian Meatballs
Teaspoons Sugar	0.6	0.8	0.6
Portions Protein	1	1.5	3
	Breakfast	Snack	Lunch

Snack	Dinner	DAILY TOTALS	
1/2 Avocado 1/4 cup salsa	Chicken Milanese with Arugula Salad		**Sunday**
1.6 0.5	1.2 5	8.5 12.5	Teaspoons Sugar Portions Protein
Turkey jerky, 3 pieces	Persian Beef Kebabs, Warm Spinach Salad with Miso Mushrooms		**Monday**
0.4 1	1.6 3	7 12	Teaspoons Sugar Portions Protein
Cottage cheese, 4 ounces	Unstuffed Cabbage		**Tuesday**
0.6 2	3.4 2	8 12	Teaspoons Sugar Portions Protein
1/2 Avocado 1/4 cup salsa	Beef and Garden Vegetable Bolognese		**Wednesday**
1.6 0.5	2.2 2	9.1 12.5	Teaspoons Sugar Portions Protein
Baby carrots and hummus, 1/2 cup of each	Lemongrass Chicken over Chard Nests		**Thursday**
2 1	1.6 3	7 13	Teaspoons Sugar Portions Protein
Veggies and guacamole (use 1 avocado, and add veggies such as celery, bell pepper, baby carrots)	Roast Sicilian Pork Loin with Citrus Fennel		**Friday**
3.4 1	0.6 5	7.7 12	Teaspoons Sugar Portions Protein
Turkey jerky, 3 pieces	Ligurian Stuffed Chicken		**Saturday**
0.4 1	3.6 6	6 12.5	Teaspoons Sugar Portions Protein
Snack	Dinner	DAILY TOTALS	

When you want a sweet treat for an occasional dessert, add 2 tablespoons of whipping cream and a few berries (blackberries, blueberries, or strawberries) to a container of low-fat Greek yogurt. Delish.

WARM SHROOMS-N-SPINACH

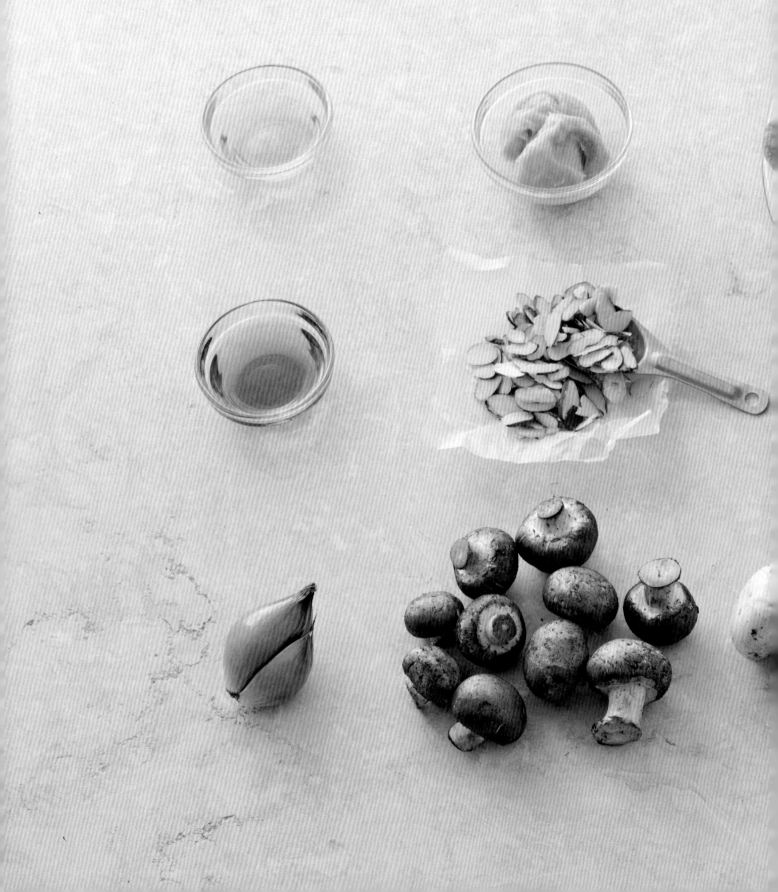

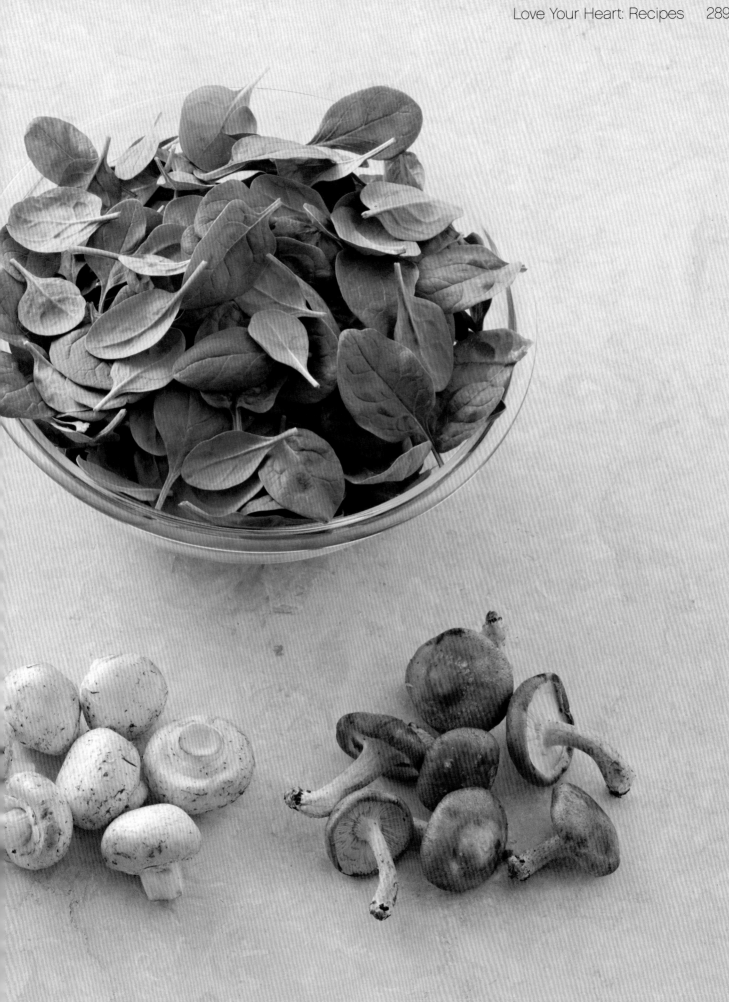

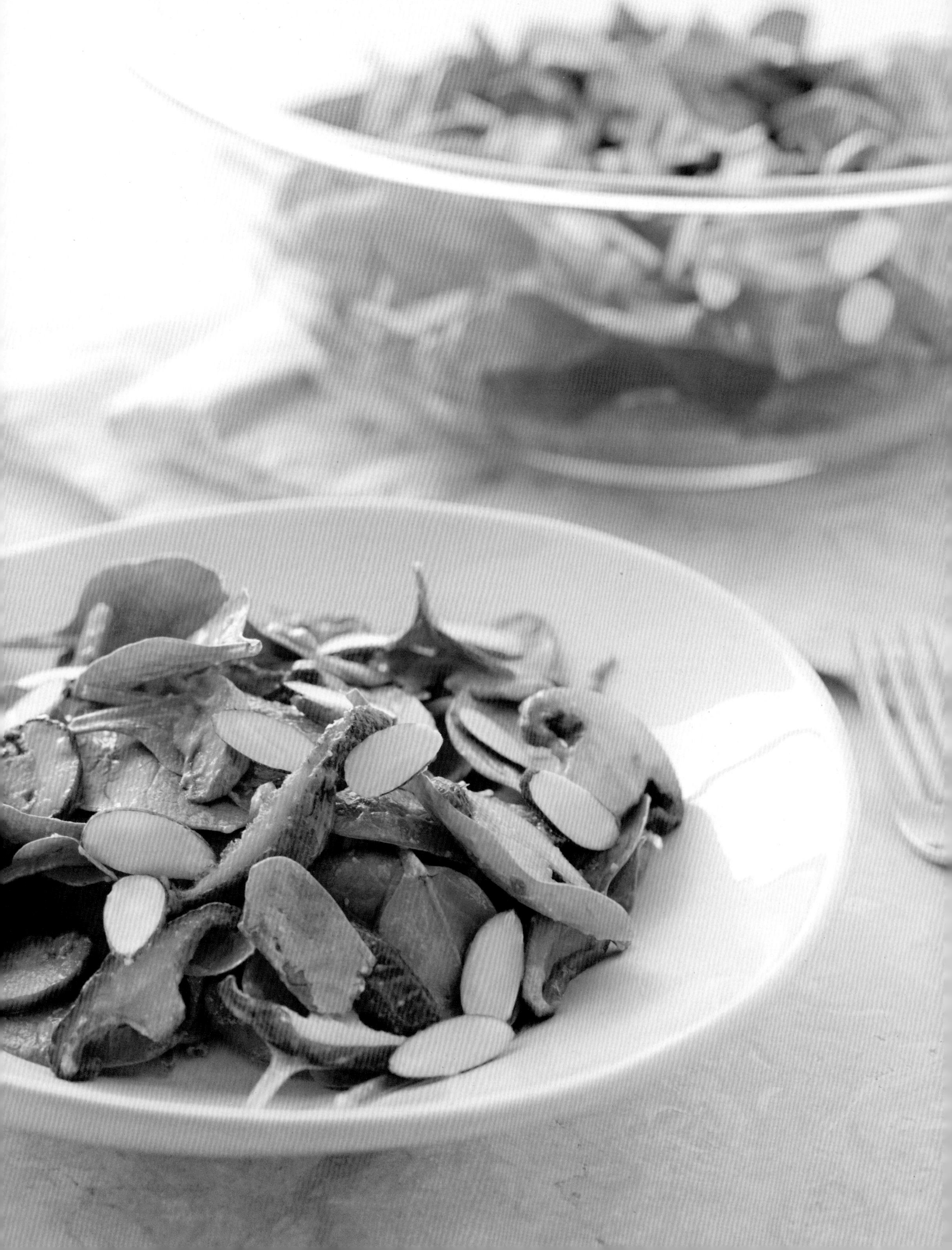

WARM SHROOMS-N-SPINACH

SUGAR 2.2 tsp

TIME 15 minutes

SERVES four

INGREDIENTS

2 tablespoons white miso

2 tablespoons rice vinegar
(sugar-free)

1 tablespoon extra virgin olive oil

1 cup sliced button mushrooms

1 cup sliced shiitake mushroom caps

1 cup sliced cremini (baby bella)
mushrooms

1 large shallot, minced (optional)

One 14-ounce bag spinach leaves or
baby spinach

2 tablespoons sliced almonds

1 In a small bowl, whisk the miso with the vinegar.

2 Heat the olive oil in a large skillet over medium-high heat. Add the mushrooms and shallot and sauté for 3 minutes, or until mushrooms begin to brown.

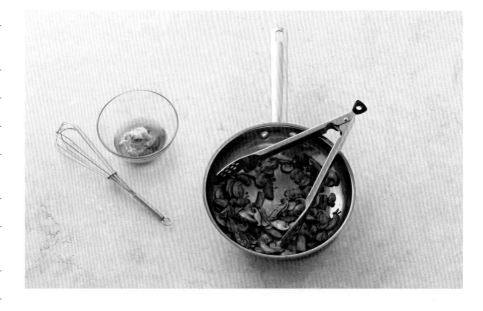

3 Pour the miso mixture over the mushrooms and cook for an additional minute.

4 Place the spinach in a serving bowl. Pour the mushroom mixture over the spinach, add the almonds, and toss. Serve warm.

EGGPLANT ROULADES

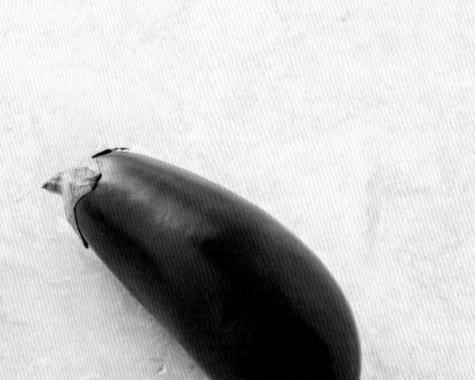
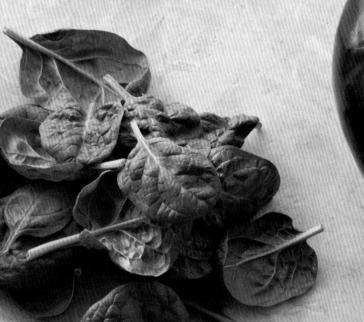
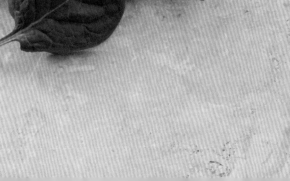

EGGPLANT ROULADES

SUGAR 𝄞𝄞𝄞𝄞𝄞 4.2 tsp

TIME 60 minutes

SERVES six

INGREDIENTS

2 medium eggplants

2 teaspoons extra virgin olive oil

One 15-ounce container part-skim ricotta

½ cup grated Parmesan cheese

½ cup part-skim shredded mozzarella cheese

1 large egg, lightly beaten

1 cup fresh spinach leaves

¼ cup fresh basil

2 cups tomato puree (or 3 medium tomatoes, pulsed in a food processor)

1 Preheat the oven to 375°F. Slice the eggplant lengthwise about ¼ inch thick. Put on a baking pan and coat lightly on both sides with olive oil. Place in the oven and bake for 5 to 6 minutes, until lightly softened and flexible. Remove from the oven and cool to room temperature.

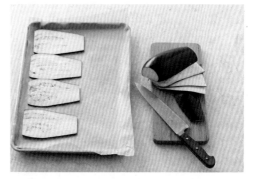

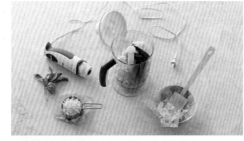

2 Combine the ricotta, ¼ cup of the Parmesan, ¼ cup of the mozzarella, the egg, spinach, and basil in a food processor with a standard S blade, or mix by hand with a whisk in a large mixing bowl (chop spinach first).

3 Pour half of the tomato puree in the bottom of a 9 x 12-inch baking dish. Place a large spoonful of the cheese mixture on the end of each slice of eggplant and roll it up. Place the rolled eggplant in the pan, seam side down, then cover with the remaining tomatoes and top with the remaining Parmesan and mozzarella cheeses.

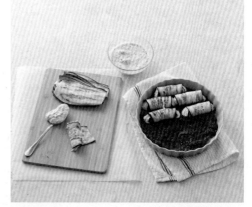

4 Cover with foil and bake for 25 to 30 minutes, until the eggplant rolls are heated through. Remove the foil and bake for 5 to 10 minutes, until the cheese begins to brown. Remove from the oven and let stand for 5 to 10 minutes before serving.

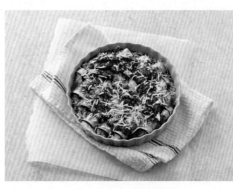

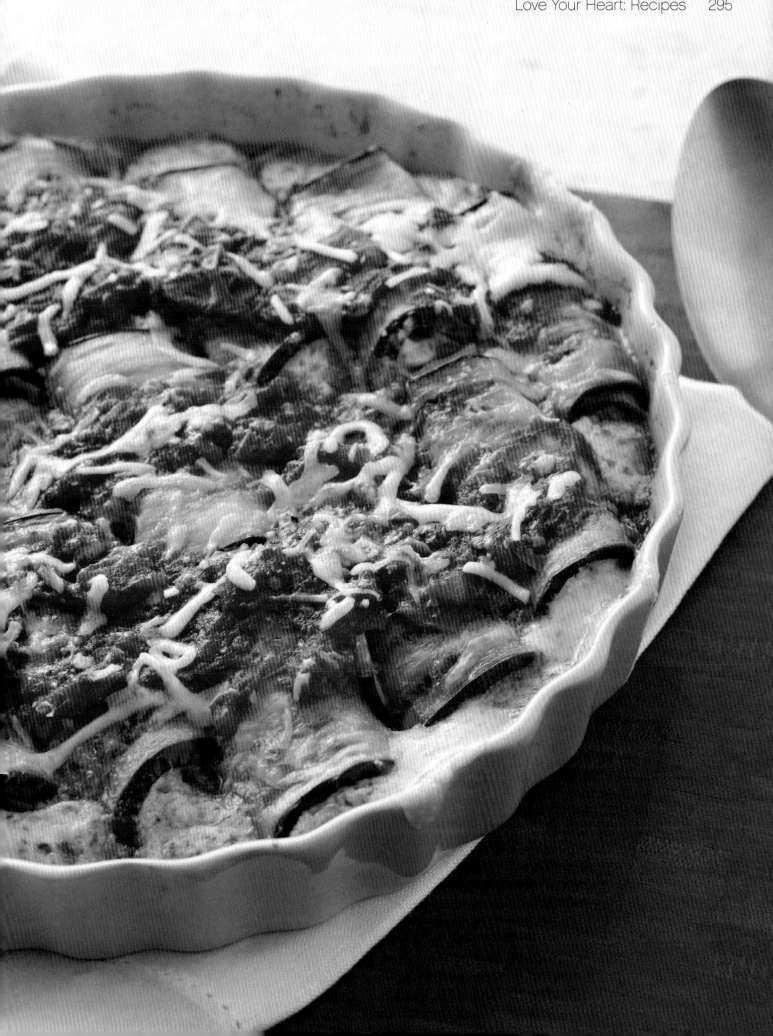

CHICKEN LIME COBB

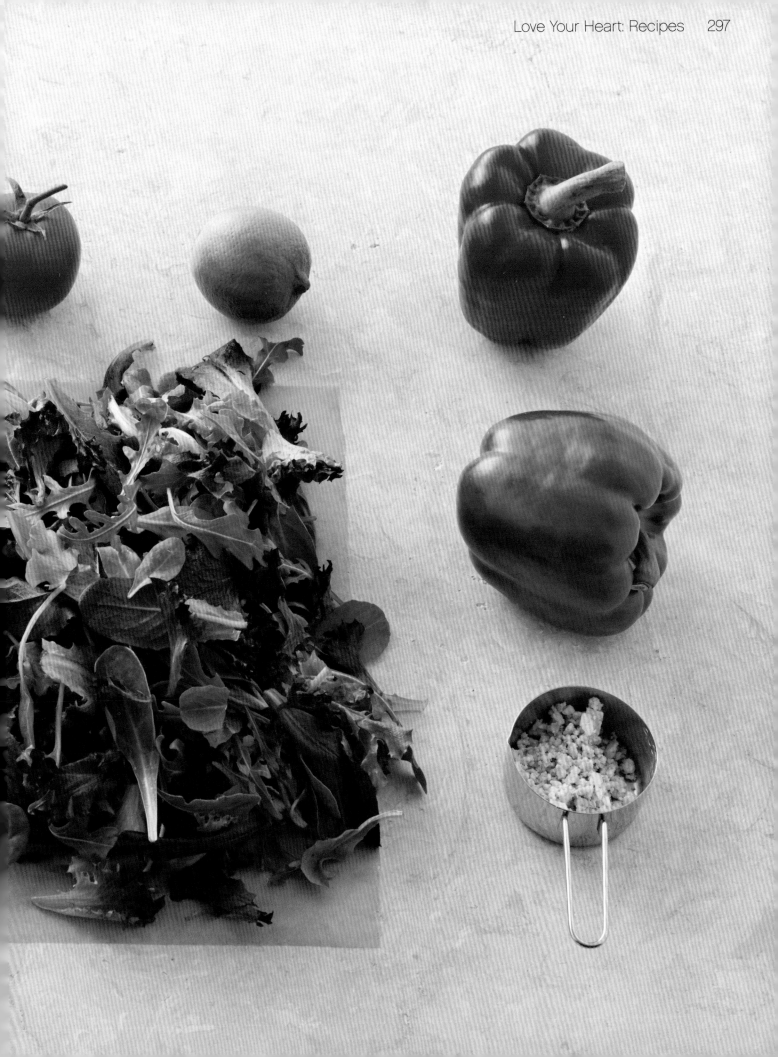

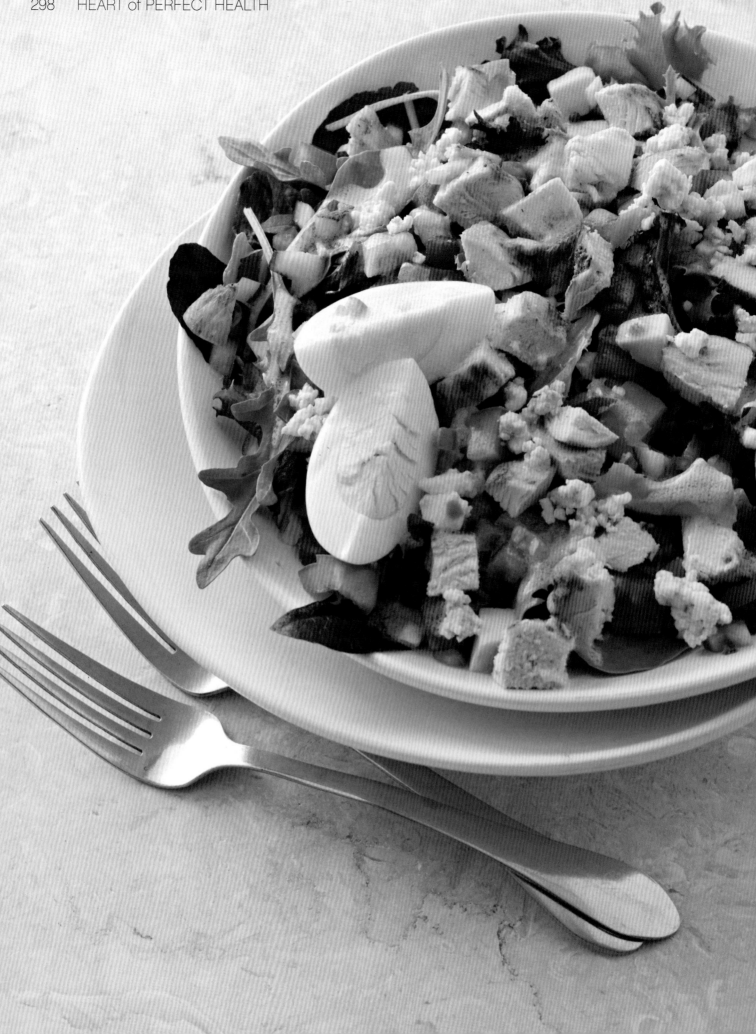

CHICKEN LIME COBB

SUGAR 2 tsp

TIME 15 minutes

SERVES two

INGREDIENTS

Dressing

2 teaspoons extra virgin olive oil

¼ cup low-fat buttermilk

2 teaspoons minced jarred pickled jalapeño pepper

Juice of 1 lime

2 teaspoons Dijon-style mustard

Salad

8 ounces cooked chicken breast, chopped

½ red bell pepper, chopped

½ green bell pepper, chopped

¼ red onion, chopped

1 medium tomato, chopped

½ avocado, chopped

¼ cup reduced-fat blue cheese crumbles

1 hard-boiled egg, chopped

2 cups mixed salad greens

1 In a small bowl, whisk together dressing ingredients.

2 In a large bowl, combine all the salad ingredients. Drizzle on the dressing and serve.

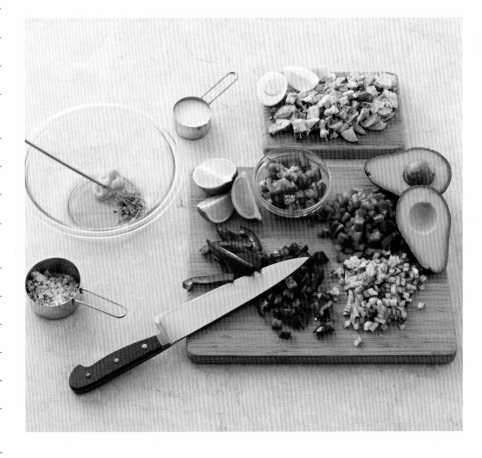

INDIAN SPICED GARBANZOS

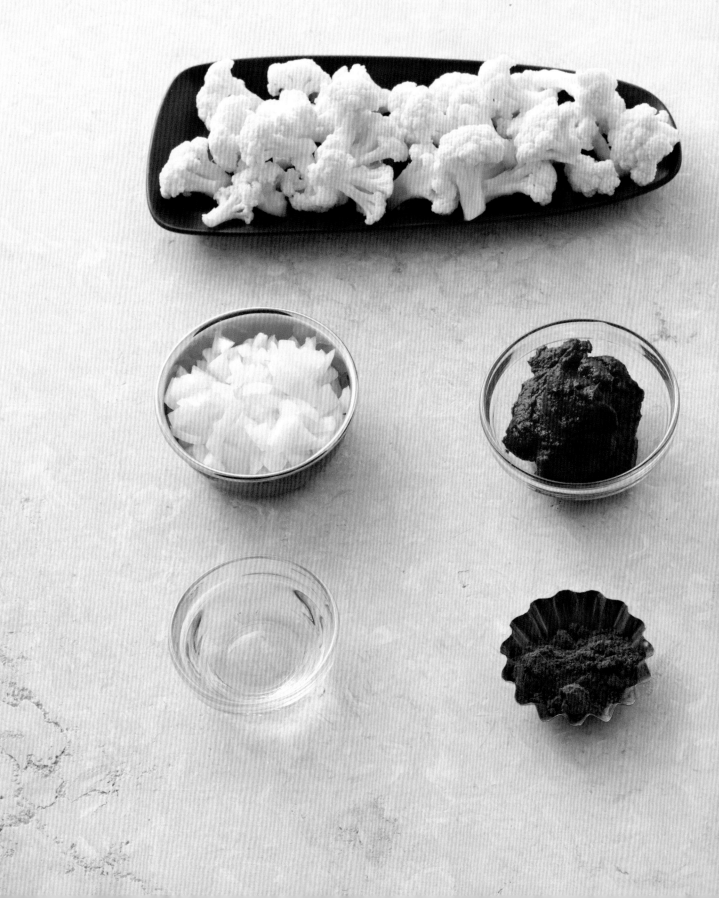

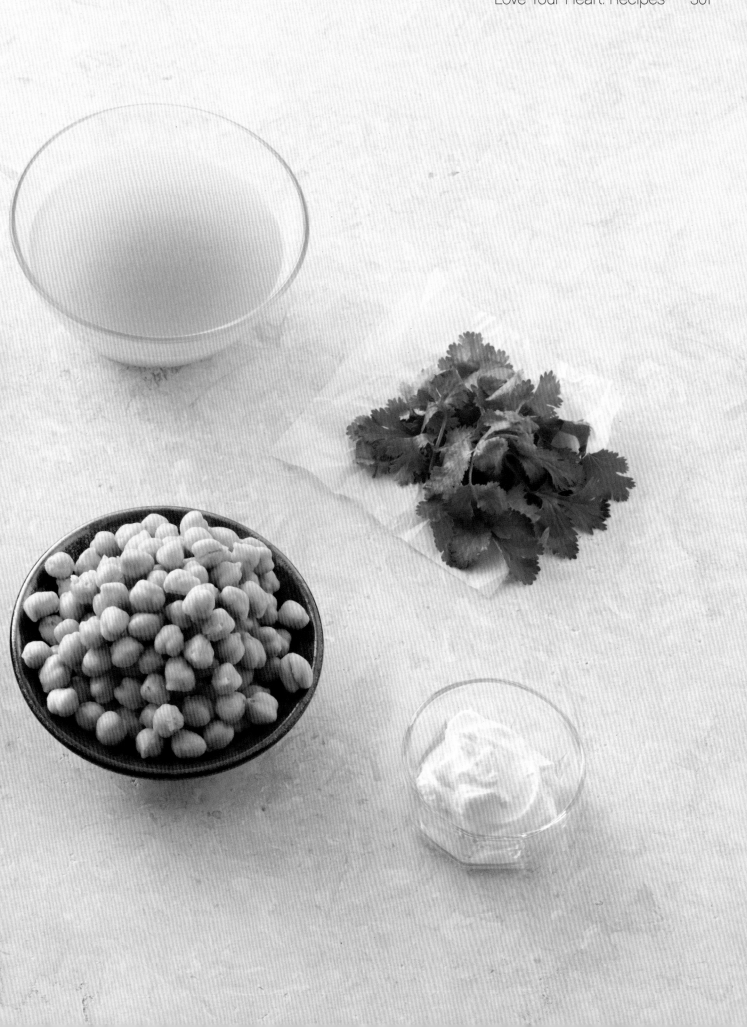

INDIAN ƒPICED GARBANZOƒ

SUGAR 3.5 tsp

TIME 25 minutes

SERVES four

INGREDIENTS

2 teaspoons extra virgin olive oil or canola oil

½ medium onion, diced

1 tablespoon garam masala (or substitute a high-quality curry powder)

2 tablespoons tomato paste

One 15-ounce can chickpeas, drained and rinsed

1 cup cauliflower florets

14 ounces low-sodium vegetable stock

¼ cup fresh cilantro leaves, chopped

¼ cup plain fat-free Greek yogurt

1 Heat the oil in a large saucepan over medium-high heat. Add the onion, and garam masala and sauté for 2 to 3 minutes, until the onion is softened and the seasonings are aromatic. Add the tomato paste and sauté for 1 minute.

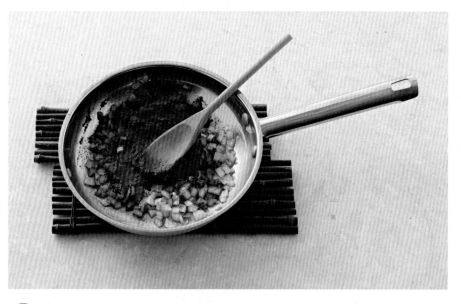

2 Add the chickpeas, cauliflower, and vegetable stock. Bring to a boil, then lower the heat and simmer for 10 to 12 minutes, until the cauliflower is tender and a sauce is formed. If the sauce appears too thick, add a little water or additional vegetable stock.

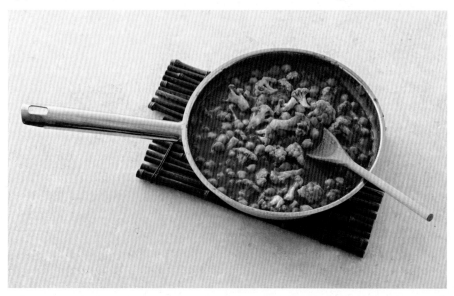

3 Garnish each serving with cilantro and a dollop of the yogurt.

BUTTERNUT CHOWDER

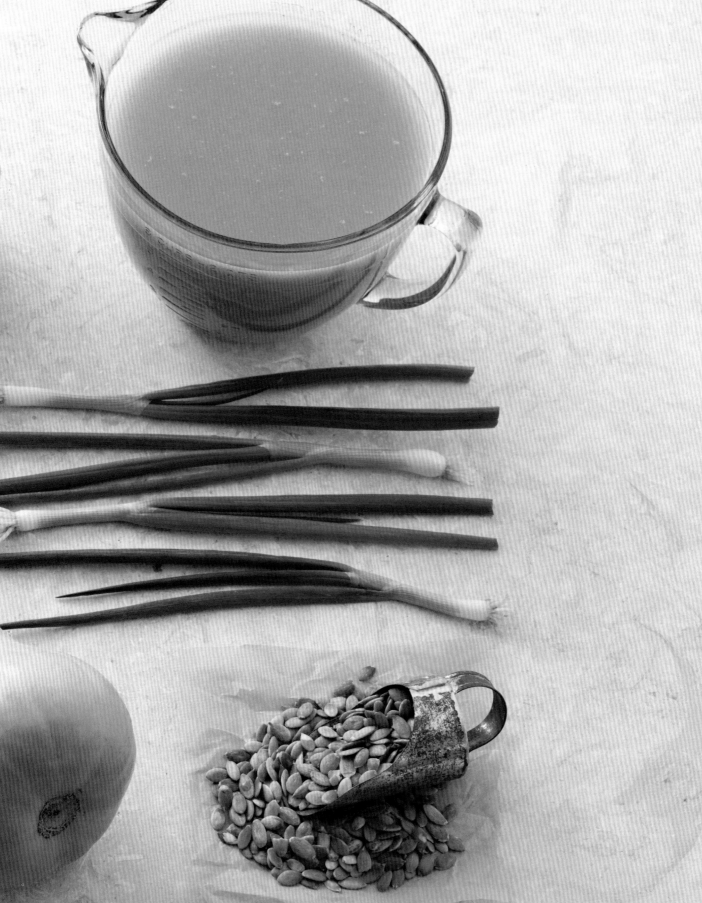

BUTTERNUT CHOWDER

SUGAR 2.6 tsp

TIME 60 minutes

SERVES four

INGREDIENTS

2 teaspoons canola oil

1 cup hulled unsalted pumpkin seeds
(pepitas)

2 pounds butternut squash, peeled
and cut into 1-inch cubes

8 cups low-sodium vegetable stock

1 large tomato, chopped

1 medium onion, chopped

1 medium green bell pepper,
chopped

1 jalapeño pepper or Scotch bonnet
chile, seeded and minced (optional)

1 tablespoon minced fresh ginger

8 scallions, chopped

3 sprigs fresh thyme, stems removed

¼ cup chopped fresh cilantro, plus
cilantro sprigs for garnish

1 Heat the oil in medium skillet over medium heat. Add the pepitas and stir frequently for 5 to 7 minutes, until they begin to brown and pop. Remove from the heat and set aside.

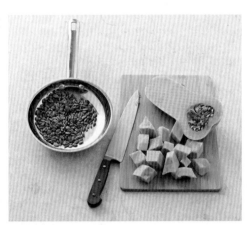

2 Combine the squash, stock, tomato, onion, peppers, ginger, scallions, and thyme in a large pot. Place over high heat and bring to a boil, then reduce the heat and simmer uncovered for about 45 minutes, stirring occasionally, until the vegetables are tender.

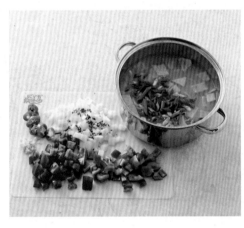

3 Remove from the heat and blend with an immersion blender for 2 to 4 minutes, until smooth. Add the cilantro and lime juice.

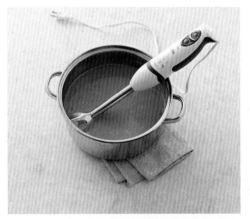

4 Serve with a sprinkle of pepitas and a sprig of cilantro.

GROUPER-N-GREENS

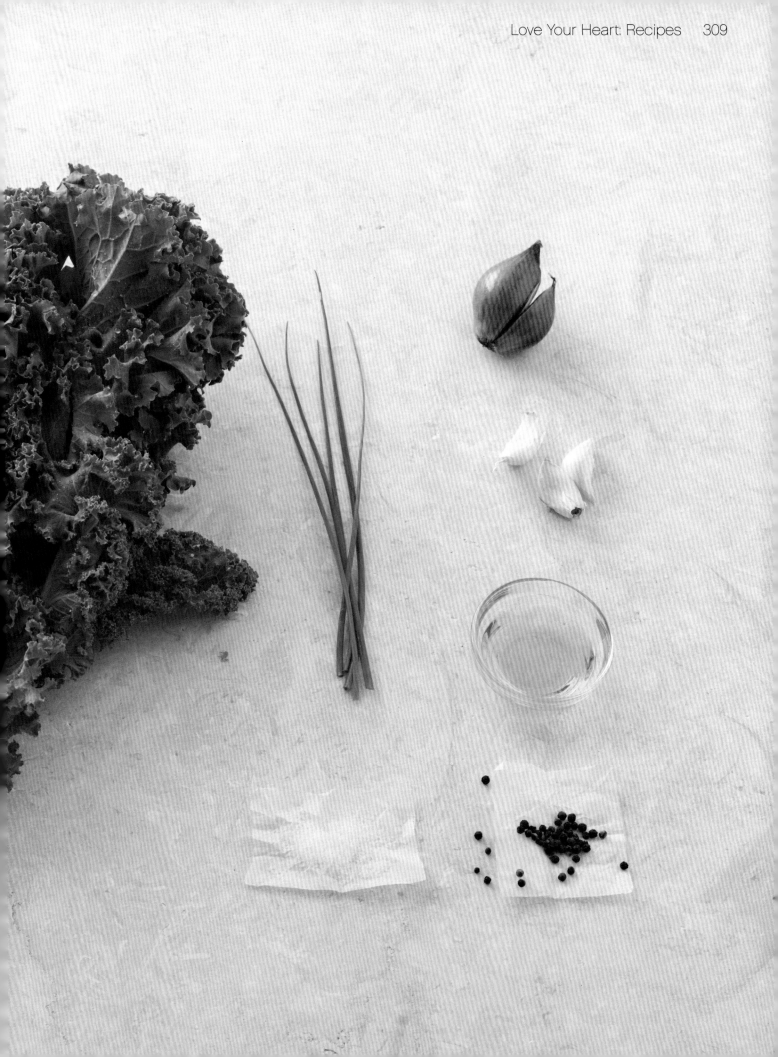

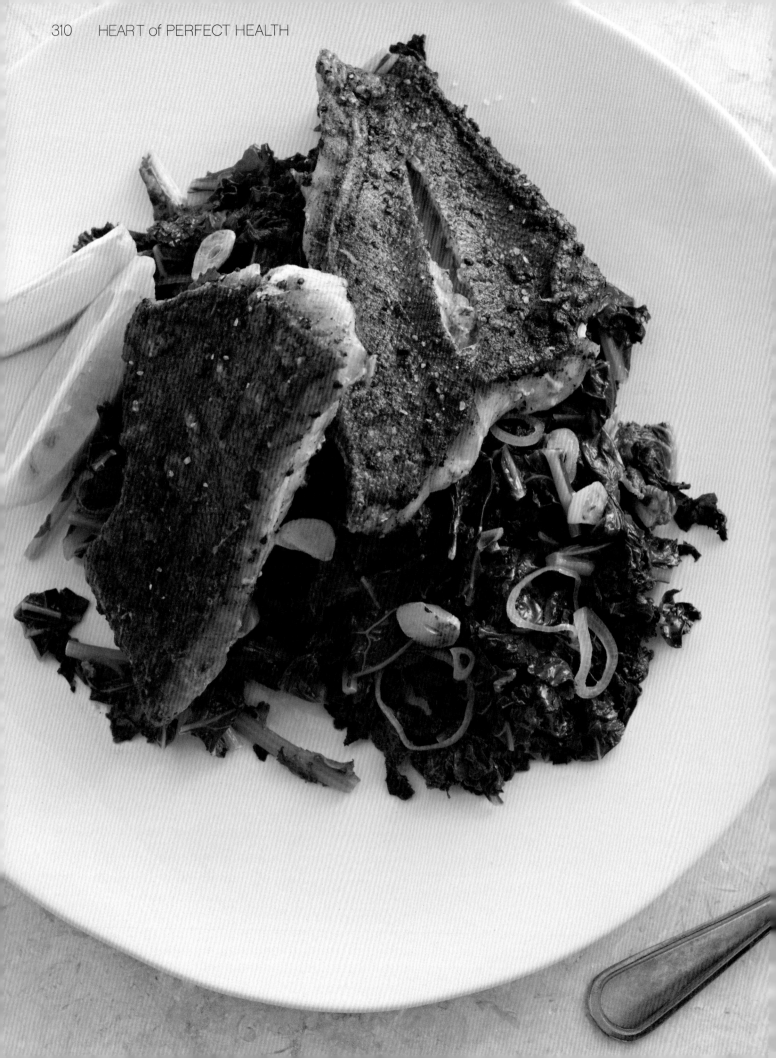

GROUPER-N-GREENS

SUGAR 1.6 tsp

TIME 20 minutes

SERVES four

INGREDIENTS

2 tablespoons extra virgin olive oil

4 cups chopped kale or Swiss chard leaves

1 shallot, thinly sliced

3 cloves garlic, sliced

Two 8-ounce grouper fillets (or other large whitefish)

Salt and freshly ground pepper

1 lemon

4 fresh chives, thinly sliced

1 Heat half the olive oil in a large sauté pan over medium heat.

2 Add the kale, shallot, and garlic and sauté, stirring occasionally, for 5 to 7 minutes, until the vegetables are slightly softened. Add 2 tablespoons water, cover, and steam for about 1 minute, until the water has cooked off. Remove from the pan and set aside.

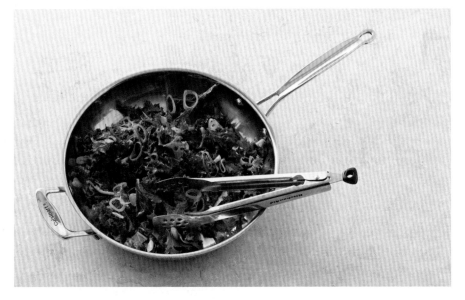

3 Wipe out the pan with a paper towel and reheat it with the remaining oil over medium-high heat. Season the fish with salt and pepper and place it in the pan, skin side down. Cook for 5 to 6 minutes, until the skin is browned and crisp. Turn the fish flesh side down and cook for another 4 minutes.

4 Serve the fish over the kale; squeeze over the lemon and garnish with the chives.

SEARED SESAME TUNA

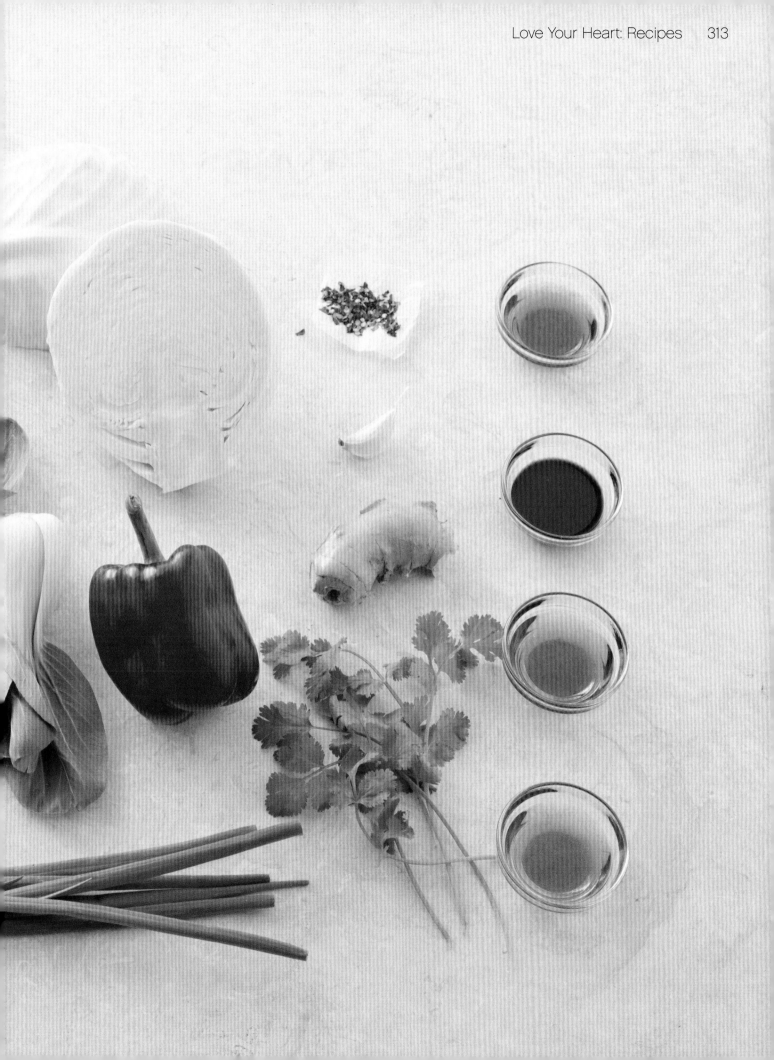

SEARED SESAME TUNA

SUGAR 1 tsp

TIME 45 minutes

SERVES four

INGREDIENTS

Slaw 0.8 tsp

1 tablespoon sesame oil

1 tablespoon low-sodium tamari

1 tablespoon mirin

1 tablespoon rice vinegar (sugar-free)

2 teaspoons minced fresh ginger

1 clove garlic, minced

½ teaspoon crushed red chili flakes

3 cups thinly sliced green cabbage

1 cup thinly sliced Napa cabbage

1 cup thinly sliced bok choy

½ red bell pepper, thinly sliced

1 carrot, thinly sliced

3 scallions, thinly sliced

Tuna 0.2 tsp

1 tablespoon tan sesame seeds

½ tablespoon black sesame seeds

¼ teaspoon wasabi powder

1 pound tuna steak, about 2 inches thick

1 teaspoon extra virgin olive oil

1 tablespoon minced fresh cilantro

1 In a small bowl, whisk together the sesame oil, tamari, mirin, vinegar, ginger, garlic, and red chili flakes.

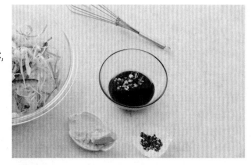

2 In a large bowl, combine the green cabbage, Napa cabbage, bok choy, red pepper, carrot, and scallions. Add the dressing and mix well. Set aside for at least 20 minutes before serving.

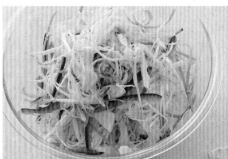

3 In a shallow bowl, combine the sesame seeds and wasabi powder. Coat the tuna steaks, in sesame seed mixture, making sure both sides are covered.

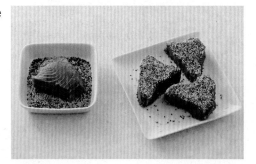

4 Heat the olive oil in a large skillet over medium-high heat. Sear the tuna in pan for 2 to 3 minutes per side, until both sides are well browned but the tuna is still very rare in center.

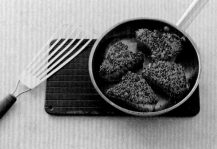

5 Serve garnished with the cilantro.

GARLIC-N-LEMON SHRIMP

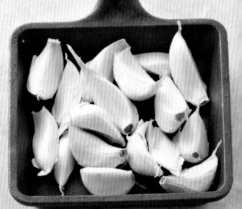

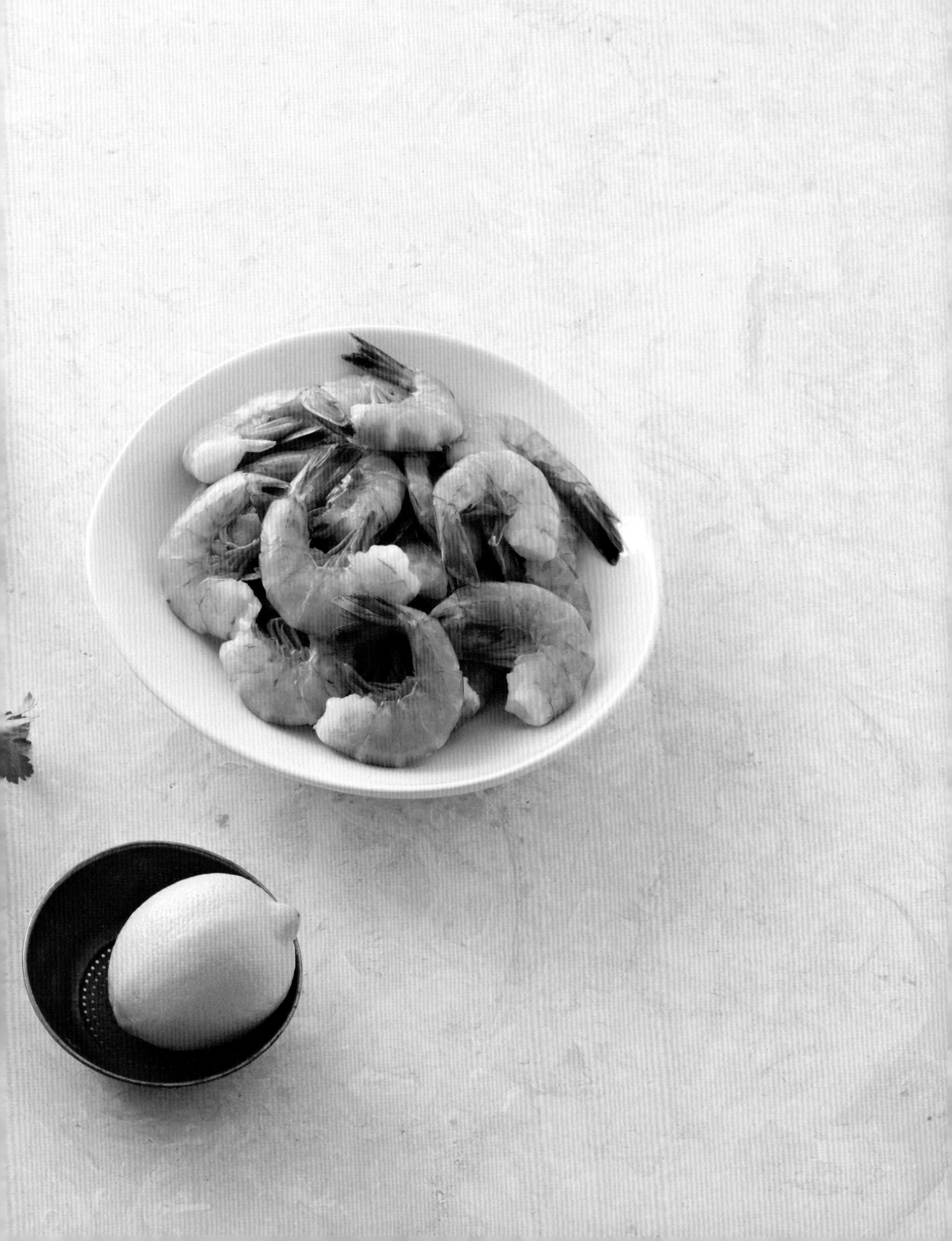

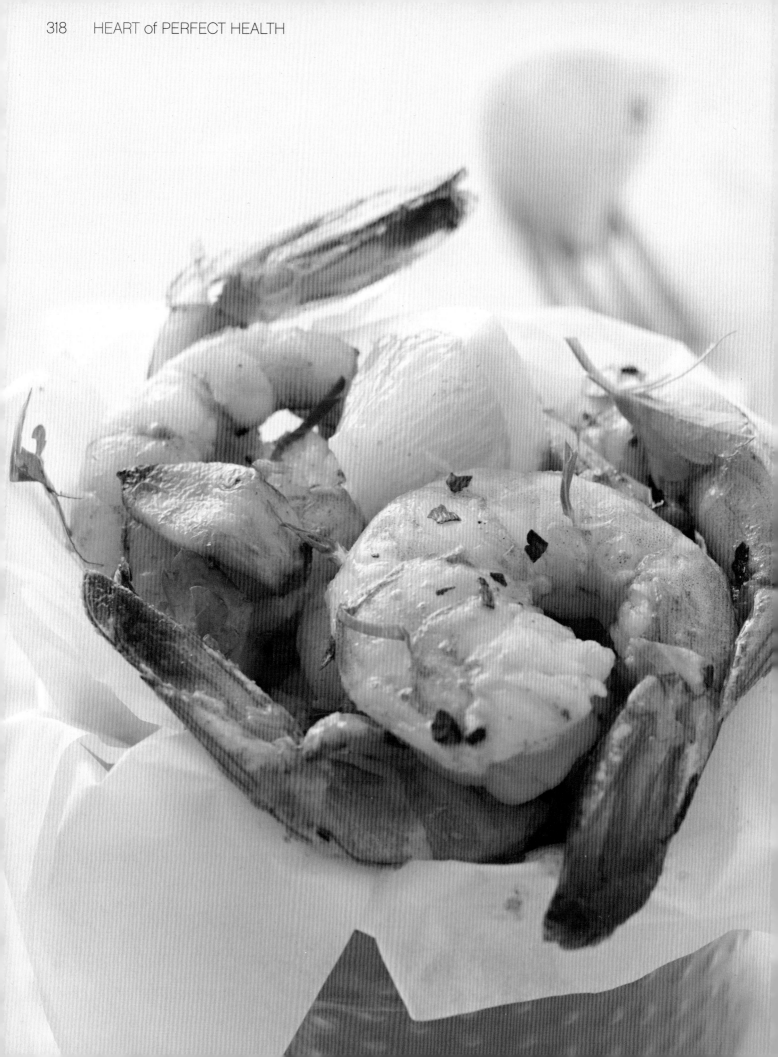

GARLIC-N-LEMON SHRIMP

SUGAR 1.4 tsp

TIME 30 minutes

SERVES two

INGREDIENTS

12 whole cloves garlic, peeled

1 tablespoon extra virgin olive oil

1 pound large shrimp (21 to 25 count), peeled and deveined

½ teaspoon smoked paprika

¼ teaspoon red chili flakes

Juice of 1 lemon

1 tablespoon chopped fresh parsley

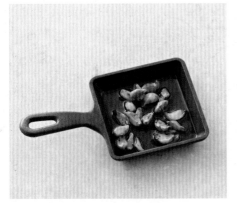 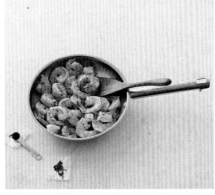 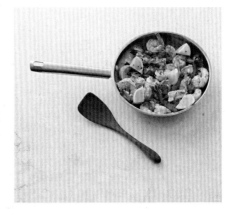

1 Preheat the oven to 375°F. Combine the garlic and oil in a small ovenproof skillet and bake, uncovered, for 15 to 20 minutes, stirring occasionally, until golden brown. Set aside.

2 Remove the garlic from the oil and set aside. Transfer remaining oil into a large sauté pan and heat it over medium-high heat. Add the shrimp, paprika, and chili flakes and sauté the shrimp for about 3 minutes per side, until they turn pink. Add the baked garlic and sauté for 1 minute.

3 Remove from the heat and toss with the lemon juice and parsley.

SEAFOOD GUMBO

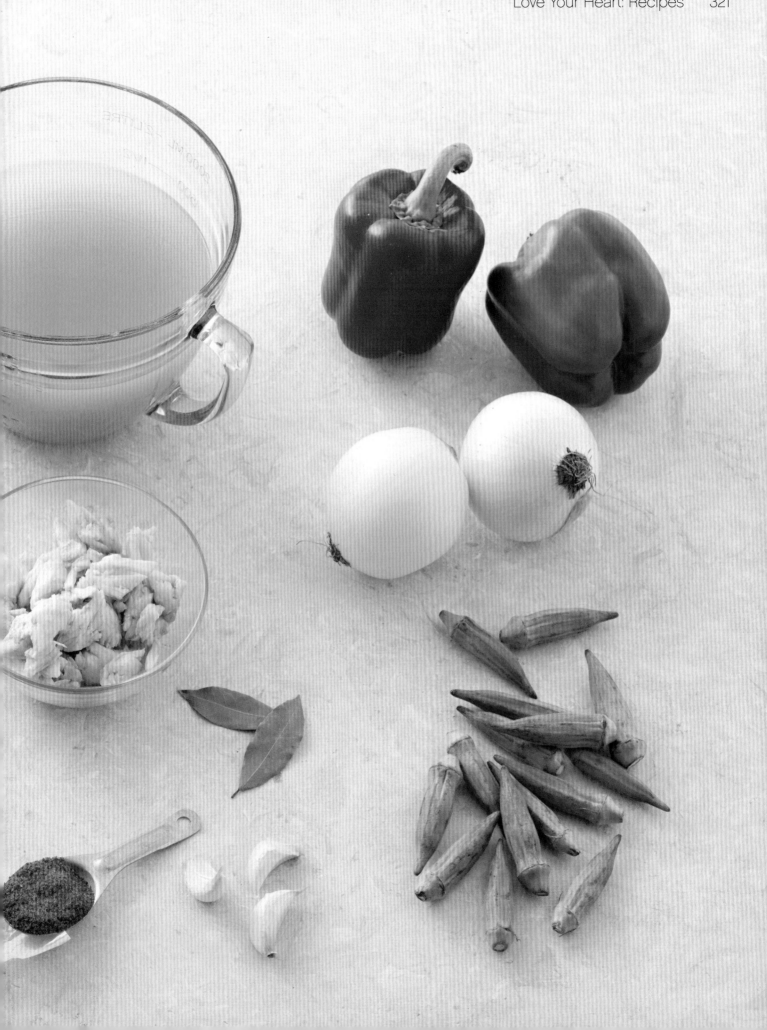

SEAFOOD GUMBO

SUGAR 1.8 tsp

TIME 60 minutes

SERVES eight

INGREDIENTS

1 tablespoon extra virgin olive oil

2 cups chopped onions

2 cups chopped celery

1 cup chopped green bell tpepper

1 cup chopped red bell pepper

3 cloves garlic, minced

1 tablespoon Cajun seasoning mix or similar Creole spice blend

2 bay leaves

6 cups low-sodium vegetable or chicken stock

One 14.5-ounce can low-sodium chopped tomatoes

1 pound medium shrimp (30 count), peeled and deveined

1 cup fresh crabmeat

2 tablespoons hot sauce

1 cup sliced fresh or frozen okra (optional)

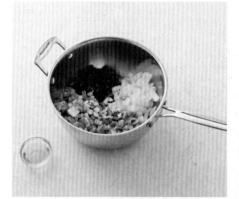 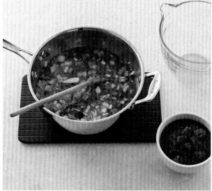 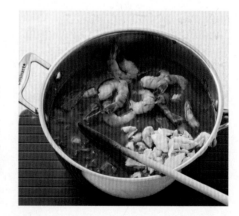

1 Heat the oil in a heavy-bottom 5-quart saucepan over medium heat. Add the onions, celery, peppers, garlic, Cajun seasoning, and bay leaves. Sauté for 5 to 7 minutes, until the onions and peppers are softened.

2 Add the stock and tomatoes with their juices and bring to a boil. Reduce the heat and simmer for 40 minutes.

3 Add the shrimp, crabmeat, hot sauce, and okra. Return the mixture to a boil, cover, and remove from the heat; let stand for 10 minutes, or until the shrimp turn pink.

4 Remove the bay leaves before serving.

'CRESS STUFFED STEAK

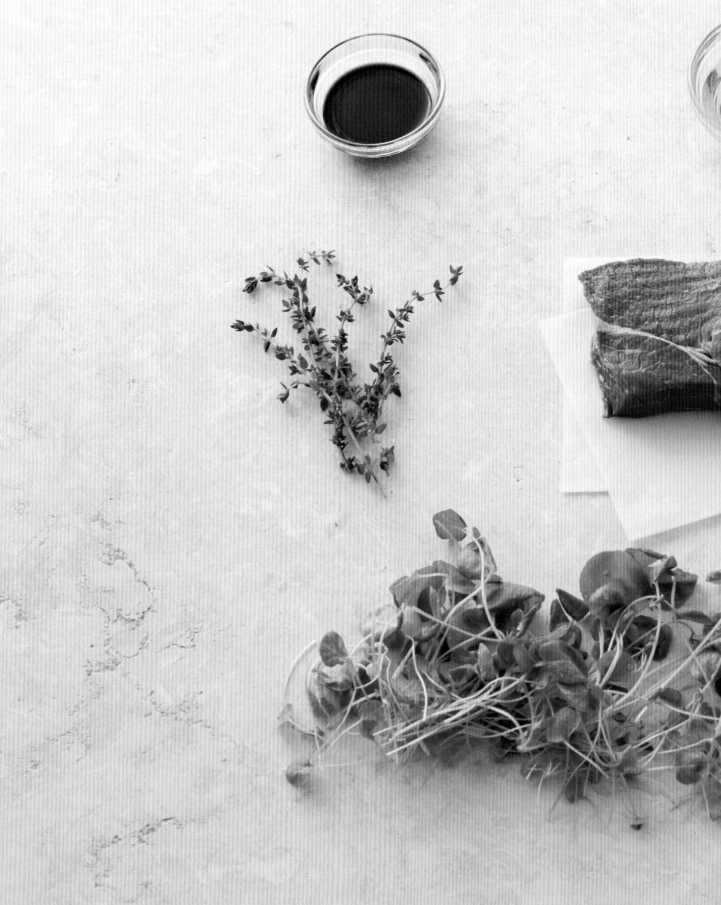

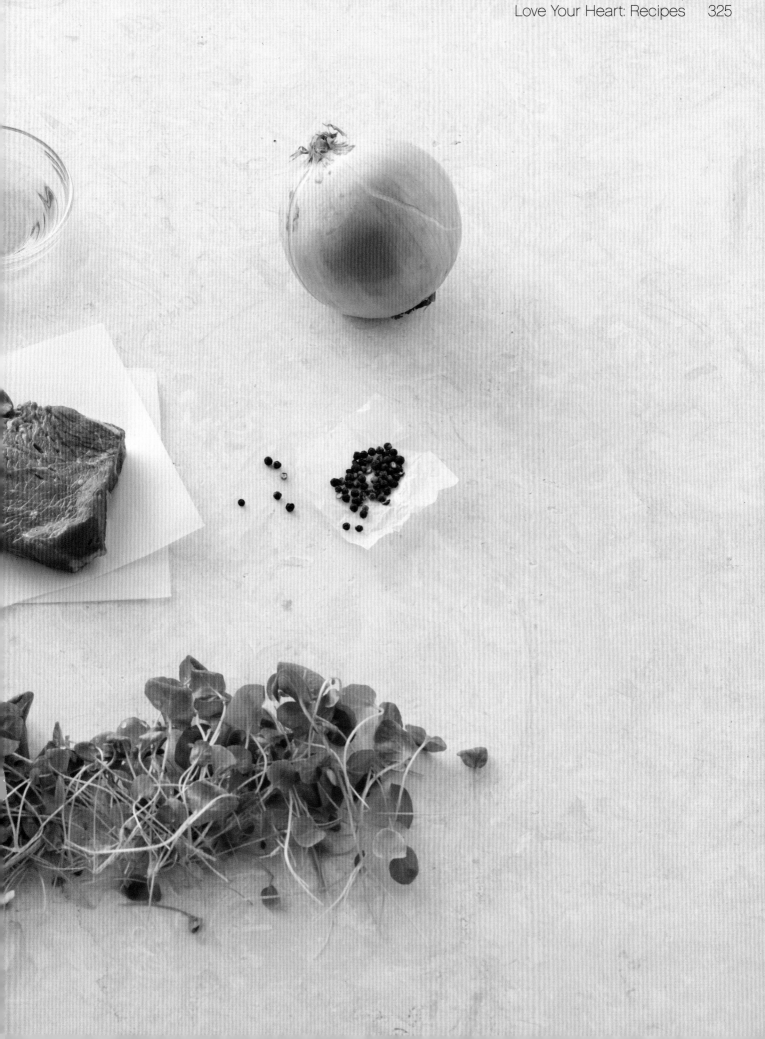

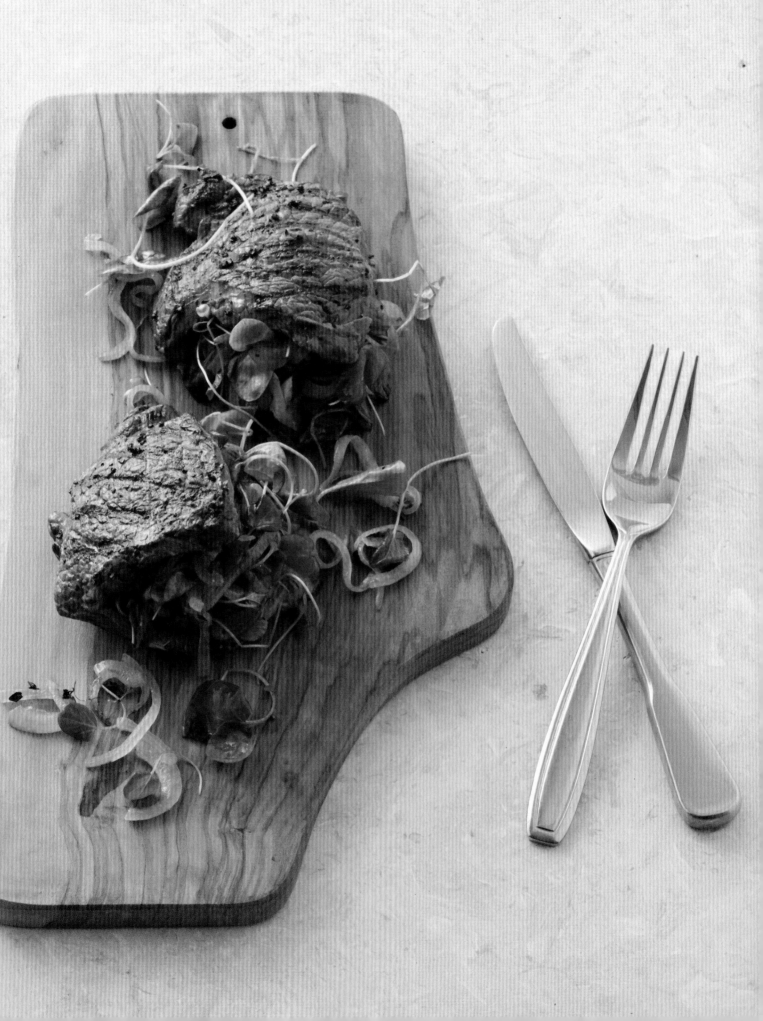

'CRESS STUFFED STEAK

SUGAR 1.4 tsp

TIME 30 minutes

SERVES two

INGREDIENTS

8 ounces lean beef, such as top round or sirloin

2 teaspoons extra virgin olive oil

1 medium sweet onion, thinly sliced

Leaves from 2 sprigs fresh thyme

1 cup watercress leaves, stems removed

½ teaspoon cracked black peppercorns

1 tablespoon balsamic vinegar

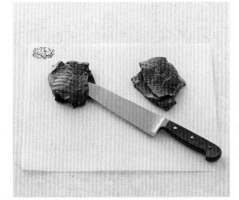

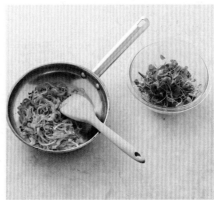

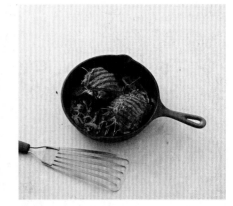

1 Cut the beef into 2 equal portions, then slice a pocket into each. Set aside.

2 Heat the oil in a large sauté pan over medium-high heat. Add the onion and thyme leaves and sauté for 4 to 6 minutes, stirring occasionally, until the onion is well browned and tender. Remove from the heat and add the watercress leaves. Cool to room temperature.

3 Stuff the steaks with the onion mixture, securing the flaps with a toothpick. Season the steak with cracked peppercorns. Preheat a grill pan over medium-high heat. Place the stuffed steaks on the grill pan and cook for 3 to 4 minutes per side, until brown. Remove from the heat and rest for 3 to 5 minutes. Drizzle with the balsamic vinegar and serve, over a bed of fresh watercress.

PERSIAN KABOB

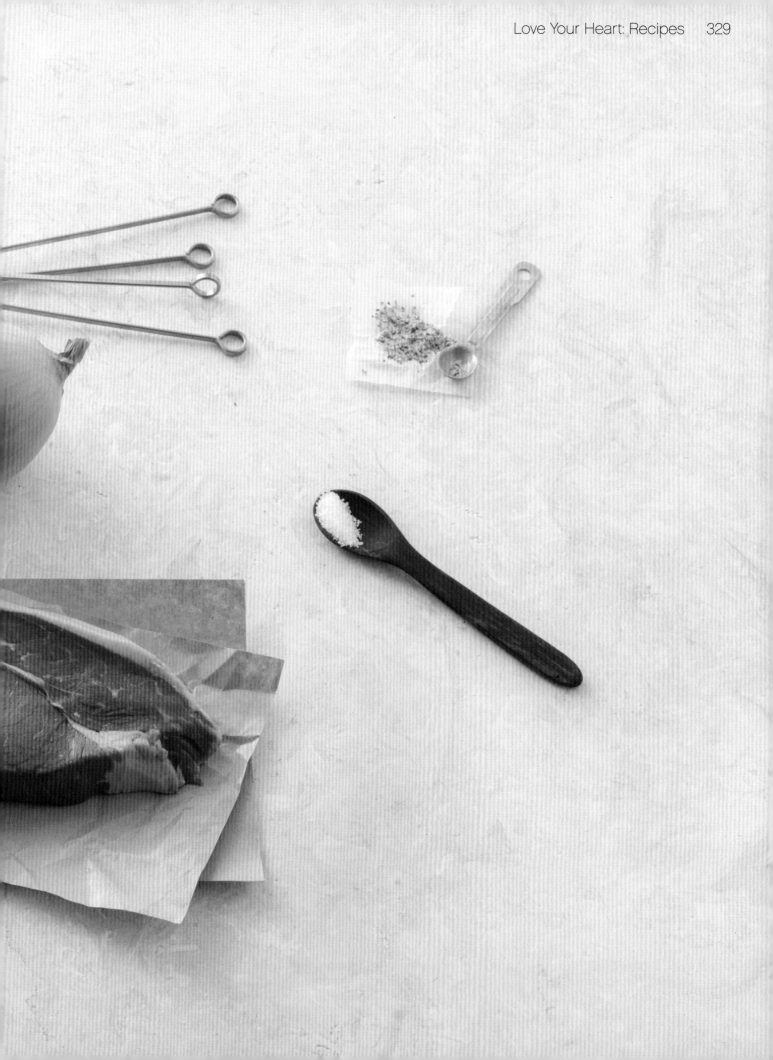

PERSIAN KABOB

SUGAR 1.6 tsp

TIME 30 minutes

SERVES two

INGREDIENTS

1 pound lean beef, such as round or sirloin, cubed

1 large onion, quartered and thickly sliced

4 firm medium plum tomatoes, thickly sliced

4 skewers (if wooden then soaked in water for 30 minutes to prevent burning)

½ teaspoon sea salt

½ teaspoon lemon pepper spice

1 tablespoon sumac (optional but recommended)

Olive oil cooking spray

1 cup raw spinach

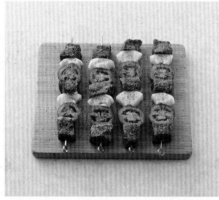

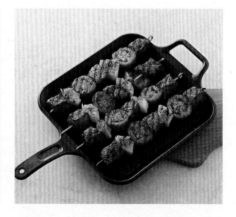

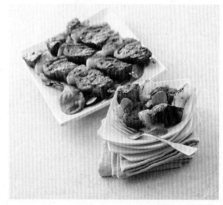

1 Arrange the beef, onion, and tomatoes on the skewers. Season both sides with the salt, lemon pepper, and sumac.

2 Coat a grill pan with olive oil spray and heat over medium-high heat. Add the skewers and cook for 4 to 6 minutes per side.

3 Serve on a bed of raw spinach.

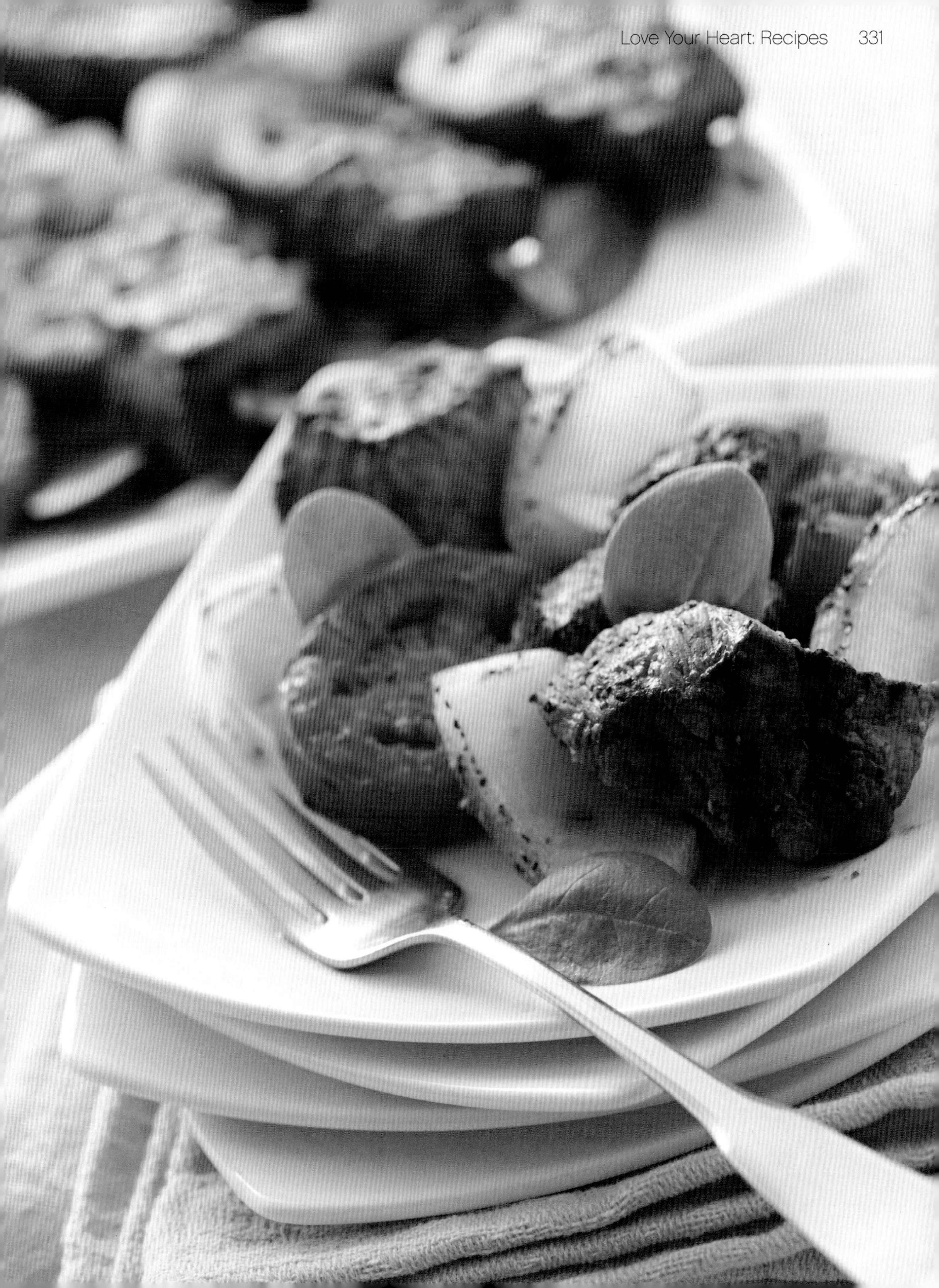

BEEF BRUSCHETTA

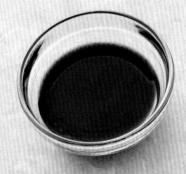

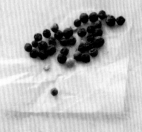

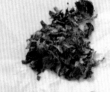

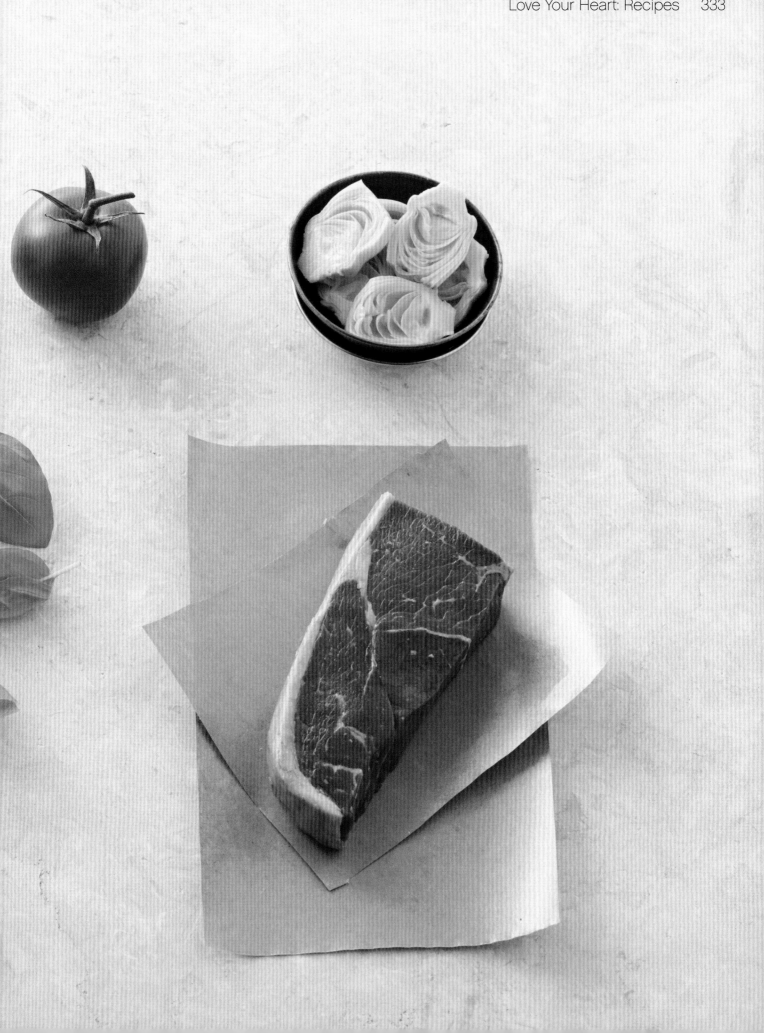

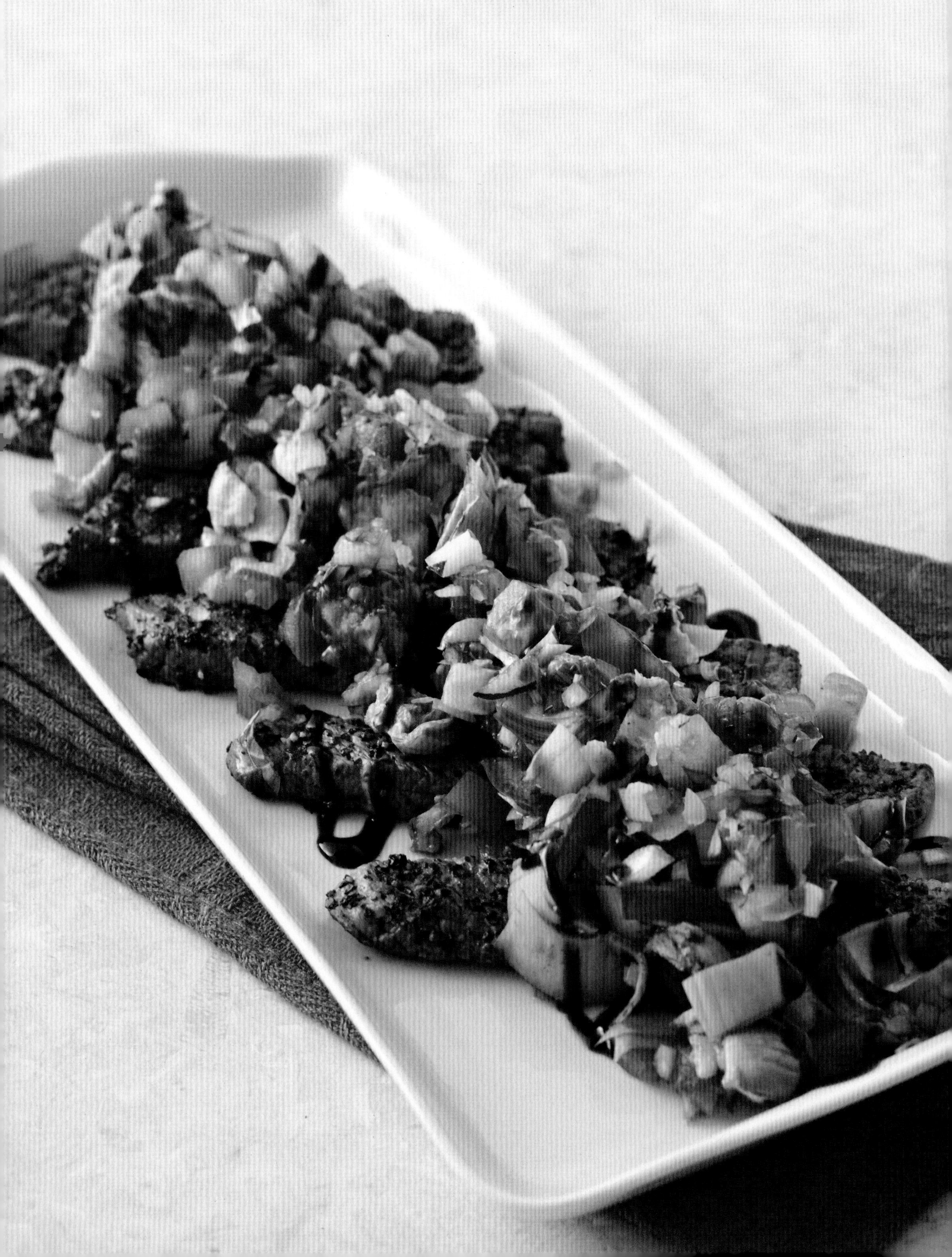

BEEF BRUSCHETTA

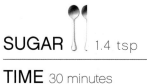

SUGAR 1.4 tsp

TIME 30 minutes

SERVES two

INGREDIENTS

Olive oil cooking spray

½ cup artichoke hearts in water, halved

¼ red onion, minced

1 ripe tomato, diced

1 teaspoon extra virgin olive oil

3 fresh basil leaves, minced

1 clove garlic, minced

1 tablespoon balsamic vinegar

8 ounces lean beef, such as top round or sirloin, cut into ½-inch slices

¼ teaspoon cracked black peppercorns

¼ teaspoon dried Italian seasoning

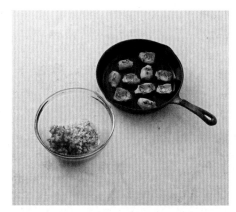

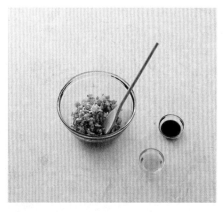

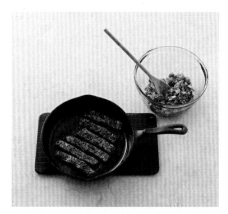

1 Coat a grill pan or cast-iron skillet with olive oil spray and heat over medium-high heat. Place the artichoke heart halves on the skillet and lightly brown them on each side for 2 to 3 minutes. Remove from the heat, cool, then cut into small pieces.

2 In a small bowl, combine the onion, tomato, artichoke hearts, olive oil, basil, garlic, and vinegar.

3 Season the beef with the cracked peppercorns and Italian seasoning. In the same grill pan or cast-iron skillet, sear the beef over medium-high heat for about 2 minutes per side, until nicely browned. Transfer to a plate and top with the artichoke bruschetta mixture.

BEEF-N-VEGGIE BOLOGNESE

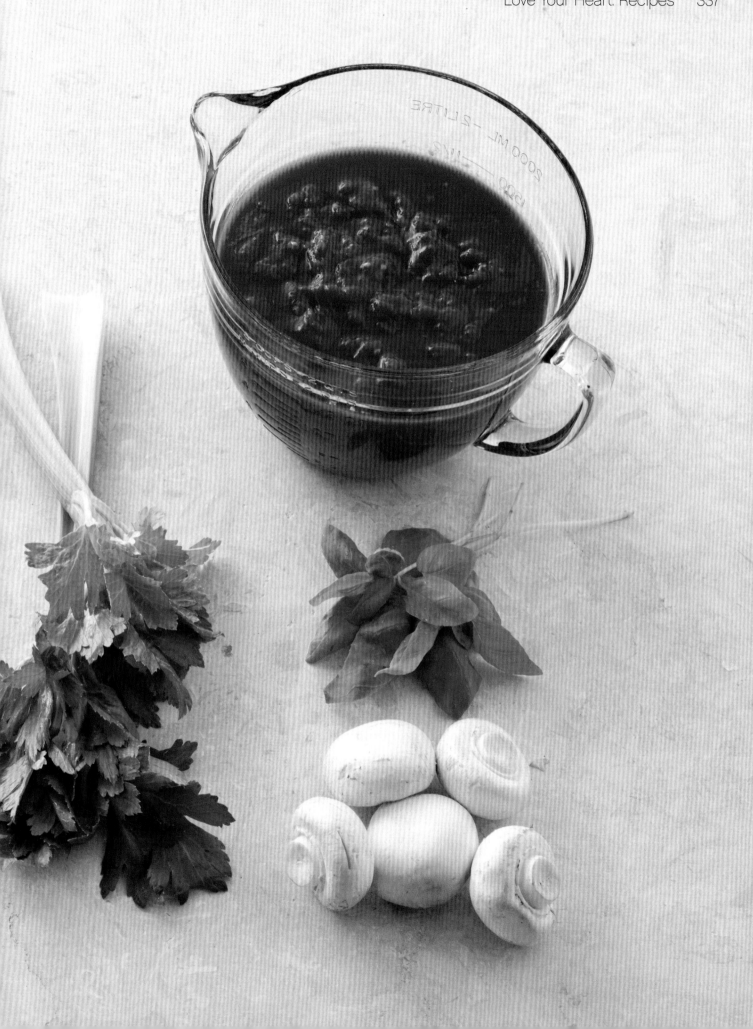

BEEF-N-VEGGIE BOLOGNESE

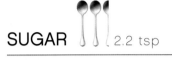

SUGAR 2.2 tsp

TIME 30 minutes

SERVES six

INGREDIENTS

2 teaspoons extra virgin olive oil

1 ½ pounds lean ground beef, such as sirloin

1 medium onion, chopped

2 stalks celery, chopped

1 carrot, chopped

1 cup button mushrooms, chopped

3 cloves garlic, minced

1 tablespoon fresh oregano

2 bay leaves

Two 28-ounce cans low-sodium chopped tomatoes

½ cup fresh basil cut into chiffonade

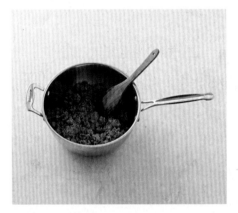

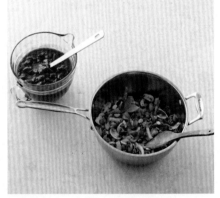

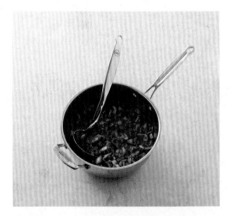

1 Heat the oil in a large heavy-bottom pot over medium heat. Add the beef and cook for 3 to 4 minutes. Drain off all excess fat, then add the onion, celery, carrot, mushrooms, garlic, Italian seasoning, and bay leaves and sauté for 3 to 4 minutes.

2 Add the tomatoes with their juices and bring to a boil. Reduce the heat, cover, and simmer for 45 minutes.

3 Serve over spaghetti sqaush (page 370) topped with the basil.

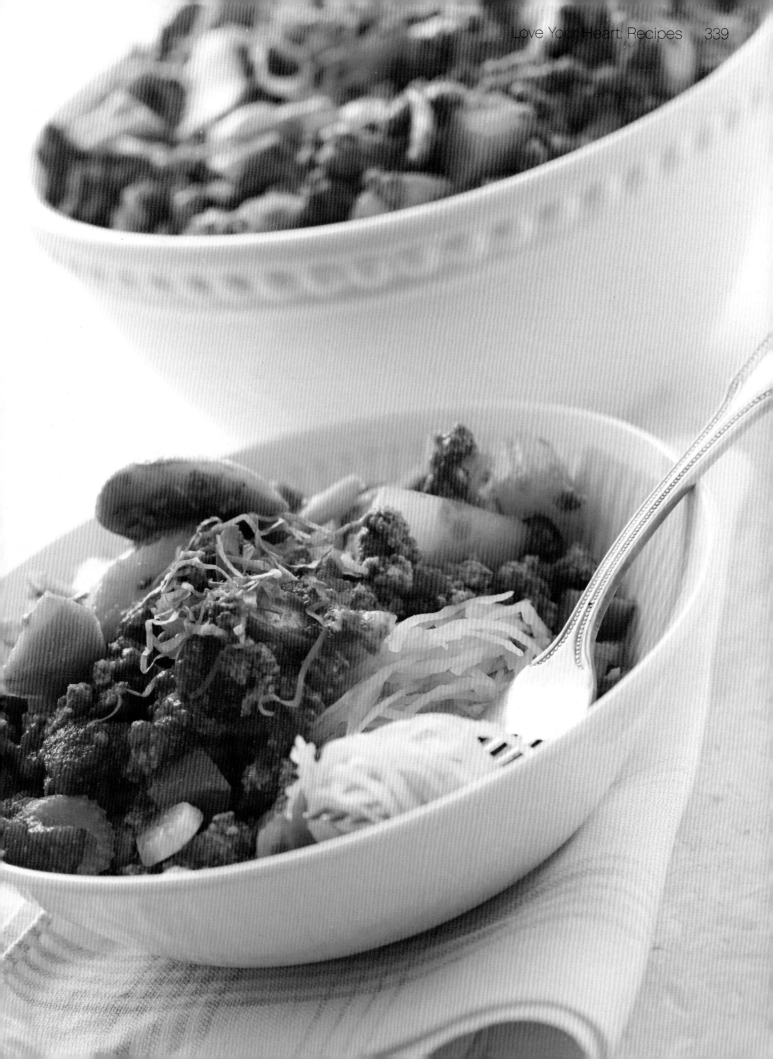

ATHENIAN MEATBALLS

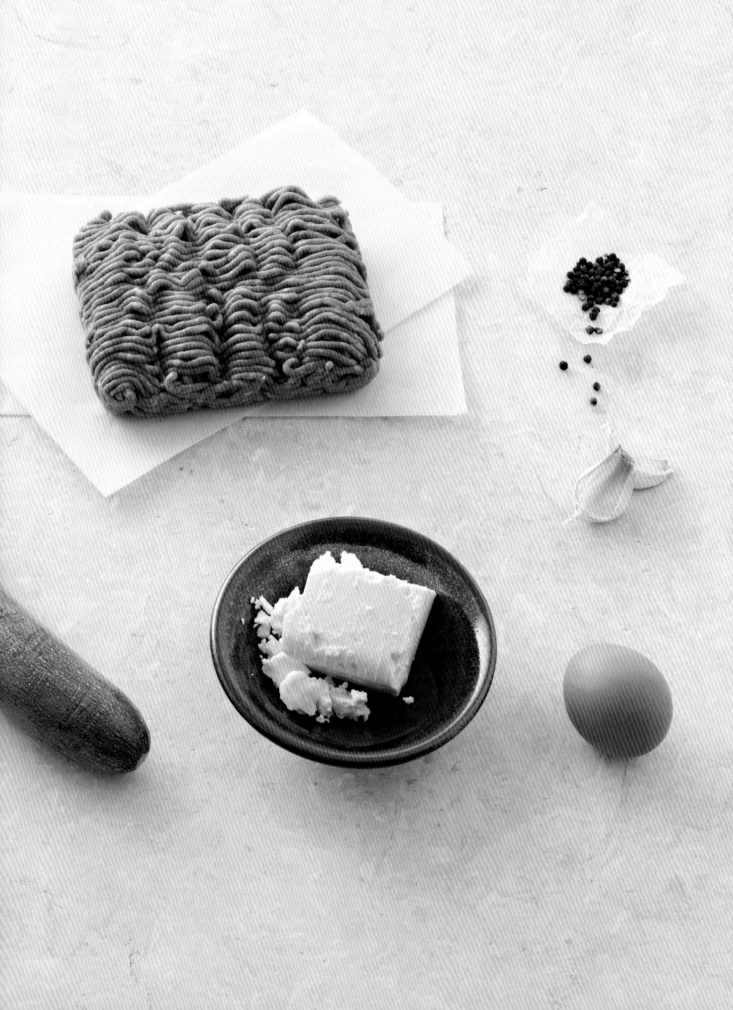

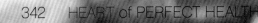

ATHENIAN MEATBALLS

SUGAR 0.6 tsp

TIME 30 minutes

SERVES six

INGREDIENTS

1 medium white onion, quartered

¼ cup fresh dill sprigs

¼ cup fresh mint leaves

2 cloves garlic

½ cup grated zucchini

1 pound ground lamb

1 large egg, beaten

¼ cup crumbled low-fat or fat-free feta cheese

¼ teaspoon ground black pepper

2 tablespoons water or skim milk

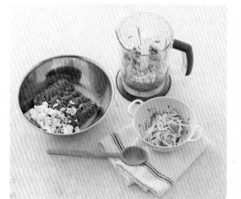
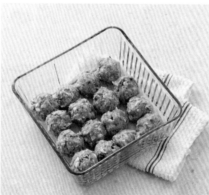
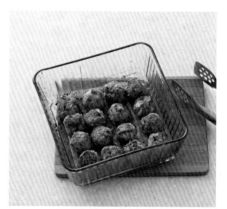

1 Peheat the oven to 375°F. Place the onion, dill, mint, and garlic in a food processor and pulse 8 to 12 times, until chopped and well mixed. Add the zucchini and pulse 2 or 3 times to combine. Transfer the mixture to a large bowl.

2 Add the lamb, egg, cheese, and black pepper and mix well with your hands until combined. Wet your hands with water or skim milk and form the mixture into balls slightly larger than a golf ball.

3 Heat a large skillet over medium-high heat. Brown the meatballs for 1 minute per side and place on an ovenproof dish or pan. Bake in the center of the oven for about 30 minutes.

SICILIAN CITRUS PORK

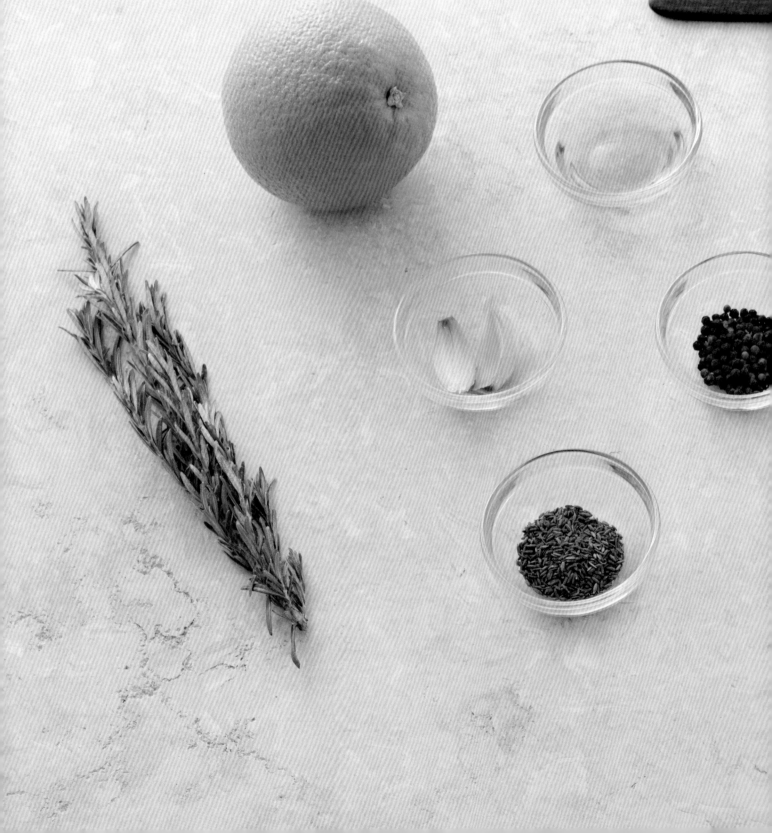

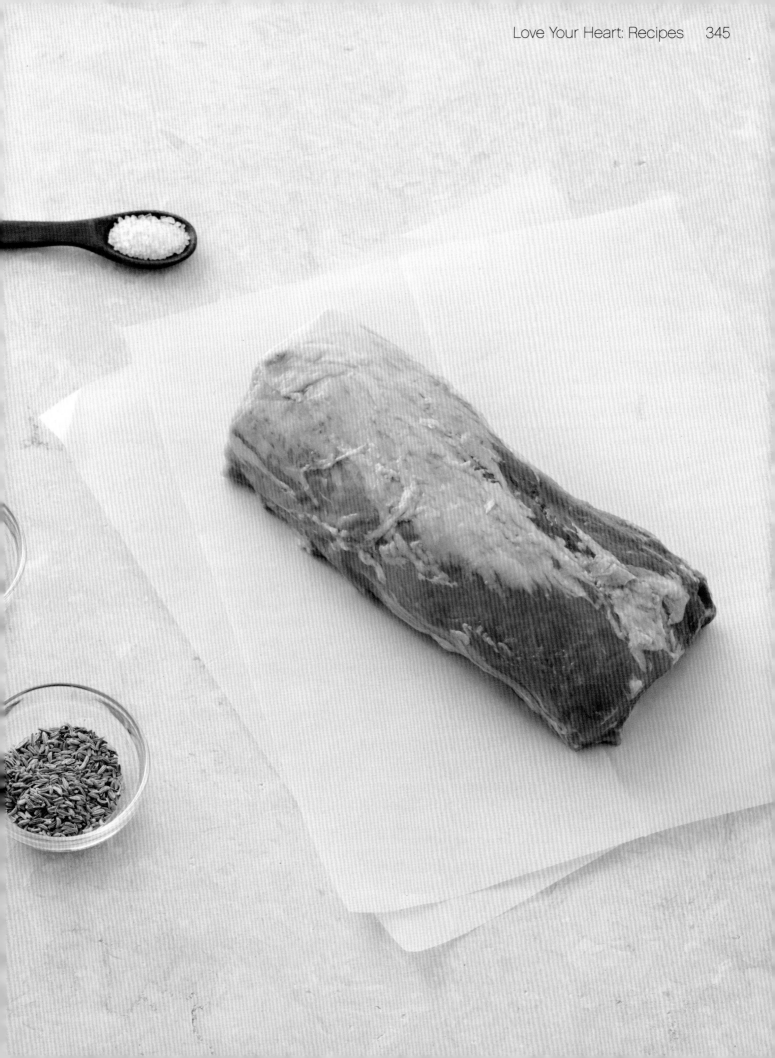

SICILIAN CITRUS PORK

SUGAR 0.6

TIME 60 minutes

SERVES six

INGREDIENTS

2 pounds center-cut pork roast, surface scored with a knife

2 cloves garlic, minced

1 teaspoon fennel seeds, crushed

½ teaspoon cumin seeds, crushed

1 tablespoon minced fresh rosemary

½ teaspoon black peppercorns, crushed

1 tablespoon extra virgin olive oil

1 orange, cut into thin slices

1 Cover the top of the scored pork with the garlic, fennel, cumin, rosemary, and peppercorns; rub gently and brush with the oil. Transfer the pork to a zip-top bag and add the orange slices. Seal tightly and marinate for at least an hour or overnight in the refrigerator.

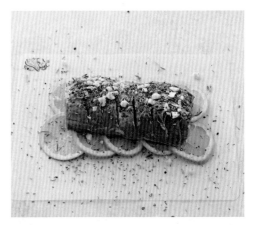

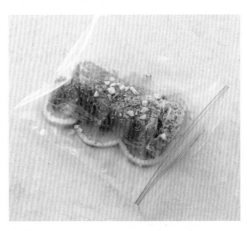

2 Preheat the oven to 375°F. Remove the pork and orange slices from the bag and place in a roasting pan. Add ½ cup water and cover with foil; cook for about 40 minutes.

3 Remove the foil and cook for about 15 minutes, basting the roast occasionally with the pan juices, until the internal temperature reads 160°F on a meat thermometer.

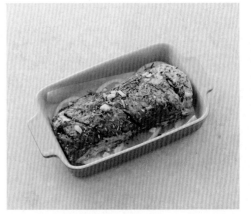

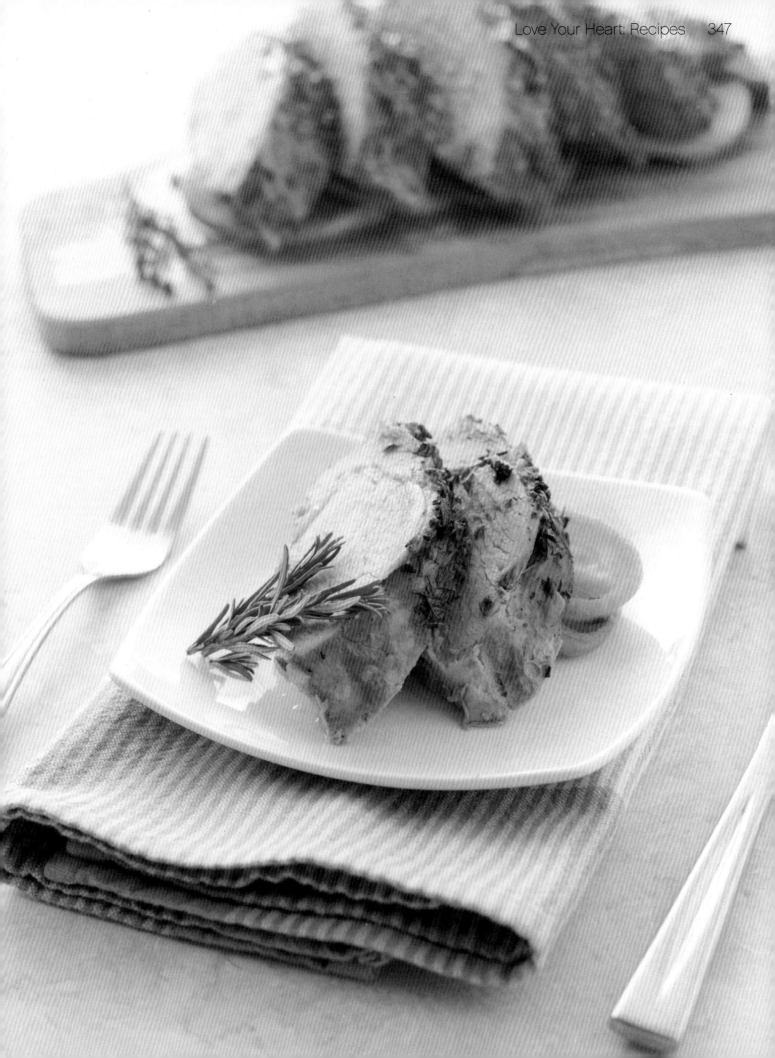

LEMONGRASS CHICKEN

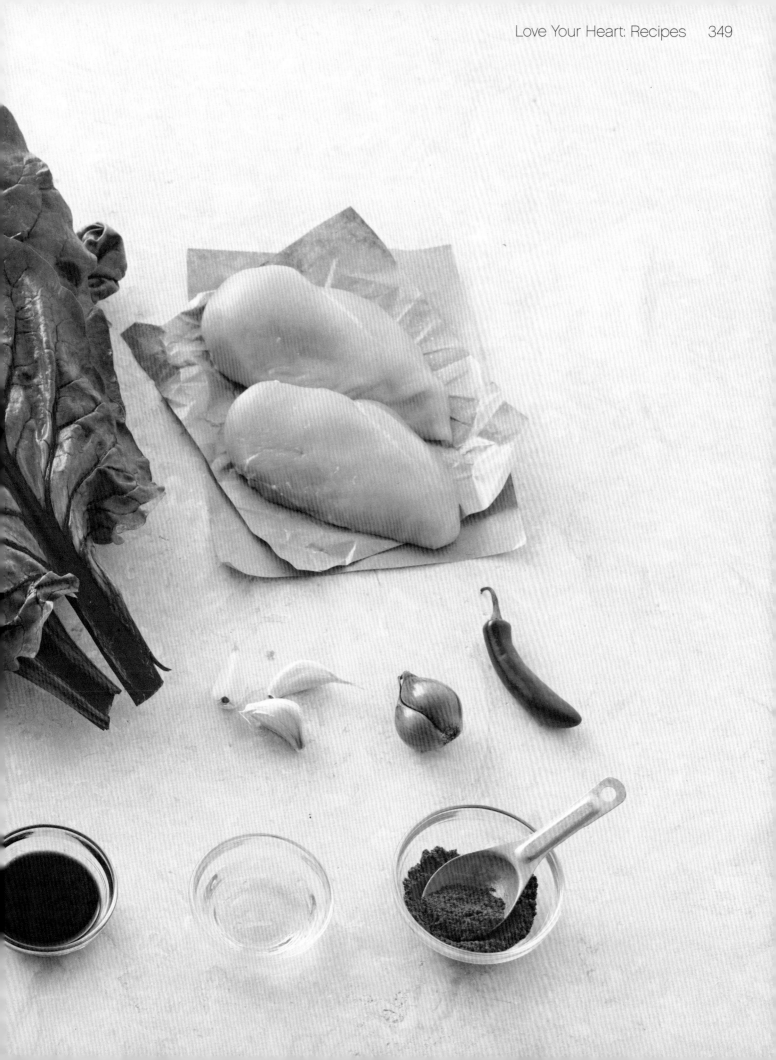

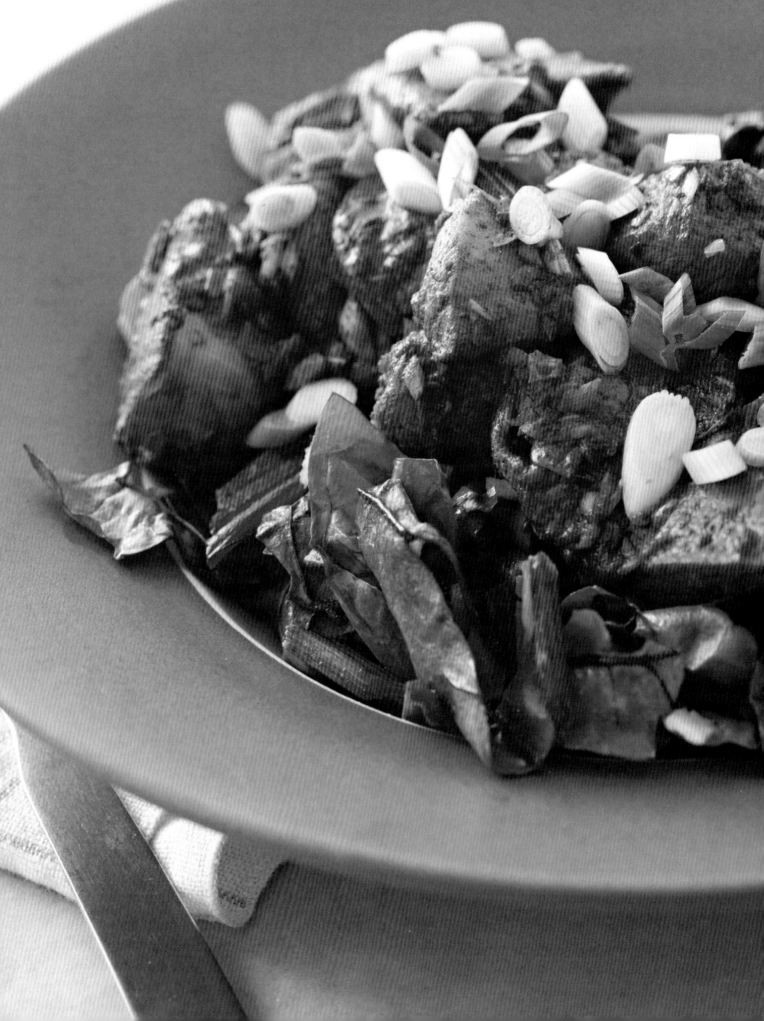

LEMONGRASS CHICKEN

SUGAR 1.6 tsp

TIME 25 minutes

SERVES four

INGREDIENTS

3 cloves garlic, minced

1 large shallot, minced

1 tablespoon curry powder

1 chile, such as serrano or jalapeño, seeds removed, minced

2 fresh lemongrass stalks, outer layer removed, minced

1 1/2 pounds boneless skinless chicken breast, cut into 2-inch chunks

1 tablespoon reduced-sodium tamari

1 tablespoon extra light virgin olive oil

1 tablespoon minced fresh ginger

1 bunch (about 1 pound) Swiss chard, chopped

4 scallions, thinly sliced

1 In a medium bowl, combine the garlic, shallot, curry powder, chile, and lemongrass. Add the chicken and tamari and stir to coat well; set aside to marinate.

2 Heat half the oil in a large sauté pan or wok over high heat. Add the marinated chicken pieces and stir-fry, turning every few minutes, until well browned on all sides. Add 2 tablespoons water and continue to cook until the chicken is fragrant, appears glazed, and is cooked through when pierced with a fork or knife. Remove from the pan and set aside.

3 Wipe out the pan with a paper towel and heat the remaining oil in the same pan. Add the ginger and stir-fry for 1 minute. Add the chard and stir-fry for 2 minutes, or until the chard is wilted and the ginger is fragrant.

4 Place the chard on a serving plate and top with the chicken pieces. Serve garnished with the scallions.

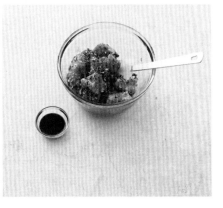

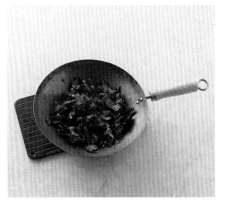

CHICKEN MILANE/E

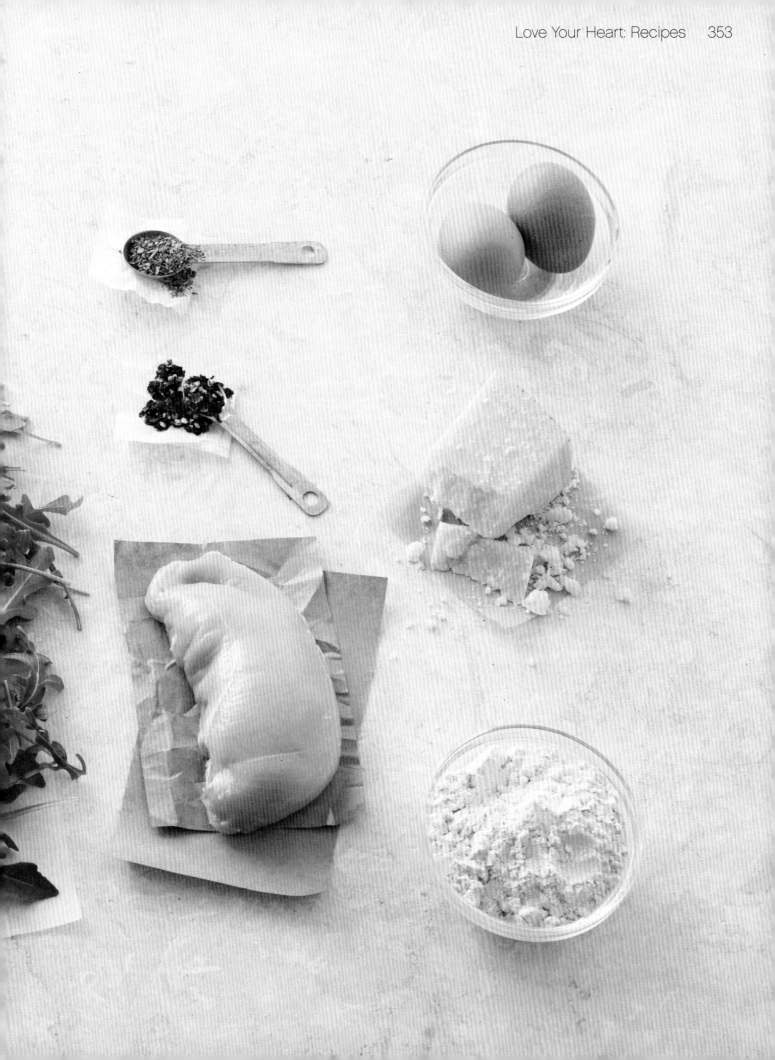

CHICKEN MILANESE

SUGAR 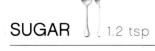 1.2 tsp

TIME 30 minutes

SERVES two

INGREDIENTS

One 8-ounce boneless skinless chicken breast, cut in half

½ cup chickpea flour

1 tablespoon minced fresh parsley

1 teaspoon dried Italian seasoning

¼ teaspoon crushed red chili flakes

2 large egg whites, lightly beaten

2 tablespoons extra virgin olive oil

2 cups loosely packed baby arugula leaves

¼ red onion, thinly sliced

Juice of 1 lemon

1 tablespoon shaved Parmesan cheese

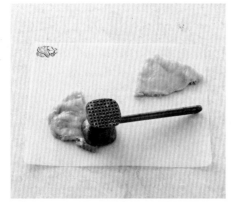

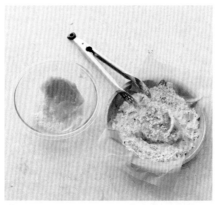

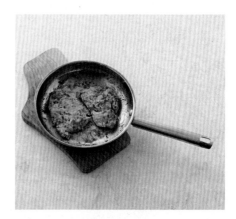

1 Place chicken breast halves between sheets of wax paper or plastic wrap and lightly flatten with a meat mallet or rolling pin.

2 In a low flat bowl or pie pan, combine the chickpea flour, parsley, Italian seasoning, and red chili flakes. Place the egg whites in a medium bowl. Moisten the chicken breasts in the egg whites, then dredge in the chickpea flour mixture, covering all areas.

3 Heat half the oil a large ovenproof skillet over medium-high heat. Place the chicken breasts in the skillet and cook for 3 to 5 minutes per side, until golden. If necessary, transfer the pan with chicken to a 375°F oven for 5 to 10 minutes, until the chicken reaches an internal temperature of 160°F.

4 Serve the chicken breasts warm over the arugula and red onion. Drizzle the remaining olive oil and the lemon juice on top and sprinkle with the cheese.

LIGURIAN CHICKEN

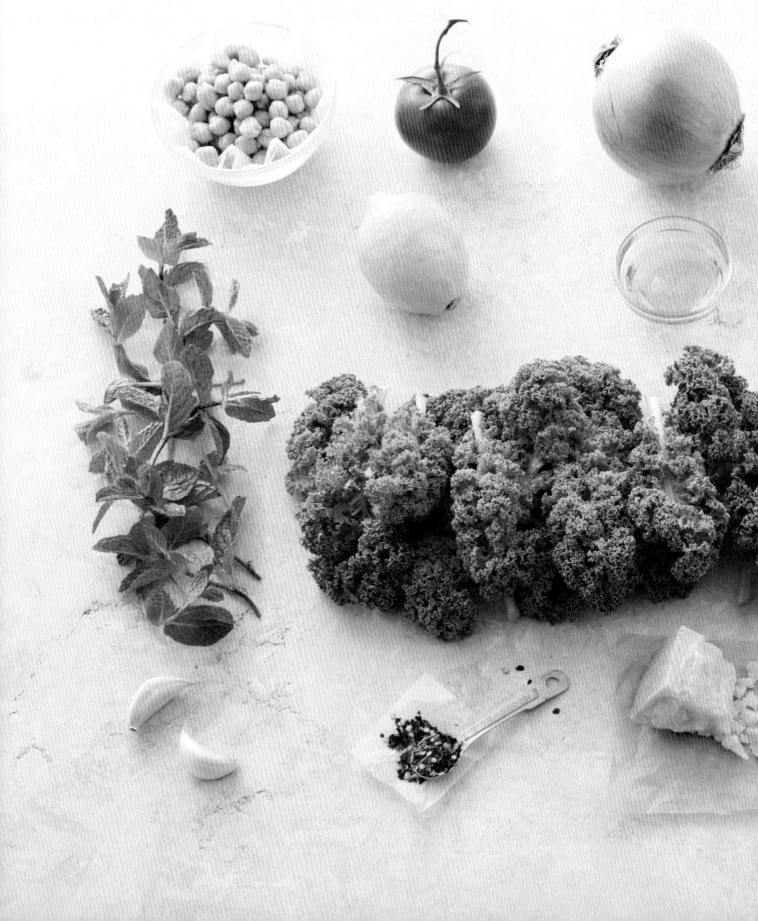

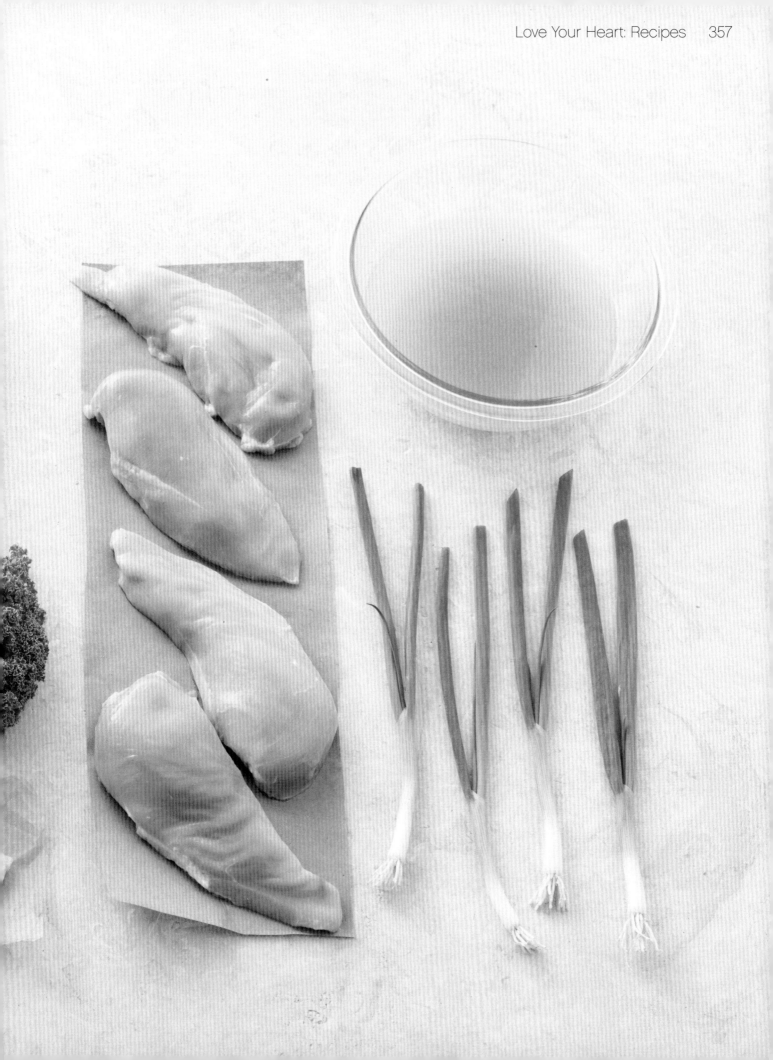

5 Lightly cover with foil and bake for 30 to 35 minutes. Remove the foil and bake for an additional 10 to 15 minutes, until the chicken breasts are completely cooked through. Serve with the pan juices.

LIGURIAN CHICKEN

SUGAR 3.6 tsp

TIME 60 minutes

SERVES four

INGREDIENTS

1 cup cooked chickpeas

1 tablespoon extra virgin olive oil

3 cups chopped kale leaves

2 cloves garlic, minced

4 scallions, minced

2 tablespoons grated Parmesan cheese

1 large onion, sliced

1 large tomato, chopped

Leaves from 1 bunch fresh mint

Four 6-ounce boneless, skinless chicken breasts, pounded lightly

1 lemon, sliced

½ teaspoon crushed red chili flakes

2 cups water or low-sodium chicken stock

1 Preheat the oven to 400° F. In a medium bowl, lightly mash the chickpeas with a fork.

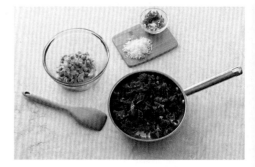

2 Heat the oil in large sauté pan over medium-high heat. Add the kale and garlic and sauté for 2 minutes. Remove from the heat. Add the cooked kale to the chickpeas, then add the scallions and cheese. Cool.

3 Scatter the onion and the tomato on the bottom of a 9 x 12-inch baking dish. Layer on the mint leaves.

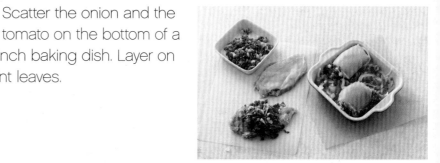

4 Gently fold the chicken breasts around the chickpea mixture and add to the baking dish. Top with the lemon slices and chili flakes and pour in the stock.

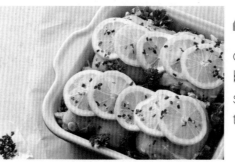

UNSTUFFED CABBAGE

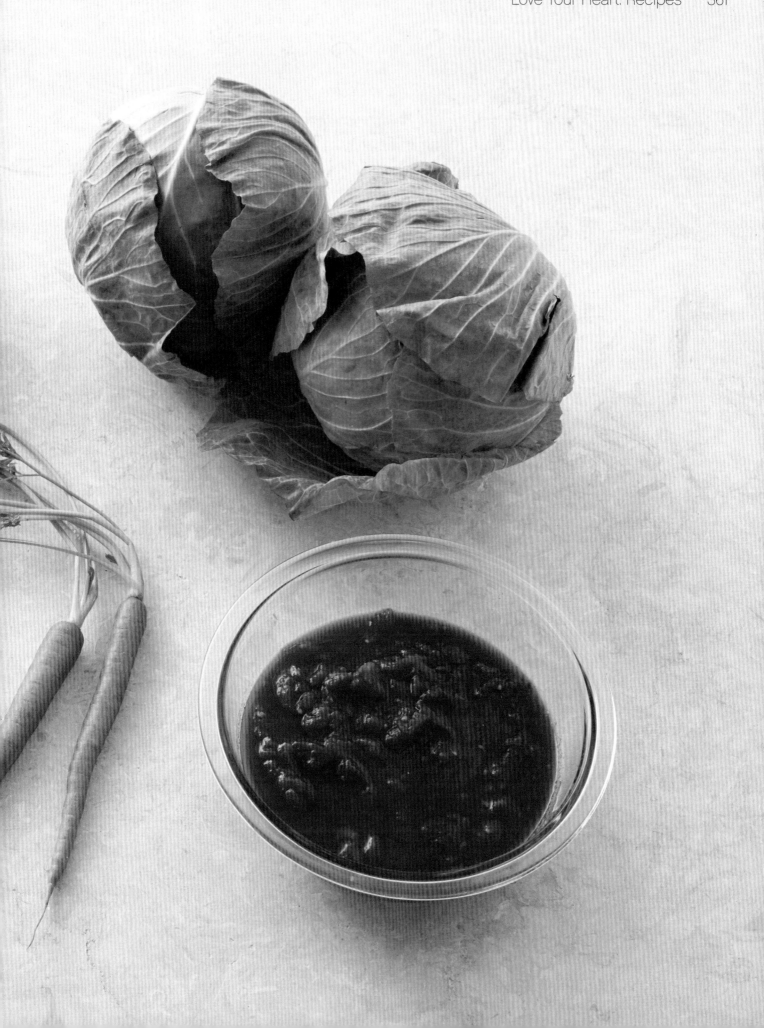

UNSTUFFED CABBAGE

SUGAR 3.4 tsp

TIME 60 minutes

SERVES four

INGREDIENTS

2 teaspoons extra virgin olive oil

1 medium onion, chopped

2 small carrots, shredded

1 pound lean ground turkey

4 cups shredded green cabbage

One 28-ounce can low-sodium chopped tomatoes

1 cup tomato puree

¼ cup apple cider vinegar

1 Heat the oil in a large skillet over medium heat. Add the onion and carrots and sauté for 2 minutes. Add the turkey and sauté for 5 minutes. Add the cabbage and sauté for 2 minutes.

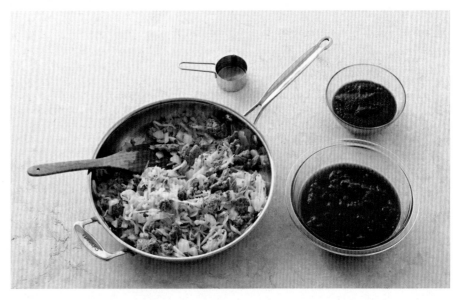

2 Add the tomatoes with their juices, the tomato puree, and vinegar. Bring to a boil, then reduce the heat, cover, and simmer for 45 minutes.

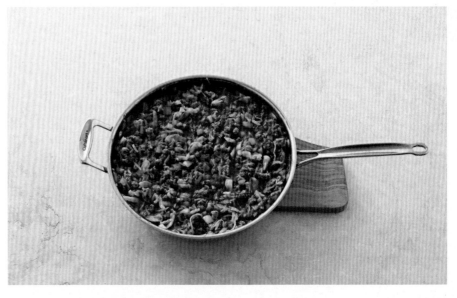

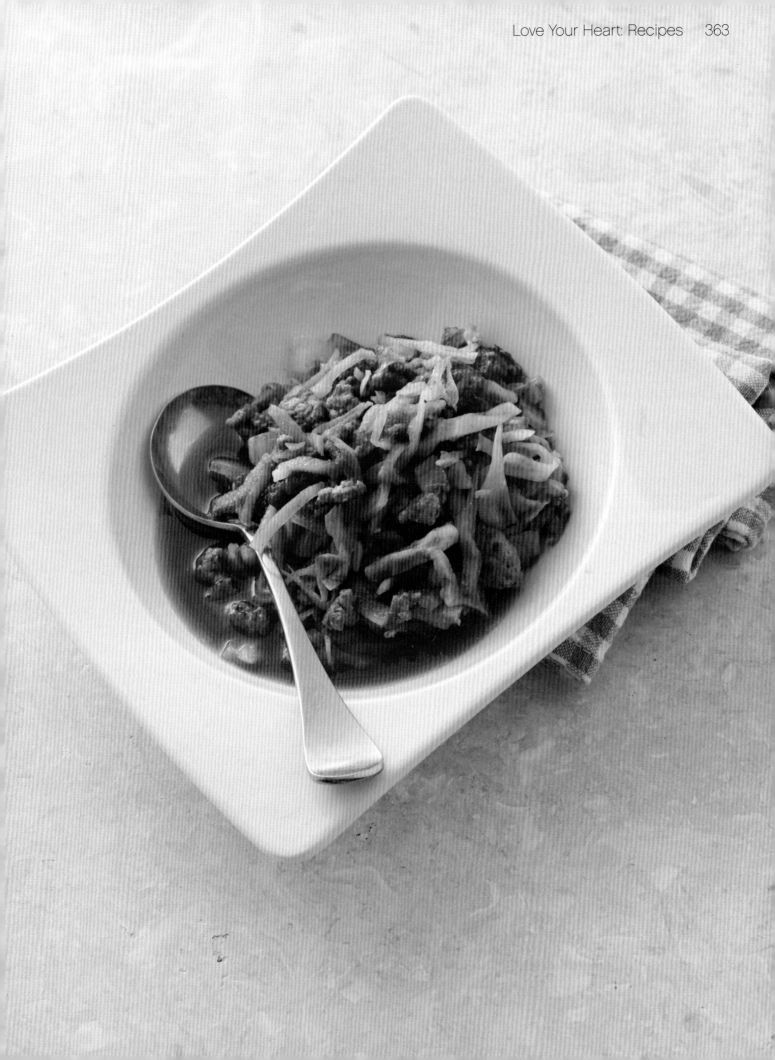

NON-OAT NUTMEAL

SUGAR 2.3 tsp

TIME 15 minutes

SERVES three

INGREDIENTS

¼ cup raw cashews

¼ cup walnut halves

¼ cup pecan halves

3 tablespoons ground flaxseed

1 teaspoon ground cinnamon

¼ teaspoon ground ginger

1 large egg

½ cup unsweetened almond milk

1 tablespoon almond butter

1 teaspoon butterlike spread

Handful of fresh blackberries

1 Combine the nuts, flaxseed, cinnamon, and ginger in a food processor or blender. Process until the nuts are coarsely ground.

2 In a medium bowl, whisk the egg with the almond milk and almond butter.

3 Stir the ground nuts into the egg mixture.

4 Transfer to a medium saucepan, place over medium heat, and cook, stirring frequently, until it reaches your desired consistency, about 5 minutes

5 Divide among serving bowls and top with the butterlike spread and the blackberries.

VEGGIE-EGG PATTIES

SUGAR 0.6 tsp

TIME 30 minutes

SERVES three

INGREDIENTS

1 zucchini

1 red bell pepper

½ medium onion, chopped

1 large egg

Salt and freshly ground pepper

3 tablespoons canola oil

1 Grate the zucchini and bell pepper and dice the onion.

2 In a medium bowl, mix the zucchini, bell pepper, onion, and egg together. Season with salt and pepper.

3 Heat the oil in a medium skillet over medium heat.

4 Form the vegetable mixture into 2-inch balls and place in the pan. Flatten the balls with a spatula and cook until lightly browned, 6 to 8 minutes each side.

TURKEY SAUSAGE PATTIES

SUGAR 0.1 tsp

TIME 30 minutes

SERVES three

INGREDIENTS

1 pound ground turkey

1 teaspoon dried sage

½ teaspoon fennel seeds

2 cloves garlic, minced

½ teaspoon salt

Dash of ground black pepper

Dash of ground cayenne

Dash of ground allspice

1 Combine all the ingredients in a large bowl.

2 Shape into 2-inch patties, place on a plate, cover with plastic, and refrigerate for at least 1 hour.

3 Heat a large skillet over medium-high heat. Add the patties and cook for 4 to 6 minutes on each side, until the patties are cooked through.

MINI EGG FRITTATAS

SUGAR 0.5 tsp

TIME 30 minutes

SERVES eight

INGREDIENTS

3 teaspoons coconut oil

½ cup chopped onion

½ cup chopped mushrooms

1 cup chopped baby spinach

4 large eggs

2 tablespoons unsweetened almond milk

Salt and freshly ground pepper

1 Preheat the oven to 350°F. Coat two 12-hole mini muffin pans with 2 of the teaspoons coconut oil.

2 Heat the remaining 1 teaspoon coconut oil in a medium skillet over medium heat. Add the onion and mushrooms and sauté until softened, about 5 minutes.

3 Add the chopped spinach and cook until just wilted, about 2 minutes. Remove from the heat and set aside to cool.

4 In a medium bowl, whisk the eggs and almond milk. Add the cooled spinach mixture and salt and pepper to taste.

5 Pour the mixture into the muffin pans, filling the holes about halfway.

6 Bake for 15 to 20 minutes, until set. Remove the frittatas from the pans and serve.

JICAMA BEET SALAD

SUGAR 1.3 tsp

TIME 15 minutes

SERVES four

INGREDIENTS

½ large jicama

1 red beet

1 golden beet

1 tablespoon lime juice

½ teaspoon minced fresh ginger

Salt to taste

1 Peel and julienne the jicama and beets and place them in a large bowl.

2 Add the lime juice, ginger, and salt. Mix well to coat, and serve.

CAULIFLOWER "RICE" PILAF

SUGAR 0.6 tsp

TIME 30 minutes

SERVES eight

INGREDIENTS

¼ cup slivered almonds

1 medium head cauliflower

2 tablespoons extra virgin olive oil

2 tablespoons chopped onion

2 stalks of celery, chopped

1 clove garlic, minced

½ cup low-sodium chicken stock

¼ teaspoon fennel seeds

¼ teaspoon dried oregano

Dash of curry powder

1 Toast the slivered almonds in a skillet over medium heat. Remove from the heat and set aside to cool.

2 Grate the cauliflower using the large holes of a box grater or in a food processor with the grating blade.

3 Heat the oil in a large skillet over medium heat. Add the onion, celery, garlic, and cauliflower and sauté for 2 minutes.

4 Add the chicken stock, fennel, oregano, and curry powder and cook for about 10 minutes, or until desired consistency.

5 Remove from the heat, stir in the toasted almonds, and serve.

SPAGHETTI SQUASH "PASTA"

SUGAR 1.6 tsp

TIME 40 minutes

SERVES four

INGREDIENTS

1 spaghetti squash

1 Preheat the oven to 400°F.

2 Cut the squash in half lengthwise and remove the seeds. Place the halves face down on a baking dish and pour in water to come about ½ inch up the sides. Place the dish in the oven and bake for 30 minutes, or until tender.

3 Turn the squash over and cool until it is cool enough to handle. Using the tines of a fork, remove and discard the seeds and scrape out the squash. It will string like spaghetti.

CAULIFLOWER MASH

SUGAR 1 tsp

TIME 30 minutes

SERVES four

INGREDIENTS

1 pound cauliflower, trimmed

½ cup water

½ cup low-sodium chicken broth

1 tablespoon olive oil

1 Cut cauliflower, including the core, into 1-inch pieces. Bring the water and stock to a boil in a large pot. Add cauliflower pieces. Cook until tender, 20–30 minutes.

2 Drain cauliflower in colander and press with a small plate to release all the liquid in the cauliflower (this step is important for the texture of the dish).

3 Transfer cauliflower into a food processor. Add olive oil and puree the mixture until it becomes smooth and creamy.

SOUTHERN KALE

SUGAR 2.8 tsp

TIME 15 minutes

SERVES six

INGREDIENTS

1 tablespoon olive oil

2 teaspoons minced garlic

½ cup low-sodium chicken stock

15 cups rinsed, stemmed, and torn kale

¼ teaspoon crushed red pepper

Black pepper to taste

1 Heat oil in a deep skillet over medium heat. Add garlic and stock; stir. Add kale by handfuls, stirring to make room for more leaves.

2 Cover with a lid and cook, stirring occasionally for 10–15 minutes.

3 Uncover and cook until leaves are tender.

4 Add red pepper and black pepper. Toss and serve.

WILTED CABBAGE

SUGAR 0.6 tsp

TIME 10 minutes

SERVES six

INGREDIENTS

1 teaspoon olive oil

6 cups savoy cabbage or Chinese cabbage

¼ cup low-sodium chicken stock

Fresh ground black pepper

½ teaspoon cumin seeds

2 teaspoons apple cider vinegar

1 Heat oil in a Dutch oven over medium heat. Add cabbage and stock and cook about 3–4 minutes until cabbage starts to wilt, stirring occasionally. Stir in pepper.

2 Put cumin seeds in a small saucepan and toast over medium heat 1 minute, shaking pan frequently.

3 Add seeds and apple cider vinegar to cabbage and cook 3 more minutes until tender, stirring occasionally.

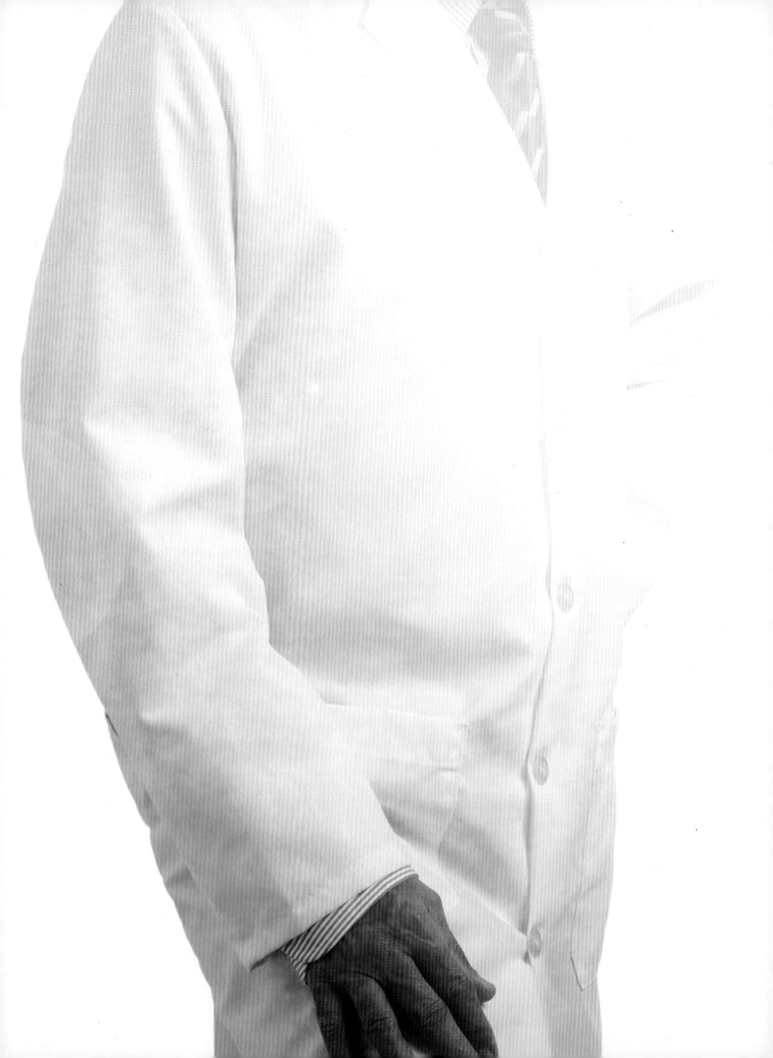

doctor bios

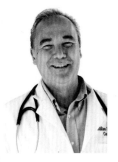

Dr. William Davis

(page 76) William Davis, MD, is a preventive cardiologist and author of the New York Times bestseller, *Wheat Belly: Lose the Wheat, Lose the Weight and Find Your Path Back to Health* whose unique wheat-free approach to diet allows him to advocate reversal, not just prevention, of heart disease. He is the medical director of Track Your Plaque, an online heart disease prevention program, and writes frequently for national publications and health Web sites. He lives with his wife and three children in Fox Point, Wisconsin, where there are no bagels or muffins in his cupboards.

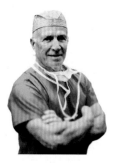

Dr. Dwight Lundell

(page 124) Dr. Lundell's experience in cardiovascular and thoracic surgery over the last 25 years includes certification by the American Board of Surgery, the American Board of Thoracic Surgery, and the Society of Thoracic Surgeons. Dr. Lundell was a pioneer in "off-pump" heart surgery, reducing surgical complications and recovery times. He's in the Beating Heart Hall of Fame and has been listed in Phoenix Magazine's Top Doctors for 10 years. Dr. Lundell has performed over 5000 coronary bypass operations.

He has been recognized by his peers as a leader and has served as Chief resident at the University of Arizona and Yale University Hospitals and later served as Chief of Staff and Chief of Surgery at Lutheran Heart Hospital.

He was one of the founding partners of the Lutheran Heart Hospital which became the second largest heart hospital in U.S. and is now owned by Banner Health.

As a recognized leader in his field, Dr. Lundell has consulted and advised for a variety of leading medical device manufacturers such as Cardio Thoracic Systems, Inc. before and after its acquisition by Guidant Corporation. He advised St. Jude Medical on tissue valve implantation and marketing. For A-Med, Inc., he consulted on, conducted, and published the first clinical study on miniature pumps for heart support. He co-authored a clinical study validating key technology for Coalescent Surgical, which was subsequently acquired by Medtronic, Inc.

Dr. Lundell now devotes his career to the prevention of heart disease and other chronic diseases; he is the author of *The Cure for Heart Disease and The Great Cholesterol Lie*, he has recently appeared on Fox and Friends three times as an expert on heart disease.

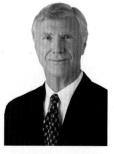

Dr. Leonard Smith

(page 144) Leonard Smith, MD is a board-certified general, gastrointestinal, and vascular surgeon. During his 25 years in private practice in Gainesville, FL not only did he maintain an active surgery practice, but he also incorporated lifestyle, diet, supplementation, exercise, detoxification, and stress management into his practice. Many of his patients with cancer, cardiovascular disease, and many other serious illnesses did so well with these programs that he began to devote most of his time to foundational health care and preventative medicine. Currently, Dr. Smith is on the volunteer faculty at the University of Miami Department of Surgery and Department of Integrative Medicine.

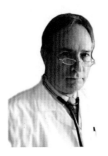

Dr. Thomas E. Levy

(page 184) Thomas E. Levy, MD, JD is a board-certified cardiologist and a bar-certified attorney. After practicing adult cardiology for 15 years, he became aware of the enormous toxicity associated with much dental work, as well as the pronounced ability of properly-administered vitamin C to neutralize much of this toxicity. He has written three books on the wide-ranging properties of vitamin C, addressing its ability to neutralize all toxins and resolve most infections, as well as its ability to resolve or substantially curtail many chronic degenerative diseases, including cancer and coronary heart disease. Additional books have addressed optimal nutrition and the specifics of dental toxicity.

Currently, Dr. Levy continues to research the impact of vitamin C and antioxidants in general on chronic degenerative diseases. His current research involves documenting that all diseases arise from increased oxidative stress, and that they all benefit from protocols that optimize the antioxidant levels in the body. His present focus centers on validating the ability of a protocol of toxin removal and antioxidant support to angiographically normalize most moderate and even much advanced atherosclerotic coronary artery disease.

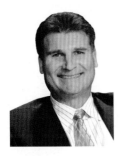

Dr. Rick Sponaugle

(page 194) Marvin "Rick" Sponaugle, MD, board certified in addiction medicine and anesthesiology, and founder of Sponaugle Wellness Center and Florida Detox, has been featured on Dr. Phil, CNN, and other national media. Dr. Sponaugle is the first addictionologist to correlate SPECT brain imaging with brain chemistry imbalances that cause specific drug craving patterns. He has also proven that hormonal imbalance in middle-aged women causes 60 percent of their addiction issues. His scientific addiction treatment stops drug craving producing only 9 percent relapse.

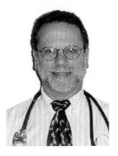

Dr. Ronald Cohn

(page 212) Dr. R. Ernest Cohn is one of the nation's few practicing physicians that have completed medical, chiropractic and naturopathic training. While he is board certified in orthopedics, he has practiced integrative medicine for more than 20 of his 35 years in practice. He presently limits his practice to the treatment of chronic and difficult conditions and the practice commonly sees cancers, Lyme disease, chronic fatigue, Epstein-Barr syndrome, cardiovascular, environmental, and nutritional dysfunctions. The practice does nutritional and IV therapies and uses conventional and integrative therapies that consist of IV and oral chelation, IV and oral nutrition, hyperbaric oxygen, colonic irrigation, lymphatic drainage, musculoskeletal medicine, and much more. His practice differs from most in that every patient is seen by multiple doctors so that multiple therapies can be applied when needed. He can be reached through his website at Holisticmedclinic@earthink.net for more information.

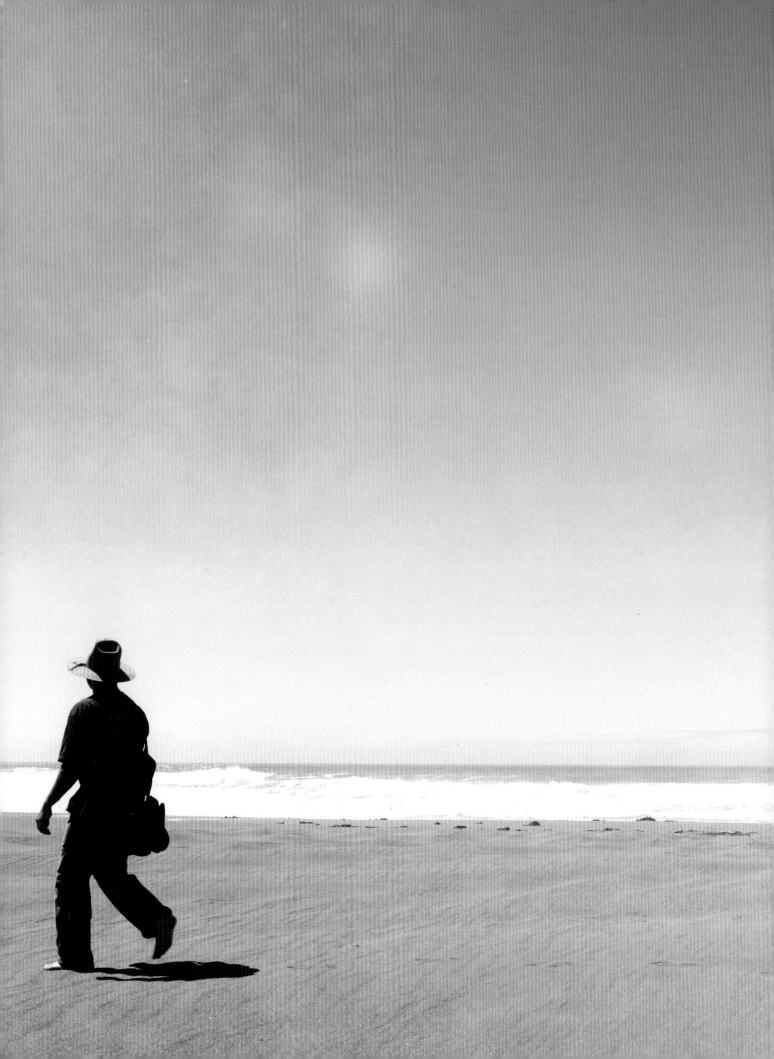

resources

Medical and Health Organizations

American Heart Association
7272 Greenville Avenue
Dallas, TX 75231
www.heart.org

Centers for Disease Control and Prevention (CDC)
Division of Nutrition, Physical Activity, and Obesity
www.cdc.gov/obesity

Vitamin D Council
1241 Johnson Avenue #134
San Luis Obispo, CA 93401
www.vitamindcouncil.org

Institute for Functional Medicine
505 South 336th Suite 500
Federal Way, WA 98003
www.functionalmedicine.org

American College for Advancement in Medicine
8001 Irvine Center Drive, Suite 825
Irvine, CA 92618
www.acam.org

American Academy of Anti-Aging Medicine
1801 North Military Trail, Suite 200
Boca Raton, FL 33431
www.a4m.com

American Chiropractic Association
1701 Clarendon Boulevard
Arlington, VA 22209
www.acatoday.org

Life Extension Foundation
P.O. Box 407198
Fort Lauderdale, FL 33340
www.lef.org

Track Your Plaque Program
Dr. William Davis
2600 North Mayfair Road, Suite 950
Wauwatosa, WI 53226
www.trackyourplaque.com
www.wheatbellyblog.com

LivOn Laboratories
Dr. Thomas Levy
4001 West Green Tree Road
Milwaukee, WI 53209
www.livonlabs.com

Holistic Medical Clinic of the Carolinas
Dr. R. Ernest Cohn
308 East Main Street
Wilkesboro, NC 28697
www.holisticmedclinic.com

Dr. Dwight Lundell
www.truthaboutheartdisease.org

Sponaugle Wellness Center
Florida Detox
Dr. Rick Sponaugle
32815 US Highway 19 North
Palm Harbor, FL 34684
www.floridadetox.com

Functional Testing Laboratories

LipoScience, Inc.
Nuclear Magnetic Resonance lipoprotein test
2500 Summer Boulevard
Raleigh, NC 27616
www.liposcience.com

Atherotech Diagnostics Lab
VAP lipoprotein test
201 London Parkway
Birmingham, AL 35211
www.atherotech.com

Berkley HeartLab
Electrophoretic lipoprotein test
468 Littlefield Avenue
South San Fransisco, CA 94080
www.bhlinc.com

OmegaQuant
Omega-3 Index
2329 North Career Avenue, Suite 113
Sioux Falls, SD 57107
www.omegaquant.com

Genova Diagnostics
63 Zillicoa Street
Asheville, NC 28801
www.gdx.net

Doctor's Data
3755 Illinois Avenue
Saint Charles, IL 60174
www.doctorsdata.com

EnteroLab
10875 Plano Road, Suite 123
Dallas, TX 75238
www.enterolab.com

Heidelberg pH Diagnostic Test
P.O. Box 529
Mineral Bluff, GA 30559
www.phcapsule.com

Real-Time Laboratories
4100 Fairway Court, Suite 600
Carrollton, TX 75010
www.real-timelabs.com

Lab Testing Direct
Online access to functional
and conventional testing.
1593 Main Street
Dunedin, FL 34698
www.labtestingdirect.com

Complementary Therapies

American Academy of Medical Acupuncture
1970 East Grand Avenue, Suite 330
El Segundo, CA 90245
www.medicalacupuncture.org

American Massage Therapy Association
500 Davis Street, Suite 900
Evanston, IL 60201-4695
www.amtamassage.org

(Complementary Therapies continued)

American Music Therapy Association
8455 Colesville Road, Suite 1000
Silver Spring, MD 20910
www.musictherapy.org

Institute of HeartMath
emWave device
14700 West Park Avenue
Boulder Creek, CA 95006
www.heartmath.org

International Association of Colon Therapists
(I-ACT)
P.O. Box 461285
San Antonio, TX 78246-1285
www.i-act.org

Yoga Alliance
1701 Clarendon Boulevard, Suite 110
Arlington, VA 22209
www.yogaalliance.org

Environmental Toxin Information

Environmental Working Group
1436 U Street Northwest, Suite 100
Washington, DC 20009
www.ewg.org

Pesticide Action Network North America
49 Powell Street, Suite 500
San Fransisco, CA 94102
www.panna.org

AIRNow
Current Air Quality Index
U.S. EPA
Office of Air Quality Planning and Standards
(OAQPA)
Mail Code E143-03
Research Triangle Park, NC 27711
www.airnow.gov

National Institute of Environmental Health
Sciences
P.O. Box 12233
Research Triangle Park, NC 27709
www.niehs.nih.gov

Dietary Supplements

ReNew Life Formulas
198 Alternate 19 South
Palm Harbor, FL 34683
www.renewlife.com

Advanced Naturals
198 Alternate 19 South
Palm Harbor, FL 34683
www.advancednaturals.com

Pure Encapsulations
490 Boston Post Road
Sudbury, MA 01776
www.purecaps.com

Source Naturals
23 Janis Way
Scotts Valley, CA 95066
www.sourcenaturals.com

LivOn Laboratories
Dr. Thomas Levy
4001 West Green Tree Road
Milwaukee, WI 53209
www.livonlabs.com

International Fish Oil Standards Program
120 Research Lane Suite 203
University of Guelph Research Park
Guelph, Ontario, Canada
N1G 4W4
www.ifosprogram.com

Comprehensive Library of Research on
Probiotics
www.probiotic-research.com

Books

By Brenda Watson, CNC and
Leonard Smith, MD
The Road to Perfect Health
The Fiber35 Diet
The Detox Strategy
Gut Solutions
Renew Your Life
Essential Cleansing
The HOPE Formula

By William Davis, MD
Wheat Belly
Track Your Plaque

By Thomas Levy, MD, JD
Stop America's #1 Killer
Curing the Incurable

By Dwight Lundell, MD
The Cure for Heart Disease

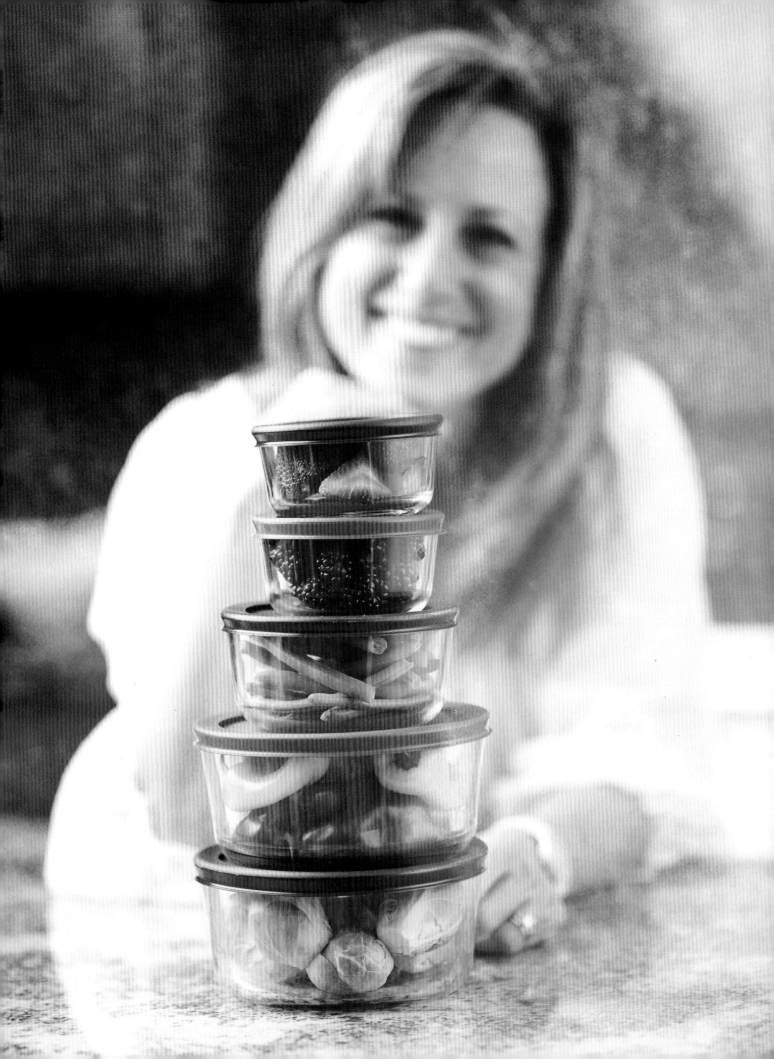

fruit and vegetable

teaspoons of sugar

$$\text{teaspoons of sugar} = (\text{carbohydrates}^{\text{total}} - \text{dietary fiber}) \div 5$$

Fruit Teaspoons of Sugar

Apple, 1 large	5.2
Apricot, 1	0.6
Avocado, 1	0.8
Banana, medium	4.8
Blackberries, 4 ounces	1.6
Blueberries, 4 ounces	2.4
Cantelope, 1 wedge	1.6
Carambola (starfruit), 1 large	1
Cherimoya, 1 cup	4.8
Cherries, sour, 1 cup	2.2
Cherries, sweet, 1 cup	3.8
Cranberries, raw, 1 cup	1.5
Fig, 1 large	2
Grapefruit, pink, ½ large	2.2
Grapefruit, white, ½ large	1.8
Grapes, 1 cup	3
Guava, 1	1
Honeydew melon, 1 cup	1.7

Kiwifruit, 1	2
Kumquat 1	0.4
Lemon, 1	1.2
Lime, 1	1
Litchi, 1	0.4
Mango, 1	6.2
Orange, 1 large	3.6
Papaya, 1 cup	2.2
Passionfruit, one	0.4
Peach, 1 large	2.8
Pear, 1 large	5.8
Pineapple, 1 cup	4
Plantain, 1	10.6
Plum, 1	1.4
Pomegranate, ½ cup arils	2.6
Raspberries, 4 ounces	0.8
Rhubarb, 1 stalk	0.2
Strawberries, ½ cup sliced	1
Tangerine, 1 large	2.8
Watermelon, 1 wedge	4.2

Vegetable Teaspoons of Sugar

Artichoke hearts, ½ cup	0.3
Arugula, ½ cup	0
Asparagus, ½ cup	0.2
Green beans, ½ cup	0.4
Beets, ½ cup	0.9
Broccoli, ½ cup	0.4
Brussels sprouts, ½ cup	0.5
Cabbage, ½ cup shredded	0.1
Carrots, ½ cup	0.8
Cassava (yucca), ½ cup	7.4
Cauliflower, ½ cup	0.2
Celery, 1 stalk	0.1
Swiss chard, ½ cup	0
Chives, 1 tablespoon	0
Collards, ½ cup	0.1
Corn, 1 large ear	4.6
Cucumber, ½ cup	0.4
Eggplant, ½ cup	0.2
Endive, ½ cup	0
Fennel, ½ cup	0.3
Kale, ½ cup	0.6
Kohlrabi, ½ cup	0.3
Lettuce, ½ cup	0
Mushrooms, ½ cup	0.4
Nopales, ½ cup	0.1
Okra, ½ cup	0.4

(measures reflect raw vegetables)

Onions, ½ cup	1.2
Parsnips, ½ cup	8.5
Snowpeas/snapeas, ½ cup	0.4
Green peas, ½ cup	1.4
Hot pepper, 1	0.2–0.6
Bell pepper, green, 1 large	1
Bell pepper, red, 1 large	1.4
Bell pepper, yellow, 1 large	2
Potato, 1 large	12
Pumpkin, ½ cup	0.7
Radicchio, ½ cup	0.2
Radish, 1 large	0
Rutabaga, ½ cup	0.7
Shallot, 1 tablespoon	0.4
Soybeans, green, ½ cup	1.7
Spinach, ½ cup	0
Summer squash, ½ cup	0.3
Zucchini, ½ cup	0.3
Acorn squash, ½ cup	1.3
Butternut squash, ½ cup	1.3
Spaghetti squash, ½ cup	0.7
Sweet potato, ½ cup	2.3
Tomatillo, 1	0.2
Tomato, green, 1 large	1.4
Tomato, red, 1 large	1
Turnip, ½ cup	0.6
Watercress, ½ cup	0
Yam, ½ cup	3.6

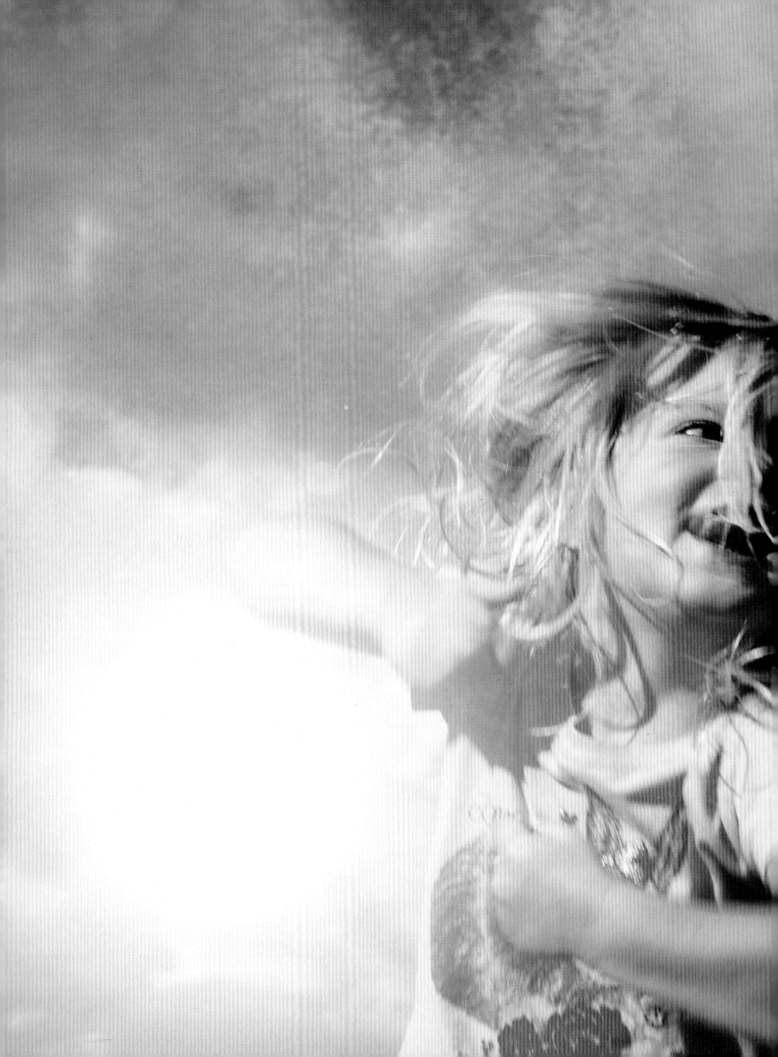

nutritional facts

Warm Shrooms-n-Spinach page 288

Yield is 4 servings

Serving size is one-quarter of recipe

2.2 teaspoons of sugar

Basic Nutritional Values:

Calories	120
Calories from Fat	55
Total Fat	6 g
Saturated Fat	0.5 g
Trans Fat	0 g
Cholesterol	0 mg
Sodium	250 mg
Total Carbohydrate	15 g
Dietary Fiber	4 g
Sugars	5 g
Protein	6 g

Eggplant Roulades page 292

Yield is 6 servings

Serving size is 2 roulades

4.2 teaspoons of sugar

Basic Nutritional Values:

Calories	285
Calories from Fat	115
Total Fat	13 g
Saturated Fat	6 g
Trans Fat	0 g
Cholesterol	65 mg
Sodium	790 mg
Total Carbohydrate	26 g
Dietary Fiber	5 g
Sugars	11 g
Protein	18 g

Chicken Lime Cobb page 296

Yield is 2 servings

Serving size is half of recipe

2 teaspoons of sugar

Basic Nutritional Values:

Calories	430
Calories from Fat	180
Total Fat	20 g
Saturated Fat	5 g
Trans Fat	0 g
Cholesterol	200 mg
Sodium	495 mg
Total Carbohydrate	17 g
Dietary Fiber	7 g
Sugars	8 g
Protein	46 g

Indian Spiced Garbanzos page 300

Yield is 4 servings

Serving size one-quarter of recipe

3.4 teaspoons of sugar

Basic Nutritional Values:

Calories	165
Calories from Fat	35
Total Fat	4 g
Saturated Fat	0.5 g
Trans Fat	0 g
Cholesterol	0 mg
Sodium	245 mg
Total Carbohydrate	24 g
Dietary Fiber	7 g
Sugars	7 g
Protein	8 g

Butternut Chowder page 304

Yield is 8 servings
Serving size is one-eighth of recipe
2.6 teaspoons of sugar
Basic Nutritional Values:

Calories	125
Calories from Fat	40
Total Fat	4.5 gm
Saturated Fat	1 g
Trans Fat	0 g
Cholesterol	0 mg
Sodium	150 mg
Total Carbohydrate	18 g
Dietary Fiber	5 g
Sugars	5 g
Protein	4 g

Toasted Pepitas page 304

Makes 1 cup.
0.2 teaspoon of sugar
Basic Nutritional Values:*

Calories	50
Calories from Fat	40
Total Fat	4.5 g
Saturated Fat	0.5 g
Trans Fat	0 g
Cholesterol	0 mg
Sodium	0 mg
Total Carbohydrate	1 g
Dietary Fiber	0 g
Sugars	0 g
Protein	2 g

Grouper-n-Greens page 308

Yield is 4 servings
Serving size is ½ fillet and about ¼ cup greens
1.6 teaspoons of sugar
Sauce Basic Nutritional Values:

Calories	208
Calories from Fat	74
Total Fat	8.4 g
Saturated Fat	1.3 g
Trans Fat	0 g
Cholesterol	41.4 mg
Sodium	114 mg
Total Carbohydrate	9.7 g
Dietary Fiber	1.5 g
Sugars	0.3 g
Protein	24.3 g

Seared Sesame Tuna page 312

Yield is 4 servings
Serving size is one-quarter of recipe
0.2 teaspoon of sugar
Basic Nutritional Values:**

Calories	175
Calories from Fat	65
Total Fat	7 gm
Saturated Fat	1.5 g
Trans Fat	0 g
Cholesterol	40 mg
Sodium	45 mg
Total Carbohydrate	1 g
Dietary Fiber	0 g
Sugars	0 g
Protein	26 g

*Recipe Comment: The analysis for this recipe is based on 1 tablespoon/serving, 16 servings/recipe

**Recipe Comment: This analysis is just for the tuna. You can substitute other fish if you cook it thoroughly.

Asian Slaw page 312

Yield is 4 to 6 servings

Serving size is one-quarter or one-sixth of recipe

0.8 teaspoon of sugar

Basic Nutritional Values:

Calories	50
Calories from Fat	20
Total Fat	2.5 g
Saturated Fat	0 g
Trans Fat	0 g
Cholesterol	0 mg
Sodium	115 mg
Total Carbohydrate	6 g
Dietary Fiber	2 g
Sugars	3 g
Protein	1 g

Caramelized Garlic
for Garlic-n-Lemon Shrimp page 316

Yield is 4 servings

Serving size is 1 tablespoon

0.6 teaspoon of sugar

Basic Nutritional Values:

Calories	40
Calories from Fat	30
Total Fat	3.5 g
Saturated Fat	0 g
Trans Fat	0 g
Cholesterol	0 mg
Sodium	0 mg
Total Carbohydrate	3 g
Dietary Fiber	0 g
Sugars	0 g
Protein	1 g

Garlic-n-Lemon Shrimp page 316

Yield is 4 servings

Serving size is one-quarter recipe

0.8 teaspoons of sugar

Basic Nutritional Values:*

Calories	170
Calories from Fat	55
Total Fat	6 g
Saturated Fat	1 g
Trans Fat	0 g
Cholesterol	185 mg
Sodium	965 mg
Total Carbohydrate	4 g
Dietary Fiber	0 g
Sugars	0 g
Protein	25 g

Seafood Gumbo page 320

Yield is 4 servings

Serving size is one-eighth recipe

1.8 teaspoons of sugar

Basic Nutritional Values:* **

Calories	125
Calories from Fat	25
Total Fat	3 g
Saturated Fat	0.5 g
Trans Fat	0 g
Cholesterol	85 mg
Sodium	640 mg
Total Carbohydrate	12 g
Dietary Fiber	3 g
Sugars	5 g
Protein	12 g

In 2011, the USDA did a survey of various species of fish in retail (supermarkets) in 12 locations around the country. They found that the fish (including shrimp) were higher in sodium than previously thought. The reason appears to be that the fish are frozen and treated with chemicals (containing sodium) that retard moisture release during thawing. Thus, for "supermarket shrimp," the gold standard USDA nutrient database (version 24, 2011) indicates that sodium is 269 mg/cooked oz.; if shrimp is not previously frozen (e.g., fresh off the trawlers), the sodium is about 80 mg/cooked ounce.

*Reflects frozen shrimp used in recipe. To lower sodium, look for fresh wild harvest shrimp.
**The optional ingredient (okra) not included in the analysis.

'Cress Stuffed Steak page 324

Yield is 2 servings

Serving size is half of recipe

1.4 teaspoons of sugar

Basic Nutritional Values:

Calories	210
Calories from Fat	70
Total Fat	8 g
Saturated Fat	2 g
Trans Fat	0 g
Cholesterol	60 mg
Sodium	40 mg
Total Carbohydrate	9 g
Dietary Fiber	2 g
Sugars	4 g
Protein	25 g

Persian Kabob page 328

Yield is 4 servings

Serving size is one-quarter of recipe

1.6 teaspoons of sugar

Basic Nutritional Values:

Calories	230
Calories from Fat	90
Total Fat	10 g
Saturated Fat	3.5 g
Trans Fat	0.5 g
Cholesterol	70 mg
Sodium	400 mg
Total Carbohydrate	11 g
Dietary Fiber	3 g
Sugars	6 g
Protein	25 g

Beef Bruschetta page 332

Yield is 2 servings

Serving size is half of recipe

1.4 teaspoons of sugar

Basic Nutritional Values:

Calories	205
Calories from Fat	55
Total Fat	6 g
Saturated Fat	1.5 g
Trans Fat	0 g
Cholesterol	60 mg
Sodium	210 mg
Total Carbohydrate	10 g
Dietary Fiber	3 g
Sugars	4 g
Protein	26 g

Beef-n-Veggie Bolognese page 336

Yield is 6 servings

Serving size one-sixth of recipe

2.2 teaspoons of sugar

Basic Nutritional Values:

Calories	220
Calories from Fat	65
Total Fat	7 g
Saturated Fat	2.5 g
Trans Fat	0 g
Cholesterol	65 mg
Sodium	195 mg
Total Carbohydrate	15 g
Dietary Fiber	4 g
Sugars	8 g
Protein	24 g

Athenian Meatballs page 340

Yield is 6 servings

Serving size is one-sixth of recipe

0.6 teaspoon of sugar

Basic Nutritional Values:

Calories	180
Calories from Fat	100
Total Fat	11 g
Saturated Fat	4.5 g
Trans Fat	0 g
Cholesterol	80 mg
Sodium	155 mg
Total Carbohydrate	4 g
Dietary Fiber	1 g
Sugars	2 g
Protein	16 g

Lemongrass Chicken page 348

Yield is 4 servings

Serving size is one-quarter recipe

1.6 teaspoons of sugar

Basic Nutritional Values:

Calories	230
Calories from Fat	65
Total Fat	7 g
Saturated Fat	1 g
Trans Fat	0 g
Cholesterol	75 mg
Sodium	365 mg
Total Carbohydrate	11 g
Dietary Fiber	3 g
Sugars	2 g
Protein	31 g

Sicilian Citrus Pork page 344

Yield is 6 servings

Serving size is one-sixth of recipe

0.6 teaspoon of sugar

Basic Nutritional Values:

Calories	240
Calories from Fat	110
Total Fat	12 g
Saturated Fat	3.5 g
Trans Fat	0 g
Cholesterol	80 mg
Sodium	50 mg
Total Carbohydrate	4 g
Dietary Fiber	1 g
Sugars	2 g
Protein	28 g

Chicken Milanese page 352

Yield is 2 servings

Serving size is half of recipe

1.2 teaspoons of sugar

Basic Nutritional Values:

Calories	280
Calories from Fat	155
Total Fat	17 g
Saturated Fat	3 g
Trans Fat	0 g
Cholesterol	55 mg
Sodium	135 mg
Total Carbohydrate	7 g
Dietary Fiber	1 g
Sugars	2 g
Protein	25 g

Ligurian Chicken page 356

Yield is 4 servings

Serving size is one-quarter of recipe

3.6 teaspoons of sugar

Basic Nutritional Values:

Calories	380
Calories from Fat	115
Total Fat	13 g
Saturated Fat	3 g
Trans Fat	0 g
Cholesterol	100 mg
Sodium	200 mg
Total Carbohydrate	24 g
Dietary Fiber	6 g
Sugars	7 g
Protein	43 g

Non-Oat Nutmeal page 364

Yield is 3 servings

Serving size is one-third of recipe

0.7 teaspoons of sugar

Basic Nutritional Values:

Calories	170
Calories from Fat	132
Total Fat	15.6 g
Saturated Fat	2.1 g
Trans Fat	0 g
Cholesterol	23.5 mg
Sodium	24.8 mg
Total Carbohydrate	6.0 g
Dietary Fiber	2.6 g
Sugars	1.3 g
Protein	4.2 g

Unstuffed Cabbage page 360

Yield is 4 servings

Serving size is one-quarter of recipe

3.4 teaspoons of sugar

Basic Nutritional Values:

Calories	295
Calories from Fat	110
Total Fat	12 g
Saturated Fat	3 g
Trans Fat	0 g
Cholesterol	85 mg
Sodium	195 mg
Total Carbohydrate	23 g
Dietary Fiber	6 g
Sugars	12 g
Protein	26 g

Veggie-Egg Patties page 365

Yield is 3 servings

Serving size is 2 patties

0.6 teaspoon of sugar

Basic Nutritional Values:

Calories	165
Calories from Fat	136
Total Fat	15.3 g
Saturated Fat	1.6 g
Trans Fat	0 g
Cholesterol	70.3 mg
Sodium	25.8 mg
Total Carbohydrate	4.5 g
Dietary Fiber	1.2 g
Sugars	2.6 g
Protein	2.8 g

Turkey Sausage Patties page 366

Yield is 3 servings
Serving size is 3 patties
0.1 teaspoon of sugar
Basic Nutritional Values:

Calories	230
Calories from Fat	113
Total Fat	12.6 g
Saturated Fat	3.4 g
Trans Fat	0 g
Cholesterol	119.3 mg
Sodium	143.7 mg
Total Carbohydrate	0.9 g
Dietary Fiber	0.2 g
Sugars	0.0 g
Protein	26.6 g

Jicama Beet Salad page 368

Yield is 4 servings
Serving size is about 1 cup
1.3 teaspoons of sugar
Basic Nutritional Values:

Calories	50
Calories from Fat	1.3
Total Fat	0.2 g
Saturated Fat	0 g
Trans Fat	0 g
Cholesterol	0 mg
Sodium	326 mg
Total Carbohydrate	11.7 g
Dietary Fiber	5.2 g
Sugars	4.3 g
Protein	1.3 g

Mini Egg Frittatas page 367

Yield is 8 servings
Serving size is 3 frittatas
0.5 teaspoon of sugar
Basic Nutritional Values:

Calories	205
Calories from Fat	129
Total Fat	14.4 g
Saturated Fat	5.2 g
Trans Fat	0 g
Cholesterol	514 mg
Sodium	219 mg
Total Carbohydrate	2.7 g
Dietary Fiber	0.3 g
Sugars	1.5 g
Protein	15.9 g

Cauliflower "Rice" Pilaf page 369

Yield is 8 servings
Serving size is about 1/2 cup
0.6 teaspoon of sugar
Basic Nutritional Values:

Calories	80
Calories from Fat	50
Total Fat	5.8 g
Saturated Fat	0.7 g
Trans Fat	0 g
Cholesterol	0 mg
Sodium	99.5 mg
Total Carbohydrate	5.6 g
Dietary Fiber	2.6 g
Sugars	2.3 g
Protein	3.0 g

Spaghetti Squash "Pasta"* page 370

Yield is 4 servings
Serving size is ibe quarter of recipe
1.6 teaspoons of sugar
Basic Nutritional Values:*

Calories	42
Calories from Fat	0
Total Fat	0 g
Saturated Fat	0 g
Trans Fat	0 g
Cholesterol	0 mg
Sodium	27.9 mg
Total Carbohydrate	10 g
Dietary Fiber	2.2 g
Sugars	3.9 g
Protein	1.0 g

Cauliflower Mash page 371

Yield is 4 servings
Serving size is one-quarter of recipe
0.6 teaspoon of sugar
Basic Nutritional Values:

Calories	95
Calories from fat	27
Total fat	3 g
Saturated Fat	0 g
Trans Fat	0 g
Cholesterol	0 mg
Sodium	50 mg
Total Carbohydrates	4 g
Dietary Fiber	1 g
Sugars	2 g
Protein	2 g

Southern Kale page 372

Yield is 6 servings
Serving size is one-sixth of recipe
2.8 teaspoons of sugar
Basic Nutritional Values:

Calories	114
Calories from fat	27
Total fat	3 g
Saturated Fat	0 g
Trans Fat	0 g
Cholesterol	0 mg
Sodium	107 mg
Total Carbohydrates	17 g
Dietary Fiber	3 g
Sugars	0 g
Protein	6 g

Wilted Cabbage page 373

Yield is 6 servings
Serving size is one-sixth of recipe
0.6 teaspoons of sugar
Basic Nutritional Values:

Calories	27
Calories from fat	9
Total fat	1 g
Saturated Fat	0 g
Trans Fat	0 g
Cholesterol	68 mg
Sodium	20 mg
Total Carbohydrates	5 g
Dietary Fiber	2 g
Sugars	2 g
Protein	1 g

* This is a great substitute for pasta. Serve with olive oil and some of your favorite spices!

notes

Heart Disease Is Killing Us

1. V. Roger, et al., "Heart Disease and Stroke Statistics—2011 Update. A Report from the American Heart Association." *Circulation.* 2011 Feb 1;123(4):e18–e209.
2. D. Lloyd-Jones, et al., "Heart Disease and Stroke Statistics—2010 Update. A Report from the American Heart Association Statistics Committee and Stroke Statistics Subcommittee." *Circulation.* 2010 Feb 23;121(7):e46–e215.
3. V. Fuster, et al., Hurst's the Heart, Book 1. 11th Edition, McGraw Hill, 2004.
4. World Health Report 1999, "Making a Difference." Geneva, Switzerland: World Health Organization, 1999.
5. C.J.L. Murray and A.D. Lopez, The Global Burden of Disease. Cambridge, MA: Harvard School of Public Health, 1996.
6. www.cdc.gov/obesity/data/trends.html
7. P. Poirier, et al., "Obesity and cardiovascular disease: pathophysiology, evaluation, and effect of weight loss: an update of the 1997 American Heart Association Scientific Statement on Obesity and Heart Disease from the Obesity Committee of the Council on Nutrition, Physical Activity, and Metabolism." *Circulation.* 2006 Feb 14;113(6):898–918.
8. C.J. Pepine, "Ischemic heart disease in women: Facts and wishful thinking." *J Am Coll Cardiol.* 2004 May 19;43(10):1727–30.
9. Ibid.
10. R. Martin, et al., "Gender disparities in common sense models of illness among myocardial infarction victims." *Health Psychology.* 2004 Jul;23(4):345–53.
11. J.C. McSweeny, et al., "Women's early warning signs of acute myocardial infarction." *Circulation.* 2003 Nov 25;108(21):2619–23.
12. A.G. Rosenfeld, "Treatment-seeking delay among women with acute myocardial infarction: decision trajectories and their predictors." *Nursing Research.* 2004 Jul–Aug;53:225–36.
13. Pepine, "Ischemic heart disease in women."
14. J.W. Hurst, The Heart, Arteries and Veins. New York: McGraw-Hill, Health Professions Division, 2002.
15. 2011 10Q Report: Advancing women's heart health through improved research, diagnosis and treatment. The National Coalition for Women with Heart Disease. June 2011, Washington, DC.
16. Roger, "Heart Disease and Stroke Statistics."
17. N.K. Wenger, "You've come a long way, baby: cardiovascular health and disease in women: problems and prospects." *Circulation.* 2004 Feb 10;109(5):558–60.
18. Roger, et al., "Heart Disease and Stroke Statistics—2011 update."
19. G. Heiss, et al., "Health risks and benefits 3 years after stopping randomized treatment with estrogen and progestin." *JAMA.* 2008 Mar 5;299(9):1036–45.
20. L.K. Curtiss, "Reversing atherosclerosis?" *N Engl J Med.* 2009 Mar 12;360(11):1144–6.
21. P. Libby, et al., "Inflammation and atherosclerosis." *Circulation.* 2002 Mar 5;105(9):1135–43.

Cholesterol Is Not All Bad

1. Life Extension Media, Disease Prevention and Treatment, Expanded Fourth Edition, Life Extension Foundation, 2003, p. 407.
2. J.M. Dietschy and S.D. Turley, "Thematic review series: brain Lipids. Cholesterol metabolism in the central nervous system during early development and in the mature animal." *J Lipid Res.* 2004 Aug;45(8):1375–97.
3. Seneff, et al., "Nutrition and Alzheimer's disease: the detrimental role of a high carbohydrate diet." *Eur J Intern Med.* 2011 Apr;22(2):134–40.
4. D.M Stocco, "StAR protein and the regulation of steroid hormone biosynthesis." *Annu Rev Physiol.* 2001;63:193–213.
5. M.K. Bogh, et al., "Vitamin D production after UVB exposure depends on baseline vitamin D and total cholesterol but not on skin pigmentation." *J Invest Dermatol.* 2010 Feb;130(2):546–53.
6. www.webmd.com/cholesterol-management/guide/understanding-numbers
7. W.T. Friedewald, et al., "Estimation of the concentration of low-density lipoprotein cholesterol in plasma, without use of the preparative ultracentrifuge." *Clin Chem.* 1972 Jun;18(6):499–502.
8. M. Miller, et al., "Triglycerides and cardiovascular disease: a scientific statement from the American Heart Association." *Circulation.* 2011 May 24;123(20):2292–333.
9. J. Hulthe, et al., "The metabolic syndrome, LDL particle size, and atherosclerosis: the Atherosclerosis and Insulin Resistance (AIR) study." *Arterioscler Thromb Vasc Biol.* 2000 Sep;20(9):2140–7.
10. S. Grundy, "Small LDL, atherogenic dyslipidemia, and the metabolic syndrome." *Circulation.* 1997;95:1–4.
11. L. Calabresi, et al., "Omacor in familial combined hyperlipidemia: effects on lipids and low density lipoprotein subclasses." *Atherosclerosis.* 2000 Feb;148(2):3879–6.
12. C.U. Choi, et al., "Statins do not decrease small, dense low-density lipoprotein." *Tex Heart Inst J.* 2010;37(4):421–8.
13. J.R. McNamara, et al., "Change in LDL particle size is associated with change in plasma triglyceride concentration." *Arterioscler Thromb.* 1992 Nov;12(11):1284–90.
14. C. Meisinger, et al., "Plasma oxidized low-density lipoprotein, a strong predictor for acute coronary heart disease events in apparently healthy, middle-aged men from the general population." *Circulation.* 2005 Aug 2;112(5):651–7.
15. J.M. Lecerf and M. de Lorgeril, "Dietary cholesterol: from physiology to cardiovascular risk." *Br J Nutr.* 2011 Jul;106(1):6–14.
16. R.M. Weggemans, et al., "Dietary cholesterol from eggs increases the ratio of total cholesterol to high-density lipoprotein cholesterol in humans: a meta-analysis." *Am J Clin Nutr.* 2001 May;73(5):885–91.
17. Simons, et al., "Effect of one egg per day on plasma cholesterol levels in moderate hypercholesterolemia." *Nutr Metab Cardiovasc Dis.* 1993;3:78–82.
18. F.B. Hu, et al., "A prospective study of egg consumption and risk of cardiovascular disease in men and women." *JAMA.* 1999 Apr 21;281(15):1387–94.
19. R. Ross, "Atherosclerosis--an inflammatory disease." *N Engl J Med.* 1999 Jan 14;340(2):115–26.

20. P.D. Cani, et al., "Changes in gut microbiota control metabolic endotoxemia-induced inflammation in high-fat diet-induced obesity and diabetes in mice." *Diabetes*. 2008 Jun;57(6):1470–81.

21. S.P. Heffron, et al., "Very-low dose endotoxemia induces high density lipoprotein remodeling and reduces cholesterol efflux in the absence of a clinical inflammatory response." *Circulation*. 2007;116:II_220.

22. P.D. Cani, et al., "Selective increases of bifidobacteria in gut microflora improve high-fat-diet-induced diabetes in mice through a mechanism associated with endotoxaemia." *Diabetologia*. 2007 Nov;50(11):2374–83.

23. H.S. Gill and F. Guarner, "Probiotics and human health: a clinical perspective." *Postgrad Med J*. 2004 Sep;80(947):516–26.

24. E. Theuwissen and R.P. Mensink, "Water-soluble dietary fibers and cardiovascular disease." *Physiol Behav*. 2008 May 23;94(2):285–92.

25. R.P. Mensink and M.B. Katan, "Effect of dietary fatty acids on serum lipids and lipoproteins: a meta-analysis of 27 trials." *Arterioscler Thromb*. 1992 Aug;12(8):911–9.

26. P.W. Siri and R.M. Krauss, "Influence of dietary carbohydrate and fat on LDL and HDL particle distributions." *Curr Atheroscler Rep*. 2005 Nov;7(6):455–9.

27. P.W. Siri-Tarino, Q. Sun, F.B. Hu, and R.M. Krauss. Meta-analysis of prospective cohort studies evaluating the association of saturated fat with cardiovascular disease. *Am J Clin Nutr*. 2010 Mar;91(3):535–46.

28. IMS Institute for Healthcare Informatics: "The Use of Medicines in the United States: Review of 2010," April 2011.

29. M.K. Jain and P.M. Ridker, "Anti-inflammatory effects of statins: clinical evidence and basic mechanisms." *Nat Rev Drug Discov*. 2005 Dec;4(12):977–87.

30. R. Kaddurah-Daouk, et al., "Enteric microbiome metabolites correlate with response to simvastatin treatment." *PLoS One*. 2011;6(10):e25482.

31. J.M. Ridlon, et al., "Bile salt biotransformations by human intestinal bacteria." *J Lipid Res*. 2006 Feb;47(2):241–59.

32. S. de Ferranti and D.S. Ludwig, "Storm over statins—the controversy surrounding pharmacologic treatment of children." *N Engl J Med*. 2008 Sep 25;359(13):1309–12.

High Blood Pressure—Take It Seriously

1. National Center for Health Statistics. Health, United States, 2008. Hyattsville, MD: National Center for Health Statistics; 2008.

2. D. Lloyd-Jones, et al., "Heart disease and stroke statistics—2010 update: a report from the American Heart Association." *Circulation*. 2010 Feb 23;121(7):e46–e215.

3. A.V. Kshirsagar, et al., "Blood pressure usually considered normal is associated with an elevated risk of cardiovascular disease." *Am J Med*. 2006 Feb;119(2):133–41.

4. S. Lewington, et al., "Age-specific relevance of usual blood pressure to vascular mortality: a meta-analysis of individual data for one million adults in 61 prospective studies." *Lancet*. 2002 Dec 14;360(9349):1903–13.

5. A.V. Chobanian, et al., "Seventh report of the joint national committee on prevention, detection, evaluation, and treatment of high blood pressure: the JNC report." *JAMA*. 2003: 2560–72.

6. F.J. He and G.A. MacGregor, "Salt reduction lowers cardiovascular risk: meta-analysis of outcome trials." *Lancet*. 2011 Jul 30;378(9789):380–2.

7. G. Jurgens and N.A. Graudal, "Effects of low sodium diet versus high sodium diet on blood pressure, renin, aldosterone, catecholamines, cholesterols, and triglyceride." *Cochrane Database Syst Rev*. 2004;(1):CD004022.

8. D. Taubert, et al., "Effects of low habitual cocoa intake on blood pressure and bioactive nitric oxide: a randomized controlled trial." *JAMA*. 2007 Jul 4;298(1):49–60.

9. C.A. Papaharalambus and K.K. Griendling, "Basic mechanisms of oxidative stress and reactive oxygen species in cardiovascular injury." *Trends Cardiovasc Med*. 2007 Feb;17(2):48–54.

10. S. Verma, et al., "A self-fulfilling prophecy: C-reactive protein attenuates nitric oxide production and inhibits angiogenesis." *Circulation*. 2002 Aug 20;106(8):913–19.

11. T. Edwards, "Inflammation, pain, and chronic disease: an integrative approach to treatment and prevention." *Altern Ther Health Med*. 2005 Nov–Dec;11(6):20–7.

12. S.M. Grundy, "Inflammation, hypertension, and the metabolic syndrome." *JAMA*. 2003 Dec 10;290(22):3000–2.

13. H.D. Sesso, et al., "C-reactive protein and the risk of developing hypertension." *JAMA*. 2003 Dec 10;290(22):2945–51.

14. L. Niskanen, et al., "Inflammation, abdominal obesity, and smoking as predictors of hypertension. Inflammation, abdominal obesity, and smoking as predictors of hypertension." *Hypertension*. 2004 Dec;44(6):859–65.

15. A. Mahmud and J. Feely, "Arterial stiffness is related to systemic inflammation in essential hypertension." *Hypertension*. 2005 Nov;46(5):1118–22.

16. P. Pauletto and M. Rattazzi, "Inflammation and hypertension: the search for a link." *Nephrol Dial Transplant*. 2006 Apr;21(4):850–3.

17. S.M. Collins, et al., "The putative role of the intestinal microbiota in the irritable bowel syndrome." *Dig Liver Dis*. 2009 Dec;41(12):850–3.

18. K. Hod, et al., "Assessment of high-sensitivity CRP as a marker of micro-inflammation in irritable bowel syndrome." *Neurogastroenterol Motil*. 2011 Dec;23(12):1105–10.

19. L.J. Appel, et al., "Effects of protein, monounsaturated fat, and carbohydrate intake on blood pressure and serum lipids: results of the OmniHeart randomized trial." *JAMA*. 2005 Nov 16;294(19):2455–64.

20. W.S. Yancy Jr, et al., "A randomized trial of a low-carbohydrate diet vs orlistat plus a low-fat diet for weight loss." *Arch Intern Med*. 2010 Jan 25;170(2):136–45.

21. C.K. Roberts, et al., "A high-fat, refined-carbohydrate diet induces endothelial dysfunction and oxidant/antioxidant imbalance and depresses NOS protein expression." *J Appl Physiol*. 2005 Jan;98(1):203–10.

22. T. Rebello, et al., "Short-term effects of various sugars on antinatriuresis and blood pressure changes in normotensive young men." *Am J Clin Nutr*. 1983 Jul;38(1):84–94.

23. Air Quality Criteria for Particulate Matter. EPA/600/P-99/002aF; U.S. Environmental Protection Agency: Washington, DC; 2004.

24. R.D. Brook, et al., "Why physicians who treat hypertension should know more about air pollution." *J Clin Hypertens* (Greenwich). 2007 Aug;9(8):629–35.

25. R.D. Brook, "You are what you breathe: evidence linking air pollution and blood pressure." *Curr Hypertens Rep.* 2005 Dec;7(6):427–34.

26. I.A. Hassan, et al., "Analysis of heavy metals in scalp hair samples of hypertensive patients by conventional and microwave digestion methods." *Spectroscopy Letters.* 2006;39(2):203–14.

27. M. Rahman, et al., "Hypertension and arsenic exposure in Bangladesh." *Hypertension.* 1999 Jan;33(1):74–8.

28. M. Tellez-Plaza, et al., "Cadmium exposure and hypertension in the 1999–2004 National Health and Nutrition Examination Survey (NHANES)." *Environ Health Perspect.* 2008 Jan;116(1):51–6.

29. M.C. Houston, "The role of mercury and cadmium heavy metals in vascular disease, hypertension, coronary heart disease, and myocardial infarction." *Altern Ther Health Med.* 2007 Mar–Apr;13(2):S128–33.

30. D. Nash, et al., "Blood lead, blood pressure, and hypertension in perimenopausal and postmenopausal women." *JAMA.* 2003 Mar 26;289(12):1523–32.

31. J.A. Staessen, et al., "The epidemiology of the association between hypertension and menopause." *J Hum Hypertens.* 1998 Sep;12(9):587–92.

32. N.D. Vaziri, et al., "Induction of oxidative stress by glutathione depletion causes severe hypertension in normal rats." *Hypertension.* 2000 Jul;36(1):142–6.

33. S.A. Sheweita, "Heavy metal-induced changes in the glutathione levels and glutathione reductase/glutathione S-transferase activities in the liver of male mice." *Inter J of Toxicol.* 1998 June;17(4):383–92.

34. www.johnshopkinshealthalerts.com/reports/hypertension_stroke/378-1.html

High Blood Sugar–Know Your Risk

1. Centers for Disease Control and Prevention. National Diabetes Fact Sheet, 2011. Atlanta, GA: U.S. Department of Health and Human Services, Centers for Disease Control and Prevention, 2011.

2. E. Selvin, et al., "Glycemic control and coronary heart disease risk in persons with and without diabetes." *Arch Intern Med.* 2005 Sep 12;165(16):1910–6.

3. diabetes.niddk.nih.gov/dm/pubs/diagnosis/

4. www.nlm.nih.gov/medlineplus/ency/article/003640.htm

5. S. Genuth, et al., "Follow-up report on the diagnosis of diabetes mellitus." *Diabetes Care.* 2003 Nov;26(11):3160–7.

6. Expert Committee on the Diagnosis and Classification of Diabetes Mellitus: Report of the Expert Committee on the Diagnosis and Classification of Diabetes Mellitus. *Diabetes Care.* 1997 20:1183–1197.

7. J.V. Bjornholt, et al., "Fasting blood glucose: an underestimated risk factor for cardiovascular death. Results from a 22-year follow-up of healthy nondiabetic men." *Diabetes Care.* 1999 Jan;22(1):45–9.

8. Life Extension Media, Disease Prevention and Treatment, Expanded Fourth Edition, Life Extension Foundation, 2003, p. 423.

9. R.A. DeFronzo, et al., "Pathogenesis of NIDDM: A balanced overview." *Diabetes Care.* 1992 Mar;15(3):318–68.

10. G. Reaven, "All obese individuals are not created equal: insulin resistance is the major determinant of cardiovascular disease in overweight/obese individuals." *Diab Vasc Dis Res.* 2005 Oct;2(3):105–12.

11. P.W. Wilson, et al., "Metabolic syndrome as a precursor of cardiovascular disease and type 2 diabetes mellitus." *Circulation.* 2005 Nov 15;112(20):3066–72.

12. S.M. de la Monte and J.R. Wands, "Alzheimer's disease is type 3 diabetes: evidence reviewed." *J Diabetes Sci Technol.* 2008 Nov;2(6):1101–13.

13. K.F. Neumann, et al., "Insulin resistance and Alzheimer's disease: molecular links and clinical implications." *Curr Alzheimer Res.* 2008 Oct;5(5):438–47.

14. S.E. Shoelson, et al., "Inflammation and insulin resistance." *J Clin Invest.* 2006 July 3; 116(7): 1793–1801.

15. H. Tilg and A.R. Moschen, "Inflammatory mechanisms in the regulation of insulin resistance." *Mol Med.* 2008 Mar–Apr; 14(3-4): 222–231.

16. A. Sjoholm and T. Nystrom, "Endothelial inflammation in insulin resistance." *Lancet.* 2005 Feb 12–18;365(9459):610–2.

17. K. Esposito, et al., "Inflammatory cytokine concentrations are acutely increased by hyperglycemia in humans: role of oxidative stress." *Circulation.* 2002 Oct 15;106(16):2067–72.

18. M. Krajcovicova-Kudlackova, et al., "Advanced glycation end products and nutrition." *Physiol Res.* 2002;51(3):313–6.

19. M. Peppa, et al., "Glucose, advanced glycation end products, and diabetes complications: what is new and what works." *Clin Diab.* 2003 Oct; 21(4):186–7.

20. J.R. Berggren, et al., "Fat as an endocrine organ: influence of exercise." *J Appl Physiol.* 2005 Aug;99(2):757–64.

21. Shoelson, et al., "Inflammation and insulin resistance."

22. P.D. Cani, et al., "Metabolic endotoxemia initiates obesity and insulin resistance." *Diabetes.* 2007 Jul;56(7):1761–72.

23. Ibid.

24. P.D. Cani, et al., "Changes in gut microbiota control metabolic endotoxemia-induced inflammation in high-fat diet-induced obesity and diabetes in mice." *Diabetes.* 2008 Jun;57(6):1470–81.

25. P.D. Cani, et al., "Changes in gut microbiota control inflammation in obese mice through a mechanism involving GLP-2-driven improvement of gut permeability." *Gut.* 2009 Aug;58(8):1091–103.

26. P.D. Cani, et al., "Selective increases of bifidobacteria in gut microflora improve high-fat-diet-induced diabetes in mice through a mechanism associated with endotoxaemia." *Diabetologia.* 2007 Nov;50(11):2374–83.

27. K. Yamashita, et al., "Effects of fructo-oligosaccharides on blood glucose and serum lipids in diabetic subjects." *Nutr Res.* 1984 Nov–Dec;4(6):961–6.

28. M.T. Streppel, et al., "Dietary fiber and blood pressure: a meta-analysis of randomized placebo-controlled trials." *Arch Intern Med.* 2005 Jan 24;165(2):150–6.

29. T.M. Wolever and J.B. Miller, "Sugars and blood glucose control." *Am J Clin Nutr.* 1995 Jul;62(1 Suppl):212S–221S; discussion 221S–227S.

30. S. Liu, et al., "A prospective study of dietary glycemic load, carbohydrate intake, and risk of coronary heart disease in US women." *Am J Clin Nutr.* 2000 Jun;71(6):1455–61.

31. N.F. Sheard, et al., "Dietary carbohydrate (amount and type) in the prevention and management of diabetes: a statement by the American Diabetes Association." *Diabetes Care.* 2004 Sep;27(9):2266–71.

32. Ibid.

33. B. Bahadori, et al., "Low-fat, high-carbohydrate (low-glycaemic index) diet induces weight loss and preserves lean body mass in obese healthy subjects: results of a 24-week study." *Diabetes Obes Metab.* 2005 May;7(3):290–3.

34. E.C. Westman, et al., "The effect of a low-carbohydrate, ketogenic diet versus a low-glycemic index diet on glycemic control in type 2 diabetes mellitus." *Nutr Metab* (Lond). 2008 Dec 19;5:36.

35. L. Stern, et al., "The effects of low-carbohydrate versus conventional weight loss diets in severely obese adults: one-year follow-up of a randomized trial." *Ann Intern Med.* 2004 May 18;140(10):778–85.

36. K.A. Meyer, et al., "Carbohydrates, dietary fiber, and incident type 2 diabetes in older women." *Am J Clin Nutr.* 2000 Apr;71(4):921–30.

37. M.B. Schulze, et al., "Glycemic index, glycemic load, and dietary fiber intake and incidence of type 2 diabetes in younger and middle-aged women." *Am J Clin Nutr.* 2004 Aug;80(2):348–56.

38. W. Davis, MD,, Wheat Belly. Rodale, 2011, p. 8.

39. C.D. Saudek, et al., "Assessing glycemia in diabetes using self-monitoring blood glucose and hemoglobin A1c." *JAMA.* 2006 Apr 12;295(14):1688–97.

The Fattening of America

1. www.cdc.gov/chronicdisease/resources/publications/AAG/obesity.htm

2. A.E. Field, et al., "Impact of overweight on the risk of developing common chronic diseases during a 10-year period." *Arch Intern Med.* 2001 Jul 9;161(13):1581–6.

3. D. Gallagher, et al., "How useful is body mass index for comparison of body fatness across age, sex, and ethnic groups?" *Am J Epidemiol.* 1996 Feb 1;143(3):228–39.

4. H.L. Walls, et al., "Comparing trends in BMI and waist circumference." *Obesity (Silver Spring).* 2011 Jan;19(1):216–9.

5. I. Janssen, et al., "Waist circumference and not body mass index explains obesity-related health risk." *Am J Clin Nutr.* 2004 Mar;79(3):379–84.

6. S. Yusuf, et al., "Obesity and the risk of myocardial infarction in 27,000 participants from 52 countries: a case-control study." *Lancet.* 2005 Nov 5;366(9497):1640–9.

7. C.J. Dobbelsteyn, et al., "A comparative evaluation of waist circumference, waist-to-hip ratio and body mass index as indicators of cardiovascular risk factors: The Canadian Heart Health Surveys." *Int J Obes Relat Metab Disord.* 2001 May;25(5):652–61.

8. K.M. Rexrode, et al., "Abdominal adiposity and coronary heart disease in women." *JAMA.* 1998 Dec 2;280(21):1843–8.

9. P. Poirier, et al., "Obesity and cardiovascular disease: pathophysiology, evaluation, and effect of weight loss." *Arterioscler Thromb Vasc Biol.* 2006 May;26(5):968–76.

10. F.X. Pi-Sunyer, "The obesity epidemic: pathophysiology and consequences of obesity." *Obes Res.* 2002 Dec;10 Suppl 2:97S–104S.

11. E.E. Kershaw and J.S. Flier, "Adipose tissue as an endocrine organ." *J Clin Endocrinol Metab.* 2004 June;89(6):2548–56.

12. T. Hampton, "Scientists study fat as endocrine organ." *JAMA.* 2006 Oct 4;296(13):1573–5.

13. Kershaw, "Adipose tissue as an endocrine organ."

14. K.E. Wellen and G.S. Hotamisligil, "Obesity-induced inflammatory changes in adipose tissue." *J Clin Invest.* 2003 Dec;112(12):1785–8.

15. A.H. Berg and P.E. Scherer, "Adipose tissue, inflammation, and cardiovascular disease." *Circ Res.* 2005 May 13;96(9):939–49.

16. A.H. Kao, et al., "Update on vascular disease in systemic lupus erythematosus." *Curr Opin Rheumatol.* 2003 Sep;15(5):519–27.

17. H.J. Rupprecht, et al., "Impact of viral and bacterial infectious burden on long-term prognosis in patients with coronary artery disease." *Circulation.* 2001 Jul 3;104(1):25–31.

18. A. Krack, et al., "The importance of the gastrointestinal system in the pathogenesis of heart failure." *Eur Heart J.* 2005 Nov;26(22):2368–74.

19. A.P. Simoloylos, "The importance of the ratio of omega-6/omega-3 essential fatty acids." *Biomed Pharmacother.* 2002 Oct;56(8):365–79.

20. P.C. Calder, "n-3 polyunsaturated fatty acids, inflammation, and inflammatory diseases." *Am J Clin Nutr.* 2006 Jun;83(6 Suppl):1505S–1519S.

21. S.M. Donahue, et al., "Prenatal fatty acid status and child adiposity at age 3 y: results from a US pregnancy cohort." *Am J Clin Nutr.* 2011 Apr;93(4):780–8.

22. Berg and Scherer, "Adipose tissue, inflammation, and cardiovascular disease."

23. M. Visser, et al., "Elevated C-reactive protein levels in overweight and obese adults." *JAMA.* 1999 Dec 8;282(22):2131–5.

24. Berg and Scherer, "Adipose tissue, inflammation, and cardiovascular disease."

25. S. Klein, et al., "Clinical implications of obesity with specific focus on cardiovascular disease: a statement for professionals from the American Heart Association Council on Nutrition, Physical Activity, and Metabolism: endorsed by the American College of Cardiology Foundation." *Circulation.* 2004 Nov 2;110(18):2952–67.

26. N.M. Delzenne, et al., "Targeting gut microbiota in obesity: effects of prebiotics and probiotics." *Nat Rev Endocrinol.* 2011 Aug 9;7(11):639-46.

27. R.E. Ley, et al., "Obesity alters gut microbial ecology." *Proc Natl Acad Sci USA.* 2005 Aug 2;102(31):11070–5.

28. R.E. Ley, et al., "Microbial ecology: human gut microbes associated with obesity." *Nature.* 2006 Dec 21;444(7122):1022–3.

29. P.J. Turnbaugh, et al., "A core gut microbiome in obese and lean twins." *Nature.* 2009 Jan 22;457(7228):480–4.

30. P.J. Turnbaugh, et al., "An obesity-associated gut microbiome with increased capacity for energy harvest." *Nature.* 2006 Dec 21;444(7122):1027–31.

31. F. Backhed, et al., "The gut microbiota as an environmental factor that regulates fat storage." *Proc Natl Acad Sci USA*. 2004 Nov 2;101(44):15718–23.

32. M. Kalliomaki, et al., "Early differences in fecal microbiota composition in children may predict overweight." *Am J Clin Nutr*. 2008 Mar;87(3):534–8.

33. E.E. Vaughan, et al., "The intestinal LABs." *Antonie Van Leeuwenhoek*. 2002 Aug;82(1-4):341–52.

34. Kalliomaki, et al., "Early differences in fecal microbiota composition in children may predict overweight."

35. M.C. Collado, et al., "Distinct composition of gut microbiota during pregnancy in overweight and normal-weight women." *Am J Clin Nutr*. 2008 Oct;88(4):894–9.

36. M.C. Collado, et al., "Effect of mother's weight on infant's microbiota acquisition, composition, and activity during early infancy: a prospective follow-up study initiated in early pregnancy." *Am J Clin Nutr*. 2010 Nov;92(5):1023–30.

37. S. Basu, et al., "Pregravid obesity associates with increased maternal endotoxemia and metabolic inflammation." *Obesity* (Silver Spring). 2011 Mar;19(3):476–82.

38. A. Gummesson, et al., "Intestinal permeability is associated with visceral adiposity in healthy women." *Obesity (Silver Spring)*. 2011 Nov;19(11):2280–2.

39. A.S. Andreasen, et al., "Effects of Lactobacillus acidophilus NCFM on insulin sensitivity and the systemic inflammatory response in human subjects." *Br J Nutr*. 2010 Dec;104(12):1831–8.

40. Y. Kadooka, et al., "Regulation of abdominal adiposity by probiotics (Lactobacillus gasseri SBT2055) in adults with obese tendencies in a randomized controlled trial." *Eur J Clin Nutr*. 2010 Jun;64(6):636–43.

41. C.L. Ogden, et al., "High body mass index for age among US children and adolescents, 2003–2006." *JAMA*. 2008 May 28;299(20):2401–5.

42. S. Devi, "Progress on childhood obesity patchy in the USA." *Lancet*. 2008 Jan 12;371(9607):105–6.

43. American Heart Association. "Obese kids' artery plaque similar to middle-aged adults." *ScienceDaily*. 11 Nov. 2008. Web. 22 Nov. 2011.

44. C.B. Ebbeling, et al., "Childhood obesity: public-health crisis, common sense cure." *Lancet*. 2002 Aug 10;360(9331):473–82.

45. K. Bibbins-Domingo, et al., "Adolescent overweight and future adult coronary heart disease." *N Engl J Med*. 2007 Dec 6;357(23):2371–9.

46. Iowa State University. "Individual Stress Linked to Adolescent Obesity." *ScienceDaily*, 14 May 2009. Web. 22 Nov. 2011.

47. M.N. Mead, "Programmed obesity?: Study links intrauterine exposures to higher BMI in toddlers." *Environ Health Perspect*. 2009 January; 117(1): A33.

48. Kalliomaki, et al., "Early differences in fecal microbiota composition in children may predict overweight."

49. S. Kersten, "Mechanisms of nutritional and hormonal regulation of lipogenesis." *EMBO Rep*. 2001 Apr;2(4):282–6.

50. W.C. Willet and R.L. Leibel, "Dietary fat is not a major determinant of body fat." *Am J Med*. 2002 Dec 30;113 Suppl 9B:47S–59S.

51. D.S. Ludwig, "The glycemic index: physiological mechanisms relating to obesity, diabetes, and cardiovascular disease." *JAMA*. 2002 May 8;287(18):2414–23.

52. L. Stern, et al., "The effects of low-carbohydrate versus conventional weight loss diets in severely obese adults: one-year follow-up of a randomized trial." *Ann Intern Med*. 2004 May 18;140(10):778–85.

53. I. Shai, et al., "Weight loss with a low-carbohydrate, Mediterranean, or low-fat diet." *N Engl J Med*. 2008 Jul 17;359(3):229–41.

54. M. Hesson, et al., "Systematic review of randomized controlled trials of low-carbohydrate vs. low-fat/low-calorie diets in the management of obesity and its comorbidities." *Obes Rev*. 2009 Jan;10(1):36–50.

55. G. Taubes, Good Calories, Bad Calories, Anchor Books, 2008.

56. R.H. Eckel, "Clinical practice. Nonsurgical management of obesity in adults." *N Engl J Med*. 2008 May 1;358(18):1941–50.

Inflammation—You Might Not Know You Have it

1. G.K. Hansson, "Inflammation, atherosclerosis, and coronary artery disease." *N Engl J Med*. 2005 Apr 21;352(16):1685–95.

2. R. Scrivo, et al., "Inflammation as 'common soil' of the multifactorial diseases." *Autoimmun Rev*. 2011 May;10(7):369–74.

3. R. Medzhitov, "Origin and physiological roles of inflammation." *Nature*. 2008 Jul 24;454(7203):428–35.

4. C.N. Serhan and J. Savill, "Resolution of inflammation: the beginning programs the end." *Nat Immunol*. 2005 Dec;6(12):1191–7.

5. R. Medzhitov, "Inflammation 2010: new adventures of an old flame." *Cell*. 2010 Mar 19;140(6):771–6.

6. S. Verma, et al., "C-reactive protein: structure affects function." *Circulation*. 2004 Apr 27;109(16):1914–7.

7. P.M. Ridker, "Cardiology Patient Page. C-reactive protein: a simple test to help predict risk of heart attack and stroke." *Circulation*. 2003 Sep 23;108(12):e81–5.

8. Ibid.

9. Verma, et al., "C-reactive protein: structure affects function."

10. www.metametrix.com/test-menu/profiles/oxidative-stress-indicators/lipid-peroxides?t=clinicianInfo

11. M.D. Stringer, et al., "Lipid peroxides and atherosclerosis." *BMJ*. 1989 February 4; 298(6669): 281–4.

12. D. Giugliano, et al., "The effects of diet on inflammation: emphasis on the metabolic syndrome." *J Am Coll Cardiol*. 2006 Aug 15;48(4):677–85.

13. A.P. Simopoulos, "The importance of the omega-6/omega-3 fatty acid ratio in cardiovascular disease and other chronic diseases." *Exp Biol Med* (Maywood). 2008 Jun;233(6):674–88.

14. E. Lopez-Garcia, et al., "Consumption of (n-3) fatty acids is related to plasma biomarkers of inflammation and endothelial activation in women." *J Nutr*. 2004 Jul;134(7):1806–11.

15. P.D. Tsitouras, et al., "High omega-3 fat intake improves insulin sensitivity and reduces CRP and IL6, but does not affect other endocrine axes in healthy older adults." *Horm Metab Res*. 2008 Mar;40(3):199–205.

16. C.N. Serhan, "Systems approach to inflammation resolution: identification of novel anti-inflammatory and pro-resolving mediators." *J Thromb Haemost*. 2009 Jul;7 Suppl 1:44–8.

17. M.B. Schultz, et al., "Dietary pattern, inflammation, and incidence of type 2 diabetes in women." *Am J Clin Nutr.* 2005 Sep;82(3):675-84; quiz 714–5.

18. I. Aeberli, et al., "Low to moderate sugar-sweetened beverage consumption impairs glucose and lipid metabolism and promotes inflammation in healthy young men: a randomized controlled trial." *Am J Clin Nutr.* 2011 Aug;94(2):479–85.

19. M.J. James, et al., "Dietary polyunsaturated fatty acids and inflammatory mediator production." *Am J Clin Nutr.* 2000 Jan;71(1 Suppl):343S–8S.

20. R.J. Wood, et al., "Effects of a carbohydrate-restricted diet on emerging plasma markers for cardiovascular disease." *Nutr Metab (Lond).* 2006 May 4;3:19.

21. D.E. King, "Dietary fiber, inflammation, and cardiovascular disease." *Mol Nutr Food Res.* 2005 Jun;49(6):594–600.

22. Y. Ma, et al., "Association between dietary fiber and serum C-reactive protein." *Am J Clin Nutr.* 2006 Apr;83(4):760–6.

23. D.S. Jones, M.D. (editor), Textbook of Functional Medicine. The Institute for Functional Medicine, 2005, p. 611.

24. P.H. Black and L.D. Garbutt, et al., "Stress, inflammation and cardiovascular disease." *J Psychosom Res.* 2002 Jan;52(1):1–23.

25. A.H. Berg and P.E. Scherer, "Adipose tissue, inflammation, and cardiovascular disease." *Circ Res.* 2005 May 13;96(9):939–49.

26. A.M. O'Hara and F. Shanahan, "The gut flora as a forgotten organ." *EMBO Rep.* 2006 Jul;7(7):688–93.

27. J.L. Round and S.K. Mazmanian, "The gut microbiota shapes intestinal immune responses during health and disease." *Nat Rev Immunol.* 2009 May;9(5):313–23.

28. M. Camilleri and H. Gorman, "Intestinal permeability and irritable bowel syndrome." *Neurogastroenterol Motil.* 2007 Jul;19(7):545–52.

29. J. Mankertz and J.D. Schulzke, "Altered permeability in inflammatory bowel disease: pathophysiology and clinical implications." *Curr Opin Gastroenterol.* 2007 Jul;23(4):379–83.

30. A. Sandek, et al., "Altered intestinal function in patients with chronic heart failure." *J Am Coll Cardiol.* 2007 Oct 16;50(16):1561–9.

31. A. Krack, et al., "The importance of the gastrointestinal system in the pathogenesis of heart failure." *Eur Heart J.* 2005 Nov;26(22):2368–74.

32. E. Bosi, et al., "Increased intestinal permeability precedes clinical onset of type 1 diabetes." *Diabetologia.* 2006 Dec;49(12):2824–7.

33. O. Vaarala, "Leaking gut in type 1 diabetes." *Curr Opin Gastroenterol.* 2008 Nov;24(6):701–6.

34. L. Miele, et al., "Increased intestinal permeability and tight junction alterations in nonalcoholic fatty liver disease." *Hepatology.* 2009 Jun;49(6):1877–87.

35. J.D. Soderholm and M.H. Perdue, "Stress and gastrointestinal tract. II. Stress and intestinal barrier function." *Am J Physiol Gastrointest Liver Physiol.* 2001 Jan;280(1):G7–G13.

36. M. Maes, "Increased serum IgA and IgM against LPS of enterobacteria in chronic fatigue syndrome (CFS): indication for the involvement of gram-negative enterobacteria in the etiology of CFS and for the presence of an increased gut-intestinal permeability." *J Affect Disord.* 2007 Apr;99(1-3):237–40.

37. A. Goebel, et al., "Altered intestinal permeability in patients with primary fibromyalgia and in patients with complex regional pain syndrome." *Rheumatology (Oxford).* 2008 Aug;47(8):1223–7.

38. P. D'Eufemia, et al., "Abnormal intestinal permeability in children with autism." *Acta Paediatr.* 1996 Sep;85(9):1076–9.

39. M.G. Pike, et al., "Increased intestinal permeability in atopic eczema." *J Invest Dermatol.* 1986 Feb;86(2):101–4.

40. A. Bernard, et al., "Increased intestinal permeability in bronchial asthma." *J Allergy Clin Immunol.* 1996 Jun;97(6):1173–8.

41. A. Gummersson, et al., "Intestinal permeability is associated with visceral adiposity in healthy women." *Obesity (Silver Spring).* 2011 Nov;19(11):2280–2.

42. L. Smeeth, et al., "Risk of myocardial infarction and stroke after acute infection or vaccination." *N Engl J Med.* 2004 Dec 16;351(25):2611–8.

43. J. Zhu, et al., "Effects of total pathogen burden on coronary artery disease risk and C-reactive protein levels." *Am J Cardiol.* 2000 Jan 15;85(2):140–6.

44. J.S. Zebrack and J.L. Anderson, "The role of infection in the pathogenesis of cardiovascular disease." *Prog Cardiovasc Nurs.* 2003 Winter;18(1):42–9.

45. S. Kiechl, et al., "Chronic infections and the risk of carotid atherosclerosis: prospective results from a large population study." *Circulation.* 2001 Feb 27;103(8):1064–70.

46. C. Espinola-Klein, et al., "Impact of infectious burden on extent and long-term prognosis of atherosclerosis." *Circulation.* 2002 Jan 1;105(1):15–21.

47. K. Ericson, et al., "Relationship of Chlamydia pneumoniae infection to severity of human coronary atherosclerosis." *Circulation.* 2000 Jun 6;101(22):2568–71.

48. B.I. Byrne and M.V. Kalayoglu, "Chlamydia pneumoniae and atherosclerosis: links to the disease process." *Am Heart J.* 1999 Nov;138(5 Pt 2):S488–90.

49. Zebrack and Anderson, "The role of infection in the pathogenesis of cardiovascular disease."

50. K. Curry and L. Lawson, "Exploring the links between infectious disease and cardiovascular disease." *J Nurse Pract.* 2009;5:733–741.

51. B. Chiu, "Multiple infections in carotid atherosclerotic plaques." *Am Heart J.* 1999 Nov;138(5 Pt 2):S534–6.

52. P.J. Pussinen, et al., "Endotoxemia, immune response to periodontal pathogens, and systemic inflammation associate with incident cardiovascular disease events." *Arterioscler Thromb Vasc Biol.* 2007 Jun;27(6):1433–9.

53. N.M. Moutsopoulos and P.N. Madianos, "Low-grade inflammation in chronic infectious diseases: paradigm of periodontal infections." *Ann N Y Acad Sci.* 2006 Nov;1088:251–64.

54. Zebrack and Anderson, "The role of infection in the pathogenesis of cardiovascular disease."

55. S.E. Epstein, et al., "Infection and atherosclerosis: emerging mechanistic paradigms." *Circulation.* 1999 Jul 27;100(4):e20–8.

56. J.B. Muhlestein, et al., "Cytomegalovirus seropositivity and C-reactive protein have independent and combined predictive value for mortality in patients with angiographically demonstrated coronary artery disease." *Circulation.* 2000 Oct 17;102(16):1917–23.

57. S. Blankenberg, et al., "Cytomegalovirus infection with interleukin-6 response predicts cardiac mortality in patients with coronary artery disease." *Circulation.* 2001 Jun 19;103(24):2915–21.

58. B.J. Nicklas, et al., "Diet-induced weight loss, exercise, and chronic inflammation in older, obese adults: a randomized controlled clinical trial." *Am J Clin Nutr.* 2004 Apr;79(4):544–51.

59. Giugliano, et al., "The effects of diet on inflammation."

60. P.M. Ridker, et al., "Inflammation, aspirin, and the risk of cardiovascular disease in apparently healthy men." *N Engl J Med.* 1997 Apr 3;336(14):973–9.

61. Berg and Scherer, "Adipose tissue, inflammation, and cardiovascular disease."

The Gut Connection

1.   S. Bengmark, "Ecological control of the gastrointestinal tract. The role of probiotic flora." *Gut.* 1998 January; 42(1): 2–7.

2.   R.D. Berg, "The indigenous gastrointestinal microflora." *Trends Microbiol.* 1996 Nov;4(11):430–5.

3.   J.K. Nicholson, et al., "Gut microorganisms, mammalian metabolism and personalized health care." *Nat Rev Microbiol.* 2005 May;3(5):431–8.

4.   J. Xu and J.I. Gordon, "Honor thy symbionts." *Proc Natl Acad Sci USA.* 2003 Sep 2;100(18):10452–9.

5.   G.T. MacFarlane and S. MacFarlane, "Human colonic microbiota: ecology, physiology and metabolic potential of intestinal bacteria." *Scand J Gastroenterol Suppl.* 1997;222:3–9.

6.   P.J. Turnbaugh, et al., "The human microbiome project." *Nature.* 2007 Oct 18;449(7164):804–10.

7.   F. Backhed, et al., "Host-bacterial mutualism in the human intestine." *Science.* 2005 Mar 25;307(5717):1915–20.

8.   F. Guarner and J.R. Malagelada, "Gut flora in health and disease." *Lancet.* 2003 Feb 8;361(9356):512–9.

9.   S. Omahoney and F. Shanahan, "Enteric bacterial flora and bacterial overgrowth." In: M. Feldman, L.S. Friedman, L.J. Brant, Eds. Gastrointestinal and Liver Disease. 8th ed. Philadelphia, PA: Saunders/Elsevier;2006;2244–56.

10. FAO/WHO. Report of a Joint FAO/WHO Expert Group. Health and Nutritional Properties of Probiotics in Food Including Powder Milk with Live Lactic Acid Bacteria. Cordoba, Argentina: Food and Agricultural Organization of the United Nations, World Health Organization, 1–4 October 2001.

11. D.C. Montrose and M.H. Floch, "Probiotics used in human studies." *J Clin Gastroenterol.* 2005 Jul;39(6):469–84.

12. M.H. Floch, "Intestinal microecology." In: M.H. Floch and A.S. Kim, Eds. Probiotics: A Clinical Guide. Thoroughfare, NJ: Slack Incorporated; 2010;3–11.

13. N. Cerf-Bensussan and V. Gaboriau-Routhiau, "The immune system and the gut microbiota: friends or foes?" *Nat Rev Immunol.* 2010 Oct;10(10):735–44.

14. B. Corthesy, et al., "Cross-talk between probiotic bacteria and the host immune system." *J Nutr.* 2007 Mar;137(3 Suppl 2):781S–90S.

15. Montrose and Floch, "Probiotics used in human studies."

16. M.E. Sanders, et al., "Probiotics: their potential to impact human health." Council for Agricultural Science and Technology Issue Paper, 36. pp. 1–20.

17. E. Isolauri, et al., "Probiotics: a role in the treatment of intestinal infection and inflammation?" *Gut.* 2002 May; 50(Suppl 3): iii54–iii59.

18. H.C. Lin, "Small intestinal bacterial overgrowth: a framework for understanding irritable bowel syndrome." JAMA. 2004 Aug 18;292(7):852–8.

19. J.A. Jackson, et al., "Candida albicans: the hidden infection." *J Orthomolec Med.* 1999;14(4):198–200.

20. L. Galland, "Nutrition and Candidiasis." *J. Orthomol Psychiatry.* 1985;14(1):50–60.

21. J.A. Hawrelak and S.P. Myers, "The causes of intestinal dysbiosis: A review." *Alt Med Rev.* 2004;9(2):190–97.

22. V. Mai and P.V. Draganov, "Recent advances and remaining gaps in our knowledge of associations between gut microbiota and human health." *World J Gastroenterol.* 2009 January 7; 15(1): 81–5.

23. Hawrelak and Myers, ""The causes of intestinal dysbiosis."

24. M. Blaser, "Antibiotic overuse: stop the killing of beneficial bacteria." *Nature.* 2011 Aug 24;476(7361):393–4.

25. Hawrelak and Myers, "The causes of intestinal dysbiosis."

26. E. Bennett, et al., "Level of chronic life stress predicts clinical outcome in irritable bowel syndrome." *Gut.* 1998 August; 43(2): 256–61.

27. W. Kruis, et al., "Effect of diets low and high in refined sugars on gut transit, bile acid metabolism, and bacterial fermentation." *Gut.* 1991 April; 32(4): 367–71.

28. S.J. Lewis and K.W. Heaton, "The metabolic consequences of slow colonic transit." *Am J Gastroenterol.* 1999 Aug;94(8):2010–6.

29. P.J. Turnbaugh, et al., "The effect of diet on the human gut microbiome: a metagenomic analysis in humanized gnotobiotic mice." *Sci Transl Med.* 2009 Nov 11;1(6):6ra14.

30. M. Delzenne and P.D. Cani, "A place for dietary fibre in the management of the metabolic syndrome." *Curr Opin Clin Nutr Metab Care.* 2005 Nov;8(6):636–40.

31. K.M. Maslowski and C.R. Mackay, "Diet, gut microbiota and immune responses." Diet, gut microbiota and immune responses." *Nat Immunol.* 2011 Jan;12(1):5–9.

32. D.M. McKay, "Intestinal inflammation and the gut microflora." *Can J Gastroenterol.* 1999; Jul Aug13(6):509–16.

33. P.D. Cani, et al., "Changes in gut microbiota control metabolic endotoxemia-induced inflammation in high-fat diet-induced obesity and diabetes in mice." *Diabetes.* 2008 Jun;57(6):1470–81.

34. A. Krack, et al., "The importance of the gastrointestinal system in the pathogenesis of heart failure." *Eur Heart J.* 2005 Nov;26(22):2368–74.

35. M. Heyman and J.F. Desjeux, "Cytokine-induced alteration of the epithelial barrier to food antigens in disease." *Ann N Y Acad Sci.* 2000;915:304–11.

36. K. Fine, "Early diagnosis of gluten sensitivity: before the villi are gone." Transcript, 2003 Jun, Greater Louisville Celiac Sprue Support Group. www.enterolab.com/StaticPages/EarlyDiagnosis.aspx

37. S.M. Collins, "Stress and the gastrointestinal tract IV. Modulation of intestinal inflammation by stress: basic mechanisms and clinical relevance." *Am J Physiol Gastrointest Liver Physiol.* 2001 Mar;280(3):G315–8.

38. M. Maes, "The cytokine hypothesis of depression: inflammation, oxidative & nitrosative stress (IO&NS) and leaky gut as new targets for adjunctive treatments in depression." *Neuro Endocrinol Lett.* 2008 Jun;29(3):287–91.

39. A. Gummesson, et al., "Intestinal permeability is associated with visceral adiposity in healthy women." *Obesity (Silver Spring).* 2011 Nov;19(11):2280–2.

40. G.S. Kelly, "Hydrochloric acid: physiological functions and clinical implications." *Alt Med Rev.* 1997;2(2):116–27.

41. Ibid.

42. E.P. DiMagno, "Controversies in the treatment of exocrine pancreatic insufficiency." *Dig Dis Sci.* 1982 Jun;27(6):481–4.

43. C. Pleyer, et al., "Observer bias in the diagnosis of gastroesophageal reflux disease and functional dyspepsia." 2011 Nov. ACG Annual Scientific Meeting and Postgraduate Course, Washington, D.C.

44. D.S. Jones, M.D. (editor), Textbook of Functional Medicine, The Institute for Functional Medicine, 2005, p. 436.

45. M. Roxas, "The role of enzyme supplementation in digestive disorders." *Altern Med Rev.* 2008 Dec;13(4):307–14.

46. Jones, Textbook of Functional Medicine.

47. I. Sekirov, et al., "Gut microbiota in health and disease." *Physiol Rev.* Jul 2010;90(3):859–904.

48. P.D. Cani, et al., "Changes in gut microbiota control inflammation in obese mice through a mechanism involving GLP-2-driven improvement of gut permeability." *Gut.* 2009 Aug;58(8):1091–103.

49. N. Larsen, et al., "Gut microbiota in human adults with type 2 diabetes differs from non-diabetic adults." *PLoS One.* 2010 Feb 5;5(2):e9085.

50. F. Backhed, et al., "The gut microbiota as an environmental factor that regulates fat storage." *Proc Natl Acad Sci USA.* 2004 Nov 2;101(44):15718–23.

51. S.J. Creely, et al., "Lipopolysaccharide activates an innate immune system response in human adipose tissue in obesity and type 2 diabetes." *Am J Physiol Endocrinol Metab.* 2007 Mar;292(3):E740–7.

52. Cani, et al., "The gut microbiota as an environmental factor that regulates fat storage."

53. P.D. Cani, et al., "Metabolic endotoxemia initiates obesity and insulin resistance." *Diabetes.* 2007 Jul;56(7):1761–72.

54. M. Kalliomaki, et al., "Early differences in fecal microbiota composition in children may predict overweight." *Am J Clin Nutr.* 2008 Mar;87(3):534–8.

55. P.D. Cani, et al., "Selective increases of bifidobacteria in gut microflora improve high-fat-diet-induced diabetes in mice through a mechanism associated with endotoxaemia." *Diabetologia.* 2007 Nov;50(11):2374–83.

56. Z.M. Younossi, "Review article: current management of nonalcoholic fatty liver disease and nonalcoholic steatohepatitis." *Aliment Pharmacol Ther.* 2008 Jul;28(1):2–12.

57. L. Miele, et al., "Increased intestinal permeability and tight junction alterations in nonalcoholic fatty liver disease." *Hepatology.* 2009 Jun;49(6):1877–87.

58. A.L. Harte, et al., "Elevated endotoxin levels in non-alcoholic fatty liver disease." *J Inflamm (Lond).* 2010 Mar 30;7:15.

Interview with Dr. Leonard Smith

1. W.S. Harris and C. von Schacky, "The Omega-3 Index: a new risk factor for death from coronary heart disease?" *Prev Med.* 2004 Jul;39(1):212–20.

2. J. Qin, et al., "A human gut microbial gene catalogue established by metagenomic sequencing." *Nature.* 2010 Mar 4;464(7285):59–65.

3. S.C. Johnston, et al., "C-reactive protein levels and viable Chlamydia pneumoniae in carotid artery atherosclerosis." Stroke. 2001 Dec 1;32(12):2748–52.

4. P.D. Cani, et al., "Metabolic endotoxemia initiates obesity and insulin resistance." *Diabetes.* 2007 Jul;56(7):1761–72.

5. H.C. Gerstein, et al., "Long-term effects of intensive glucose lowering on cardiovascular outcomes." *N Engl J Med.* 2011 Mar 3;364(9):818–28.

6. A, Schweirtz, et al., "Microbiota and SCFA in lean and overweight healthy subjects." *Obesity (Silver Spring).* 2010 Jan;18(1):190–5

7. J.S. Bakken, "Fecal bacteriotherapy for recurrent Clostridium difficile infection." *Anaerobe.* 2009 Dec;15(6):285–9.

8. T.J. Borody, et al., "Treatment of ulcerative colitis using fecal bacteriotherapy." *J Clin Gastroenterol.* 2003 Jul;37(1):42–7.

9. A. Vrieze, et al., "Metabolic effects of transplanting gut microbiota from lean donors to subjects with metabolic syndrome." *EASD.* A90; 2010.

10. V. Lam, et al., "Intestinal microbiota determine severity of myocardial infarction in rats." *FASEB* J. 2012 Feb 7.

11. A. Bomba, et al., "The influence of omega-3 polyunsaturated fatty acids (omega-3 pufa) on lactobacilli adhesion to the intestinal mucosa and on immunity in gnotobiotic piglets." *Berl Munch Tierarztl Wochenschr.* 2003 Jul–Aug;116(7-8):312–6.

12. H.J. Thompson, et al., "Effect of increased vegetable and fruit consumption on markers of oxidative cellular damage." *Carcinogenesis.* 1999 Dec;20(12):2261–6.

13. C.B. Ebbeling, et al., "Effects of a low-glycemic load vs low-fat diet in obese young adults: a randomized trial." *JAMA.* 2007 May 16;297(19):2092–102.

Stress

1. M. LeFevre, et al., "Eustress, distress, and interpretation in occupational stress." *J Manager Psych.* 2003;18(7):726–44.

2. G.P. Chrousos and P.W. Gold, "The concepts of stress and stress system disorders.: overview of physical and behavioral homeostasis." *JAMA.* 1992 Mar 4;267(9):1244–52.

3. T. Chandola, et al., "Chronic stress at work and the metabolic syndrome: prospective study." *BMJ.* 2006 Mar 4;332(7540):521–5.

4. M.M. Burg, "Stress, behavior, and heart disease." www.med.yale.edu/library/heartbk/8.pdf, pp. 95–104.

5.   J. MacLeod, et al., "Psychological stress and cardiovascular disease: empirical demonstration of bias in a prospective observational study of Scottish men." *BMJ.* 2002 May 25;324(7348):1247–51.

6.   S.J. Bunker, et al., "'Stress' and coronary heart disease: psychosocial risk factors." *Med J Aust.* 2003 Mar 17;178(6):272–6.

7.   B. Ohlin, et al., "Chronic psychosocial stress predicts long-term cardiovascular morbidity and mortality in middle-aged men." *Eur Heart J.* 2004 May;25(10):867–73.

8.   T. Chandola, et al., "Work stress and coronary heart disease: what are the mechanisms?" *Eur Heart J.* 2008 Mar;29(5):640–8.

9.   Chandola, et al., "Chronic stress at work and the metabolic syndrome."

10. K. Orth-Gomer, et al., "Marital stress worsens prognosis in women with coronary heart disease: the Stockholm Female Coronary Risk Study." *JAMA.* 2000 Dec 20;284(23):3008–14.

11. Bunker, et al., "'Stress' and coronary heart disease."

12. T.G. Allison, et al., "Medical and economic costs of psychologic distress in patients with coronary artery disease." *Mayo Clin Proc.* 1995 Aug;70(8):734–42.

13. P.P. Vitaliano, et al., "A path model of chronic stress, the metabolic syndrome, and coronary heart disease." *Psychosom Med.* 2002 May-Jun;64(3):418–35.

14. E.S. Epel, et al., "Stress and body shape: stress-induced cortisol secretion is consistently greater among women with central fat." *Psychosom Med.* 2000 Sep-Oct;62(5):623–32.

15. J.L. Gordon, et al., "The effect of major depression on postexercise cardiovascular recovery." *Psychophysiology.* 2011 Nov;48(11):1605–10.

16. W. Jiang and J.R. Davidson, "Antidepressant therapy in patients with ischemic heart disease." *Am Heart J.* 2005 Nov;150(5):871–81.

17. J.H. Lichtman, et al., "Depression and coronary heart disease: recommendations for screening, referral, and treatment: a science advisory from the American Heart Association Prevention Committee of the Council on Cardiovascular Nursing, Council on Clinical Cardiology, Council on Epidemiology and Prevention, and Interdisciplinary Council on Quality of Care and Outcomes Research: endorsed by the American Psychiatric Association." *Circulation.* 2008 Oct 21;118(17):1768–75.

18. Chandola, et al., "Work stress and coronary heart disease."

19. R. McCraty, et al., "The effects of emotions on short-term power spectrum analysis of heart rate variability." *Am J Cardiol.* 1995 Nov 15;76(14):1089–93.

20. H. Tsuji, et al., "Impact of reduced heart rate variability on risk for cardiac events. The Framingham Heart Study." *Circulation.* 1996 Dec 1;94(11):2850–5.

21. M. Schledowski, et al., "Acute psychological stress increases plasma levels of cortisol, prolactin and TSH." *Life Sci.* 1992;50(17):1201–5.

22. P. Schultz, et al., "Increased free cortisol secretion after awakening in chronically stressed individuals due to work overload." *Stress Med.* 1998;14:91–7.

23. J.S. Yudkin, et al., "Inflammation, obesity, stress and coronary heart disease: is interleukin-6 the link?" *Atherosclerosis.* 2000 Feb;148(2):209–14.T

24. C. Tsigos and G.P. Chrousos, "Hypothalamic-pituitary-adrenal axis, neuroendocrine factors and stress." *J Psychosom Res.* 2002 Oct;53(4):865–71.

25. E.J. Brunner, et al., "Social inequality in coronary risk: central obesity and the metabolic syndrome. Evidence from the Whitehall II study." *Diabetologia.* 1997 Nov;40(11):1341–9.

26. D.S. Jones (editor), Textbook of Functional Medicine. The Institute for Functional Medicine, 2005, p. 670.

27. J.F. Cryan and S.M. O'Mahony, "The microbiome-gut-brain axis: from bowel to behavior." *Neurogastroenterol Motil.* 2011 Mar;23(3):187–92.

28. A. Hart and M.A. Kamm, "Review article: mechanisms of initiation and perpetuation of gut inflammation by stress." *Aliment Pharmacol Ther.* 2002 Dec;16(12):2017–28.

29. J.D. Soderhold and M.H. Perdue, "Stress and gastrointestinal tract. II. Stress and intestinal barrier function." *Am J Physiol Gastrointest Liver Physiol.* 2001 Jan;280(1):G7–G13.

30. M.T. Bailey and C.L. Coe, "Maternal separation disrupts the integrity of the intestinal microflora in infant rhesus monkeys." *Dev Psychobiol.* 1999 Sep;35(2):146–55.

31. W.E. Moore, et al., "Some current concepts in intestinal bacteriology." *Am J Clin Nutr.* 1978 Oct;31(10 Suppl):S33–42.

32. H. Eutamene and L. Bueno, "Role of probiotics in correcting abnormalities of colonic flora induced by stress." *Gut.* 2007 Nov;56(11):1495–7.

33. N. Sudo, et al., "Postnatal microbial colonization programs the hypothalamic-pituitary-adrenal system for stress response in mice." *J Physiol.* 2004 Jul 1;558(Pt 1):263–75.

34. M. Lasalandra and L.S. Friedman (eds.), The Sensitive Gut. Harvard School of Public Health, Harvard Health Publications, 2010.

Endothelial Dysfunction

1.   J. Davignon and P. Ganz, "Role of endothelial dysfunction in atherosclerosis." *Circulation.* 2004 Jun 15;109(23 Suppl 1):III27–32.

2.   P.O. Bonetti, et al., "Endothelial dysfunction: a marker of atherosclerotic risk." *Arterioscler Thromb Vasc Biol.* 2003 Feb 1;23(2):168–75.

3.   H. Cai and D.G. Harrison, "Endothelial dysfunction in cardiovascular diseases: the role of oxidant stress." *Circ Res.* 2000 Nov 10;87(10):840–4.

4.   D.S. Celemajer, et al., "Endothelium-dependent dilation in the systemic arteries of asymptomatic subjects relates to coronary risk factors and their interaction." *J Am Coll Cardiol.* 1994 Nov 15;24(6):1468–74.

5.   J. Loscalzo, "Homocysteine trials—clear outcomes for complex reasons." *N Engl J Med.* 2006 Apr 13;354(15):1629–32.

6.   M.J. Stampfer, et al., "A prospective study of plasma homocyst(e)ine and risk of myocardial infarction in US physicians." *JAMA.* 1992 Aug 19;268(7):877–81.

7.   O. Nygard, et al., "Plasma homocysteine levels and mortality in patients with coronary artery disease." *N Engl J Med.* 1997 Jul 24;337(4):230–6.

8.   R. Clarke, et al., "Lowering blood homocysteine with folic acid based supplements: meta-analysis of randomised trials." *BMJ.* 1998 March 21; 316(7135): 894–8.

9.   D.S. Wald, "Homocysteine and cardiovascular disease: evidence on causality from a meta-analysis." *BMJ.* 2002 Nov 23;325(7374):1202.

10.   L.D. Botto and Q. Yang, "5,10-Methylenetetrahydrofolate reductase gene variants and congenital anomalies: a HuGE review." *Am J Epidemiol.* 2000 May 1;151(9):862–77.

11.   Davignon and Ganz, "Role of endothelial dysfunction in atherosclerosis."

Hormones And The Heart

1.   "Hormone therapy and heart disease: is it all in the timing? Two new trials will test whether there is an 'age effect' for hormone therapy." *Harv Health Lett.* 2006 Jun;31(8):4–5.

2.   L.J. Mosca, "Contemporary management of hyperlipidemia in women." *J Womens Health Gend Based Med.* 2002 Jun;11(5):423–32.

3.   www.nhlbi.nih.gov/whi/

4.   J. Hsia, et al., "Conjugated equine estrogens and coronary heart disease: the Women's Health Initiative." *Arch Intern Med.* 2006 Feb 13;166(3):357–65.

5.   M.E. Medelsohn and R.H. Karas, "The protective effects of estrogen on the cardiovascular system." *N Engl J Med.* 1999 Jun 10;340(23):1801–11.

6.   R.K. Hermsmeyer, et al., "Cardiovascular effects of medroxyprogesterone acetate and progesterone: a case of mistaken identity?" *Nat Clin Pract Cardiovasc Med.* 2008 Jul;5(7):387–95.

7.   B.S. Apgar and G. Greenberg, "Using progestins in clinical practice." *Am Fam Physician.* 2000 Oct 15;62(8):1839–46.

8.   D. Moskowitz, "A comprehensive review of the safety and efficacy of bioidentical hormones for the management of menopause and related health risks." *Altern Med Rev.* 2006 Sep;11(3):208–23.

9.   L. Fahraeus, et al., "L-norgestrel and progesterone have different influences on plasma lipoproteins." *Eur J Clin Invest.* 1983 Dec;13(6):447–53.

10.   J.L. Toy, et al., "The comparative effects of a synthetic and a 'natural' oestrogen on the haemostatic mechanism in patients with primary amenorrhoea." *Br J Obstet Gynaecol.* 1978 May;85(5):359–62.

11.   J. Stephenson, et al., "Topical progesterone cream does not increase thrombotic and inflammatory factos in postmenopausal women." *Blood.* 2004;104:414b–415b(Abstract 5318).

12.   P. Ebling and V.A. Koivisto, "Physiological importance of dehydroepiandrosterone." *Lancet.* 1994 Jun 11;343(8911):1479–81.

13.   G.P. Bernini, et al., "Endogenous androgens and carotid intimal-medial thickness in women." *J Clin Endocrinol Metab.* 1999 Jun;84(6):2008–12.

14.   www.webmd.com/heart-disease/news/20100622/high-testosterone-may-raise-heart-risk

15.   men.webmd.com/news/20030527/low-testosterone-linked-to-heart-disease

16.   N. Makhsida, et al., "Hypogonadism and metabolic syndrome: implications for testosterone therapy." *J Urol.* 2005 Sep;174(3):827–34.

17.   K.C. Westerlind, "The role of estrogen metabolism in aging." *J Musculoskelet Neuronal Interact.* 2003 Dec;3(4):370–3; discussion 381.

18.   C.M. Masi, et al., "Estrogen metabolites and systolic blood pressure in a population-based sample of postmenopausal women." *J Clin Endocrinol Metab.* 2006 Mar;91(3):1015–20.

19.   A.T. Bentz, et al., "The relationship between physical activity and 2-hydroxyestrone, 16alpha-hydroxyestrone, and the 2/16 ratio in premenopausal women (United States)." *Cancer Causes Control.* 2005 May;16(4):455–61.

20.   C.E. Matthews, et al., "Physical activity, body size, and estrogen metabolism in women." *Cancer Causes Control.* 2004 Jun;15(5):473–81.

Toxins And Heart Disease

1.   W.J. Crinnion, "The CDC fourth national report on human exposure to environmental chemicals: what it tells us about our toxic burden and how it assist environmental medicine physicians." *Altern Med Rev.* 2010 Jul;15(2):101–9.

2.   A.E. Taylor, "Cardiovascular effects of environmental chemicals." *Otolaryngol Head Neck Surg.* 1996 Feb;114(2):209–11.

3.   R.D. Brook, et al., "Air pollution and cardiovascular disease: a statement for healthcare professionals from the Expert Panel on Population and Prevention Science of the American Heart Association." *Circulation.* 2004 Jun 1;109(21):2655–71.

4.   Ibid.

5.   B. Brunekreef and S.T. Holgate, "Air pollution and health." *Lancet.* 2002 Oct 19;360(9341):1233–42.

6.   D.W. Dockery, et al., "An association between air pollution and mortality in six U.S. cities." *N Engl J Med.* 1993 Dec 9;329(24):1753–9.

7.   J.M. Samnet, et al., "Fine particulate air pollution and mortality in 20 U.S. cities, 1987-1994." *N Engl J Med.* 2000 Dec 14;343(24):1742–9.

8.   F. Dominici, et al., "Revised analyses of the National Morbidity, Mortality, and Air Pollution Study: mortality among residents of 90 cities." *J Toxicol Environ Health A.* 2005 Jul 9-23;68(13-14):1071–92.

9.   C.R. Bartoli, et al., "Mechanisms of inhaled fine particulate air pollution-induced arterial blood pressure changes." *Environ Health Perspect.* 2009 Mar;117(3):361–6.

10.   B.Z. Simkhovich, et al., "Air pollution and cardiovascular injury epidemiology, toxicology, and mechanisms." *J Am Coll Cardiol.* 2008 Aug 26;52(9):719–26.

11.   J.A. Ambrose and R.S. Barua, "The pathophysiology of cigarette smoking and cardiovascular disease: an update." *J Am Coll Cardiol.* 2004 May 19;43(10):1731–7.

12.   A. Burton, "Secondhand smoke: Parental smoking may set up children for atherosclerosis." *Environ Health Perspect.* 2010 May; 118(5): A200.

13.   R.J. Letcher, et al., "Exposure and effects assessment of persistent organohalogen contaminants in arctic wildlife and fish." *Sci Total Environ.* 2010 Jul 1;408(15):2995–3043.

14.   P.M. Lind, et al., "Circulating levels of persistent organic pollutants (POPs) and carotid atherosclerosis in the elderly." *Environ Health Perspect.* 2011 Oct 11;120(1):38–43.

15.   D.H. Lee, et al., "Low dose of some persistent organic pollutants predicts type 2 diabetes: a nested case-control study." *Environ Health Perspect.* 2010 Sep;118(9):1235–42.

16. A. Navas-Acien, et al., "Lead exposure and cardiovascular disease--a systematic review." *Environ Health Perspect.* 2007 Mar;115(3):472–82.

17. P. Ayotte, et al., "Relation between methylmercury exposure and plasma paraoxonase activity in inuit adults from Nunavik." *Environ Health Perspect.* 2011 Aug;119(8):1077–83.

18. M. Vahter, et al., "Toxic metals and the menopause." *J Br Menopause Soc.* 2004 Jun;10(2):60–4.

19. N.E. Clarke, et al., "The in vivo dissolution of metastatic calcium; an approach to atherosclerosis." *Am J Med Sci.* 1955 Feb;229(2):142–9.

20. L.T. Chappell, "Applications of EDTA therapy." *Alt Med Rev.* 1997;2(6):426–32.

21. C. Hancke and M.D. Flytlie, "Benefits of EDTA chelation therapy in arteriosclerosis: a retrospective study of 470 patients." *J Adv Med.* 1993;6(3):161–72.

22. P.M. Kidd, "Integrative cardiac revitalization: bypass surgery, angioplasty, and chelation. Benefits, risks, and limitations." *Altern Med Rev.* 1998 Feb;3(1):4–17.

23. nccam.nih.gov/health/chelation/

Love Your Heart: The History of Diet

1. S.B. Eaton, et al., "Stone agers in the fast lane: chronic degenerative diseases in evolutionary perspective." *Am J Med.* 1988 Apr;84(4):739–49.

2. S.B. Eaton, "The ancestral human diet: what was it and should it be a paradigm for contemporary nutrition?" *Proc Nutr Soc.* 2006 Feb;65(1):1–6.

3. P.A. Cotton, et al., "Dietary sources of nutrients among US adults, 1994 to 1996." *J Am Diet Assoc.* 2004 Jun;104(6):921–30.

4. Eaton, et al., "The ancestral human diet."

5. P.M. Kris-Etherton, et al., "Polyunsaturated fatty acids in the food chain in the United States." *Am J Clin Nutr.* 2000 Jan;71(1 Suppl):179S–88S.

6. P. Trumbo, et al., "Dietary reference intakes for energy, carbohydrate, fiber, fat, fatty acids, cholesterol, protein and amino acids." *J Am Diet Assoc.* 2002 Nov;102(11):1621–30.

7. L.A. Frassetto, et al., "Dietary sodium chloride intake independently predicts the degree of hyperchloremic metabolic acidosis in healthy humans consuming a net acid-producing diet." *Am J Physiol Renal Physiol.* 2007 Aug;293(2):F521–5.

8. S. Jew, et al., "Evolution of the human diet: linking our ancestral diet to modern functional foods as a means of chronic disease prevention." *J Med Food.* 2009 Oct;12(5):925–34.

9. L. Cordain, et al., "Plant-animal subsistence ratios and macronutrient energy estimations in worldwide hunter-gatherer diets." *Am J Clin Nutr.* 2000 Mar;71(3):682–92.

10. Jew, et al., "Evolution of the human diet."

11. Anichkov NN. "A history of experimentation on arterial atherosclerosis in animals." In: Blumenthal HT, editor. Cowdry's Arteriosclerosis: A Survey of the Problem. 2nd ed. Springfield, (IL): Charles C. Thomas Publishing; 1967. p. 21–46.

12. A. Keys, et al., "Epidemiological studies related to coronary heart disease: characteristics of men aged 40–59 in seven countries." *Acta Med Scand Suppl.* 1966;460:1–392.

13. G. Taubes, "Nutrition. The soft science of dietary fat." *Science.* 2001 Mar 30;291(5513):2536–45.

14. The Lipid Research Clinics Coronary Primary Prevention Trial results. "Reduction in incidence of coronary heart disease." *JAMA.* 1984 Jan 20;251(3):351–64.

15. S.L. Weinberg, "The diet-heart hypothesis." *J Am Coll Cardiol.* 2004 Mar 3;43(5):731-3.

16. Ibid.

17. F.B. Hu, et al., "Types of dietary fat and risk of coronary heart disease: a critical review." *J Am Coll Nutr.* 2001 Feb;20(1):5–19.

18. L. Hooper, et al., "Dietary fat intake and prevention of cardiovascular disease: systematic review." *BMJ.* 2001 Mar 31;322(7289):757–63.

19. P.W. Siti-Tarino, et al., "Meta-analysis of prospective cohort studies evaluating the association of saturated fat with cardiovascular disease." *Am J Clin Nutr.* 2010 Mar;91(3):535–46.

20. R.P. Mensink and M.B. Katan, "Effect of dietary fatty acids on serum lipids and lipoproteins. A meta-analysis of 27 trials." *Arterioscler Thromb.* 1992 Aug;12(8):911–9.

21. F.B. Hu, et al., "Dietary fat intake and the risk of coronary heart disease in women." *N Engl J Med.* 1997 Nov 20;337(21):1491–9.

22. R.S. Kuipers, et al., "Saturated fat, carbohydrates and cardiovascular disease." *Neth J Med.* 2011 Sep;69(9):372–8.

23. W.S. Yancy Jr., et al., "Diets and clinical coronary events: the truth is out there." *Circulation.* 2003 Jan 7;107(1):10–6.

24. V. Jones, "The 'diabesity' epidemic: let's rehabilitate America." *MedGenMed.* 2006 May 8;8(2):34.

25. D.J. Jenkins, et al., "Glycemic index of foods: a physiological basis for carbohydrate exchange." *Am J Clin Nutr.* 1981 Mar;34(3):362–6.

26. S. Lui and W.C. Willett, "Dietary glycemic load and atherothrombotic risk." *Curr Atheroscler Rep.* 2002 Nov;4(6):454–61.

27. T.L. Cleave and G.D. Campbell, "The saccharine disease." *Am J Proctol.* 1967 Jun;18(3):202–10.

28. www.usda.gov/factbook/chapter2.htm

29. L.M. Hanover and J.S. White, "Manufacturing, composition, and applications of fructose." *Am J Clin Nutr.* 1993 Nov;58(5 Suppl):724S–732S.

30. Eaton, et al., "The ancestral human diet."

31. L. Cordain, "The paradoxical nature of hunter-gatherer diets: meat-based, yet non-atherogenic." *Eur J Clin Nutr.* 2002 Mar;56 Suppl1:S42–52.

Love Your Heart: The Whole Story

1. U.S. Department of Agriculture and U.S. Department of Health and Human Services. Report of the Dietary Guidelines Advisory Committee on the dietary guidelines for Americans, 2010. June 15, 2010. www.cnpp.usda.gov/Publications/DietaryGuidelines/2010/PolicyDoc/PolicyDoc.pdf.

2. www.hsph.harvard.edu/nutritionsource/what-should-you-eat/dietary-guidelines-2010/

3. R.M. Krauss, et al., "AHA Dietary Guidelines: revision 2000: a statement for healthcare professionals from the Nutrition Committee of the American Heart Association." *Stroke.* 2000 Nov;31(11):2751–66.

4. Centers for Disease Control and Prevention. "Trends in intake of energy and macronutrients—United States, 1971–2000. Morb Mortal Wkly Rep. 2004;53:80–2.

5. A.H. Hite, et al., "In the face of contradictory evidence: report of the Dietary Guidelines for Americans Committee." *Nutrition.* 2010 Oct;26(10):915–24.

6. Ibid.

7. B.V. Howard and J. Wylie-Rosette, "Sugar and cardiovascular disease: a statement for healthcare professionals from the Committee on Nutrition of the Council on Nutrition, Physical Activity, and Metabolism of the American Heart Association." *Circulation.* 2002 Jul 23;106(4):523–7.

8. S.L. Archer, et al., "Relationship between changes in dietary sucrose and high density lipoprotein cholesterol: the CARDIA study." Coronary Artery Risk Development in Young Adults. *Ann Epidemiol.* 1998 Oct;8(7):433–8.

9. K.N. Frayn and S.M. Kingman, "Dietary sugars and lipid metabolism in humans." *Am J Clin Nutr.* 1995 Jul;62(1 Suppl):250S-261S; discussion 261S–263S.

10. S.K. Fried and S.P. Rao, "Sugars, hypertriglyceridemia, and cardiovascular disease." *Am J Clin Nutr.* 2003 Oct;78(4):873S–880S.

11. M. Chandalia, et al., "Beneficial effects of high dietary fiber intake in patients with type 2 diabetes mellitus." *N Engl J Med.* 2000 May 11;342(19):1392–8.

12. D.S. Ludwig, et al., "Dietary fiber, weight gain, and cardiovascular disease risk factors in young adults." *JAMA.* 1999 Oct 27;282(16):1539–46.

13. I.M. Vasconcelos and J.T. Oliveira, "Antinutritional properties of plant lectins." *Toxicon.* 2004 Sep 15;44(4):385–403.

14. A. Pusztai, "Dietary lectins are metabolic signals for the gut and modulate immune and hormone functions." *Eur J Clin Nutr.* 1993 Oct;47(10):691–9.

15. D.L. Freed, "Do dietary lectins cause disease?" *BMJ.* 1999 Apr 17;318(7190):1023–4.

16. G.L. Blackburn, et al., "Physician's guide to popular low-carbohydrate weight-loss diets." *Cleve Clin J Med.* 2001 Sep;68(9):761, 765-6, 768-9, 773–4.

17. M. Hession, et al., "Systematic review of randomized controlled trials of low-carbohydrate vs. low-fat/low-calorie diets in the management of obesity and its comorbidities." *Obes Rev.* 2009 Jan;10(1):36–50.

18. A.J. Nordman, et al., "Effects of low-carbohydrate vs low-fat diets on weight loss and cardiovascular risk factors: a meta-analysis of randomized controlled trials." *Arch Intern Med.* 2006 Feb 13;166(3):285–93.

19. S.M. Nickols-Richardson, "Perceived hunger is lower and weight loss is greater in overweight premenopausal women consuming a low-carbohydrate/high-protein vs high-carbohydrate/low-fat diet." *J Am Diet Assoc.* 2005 Sep;105(9):1433–7.

20. J.S. Volek, et al., "Carbohydrate restriction has a more favorable impact on the metabolic syndrome than a low fat diet." *Lipids.* 2009 Apr;44(4):297–309.

21. G.D. Foster, et al., "A randomized trial of a low-carbohydrate diet for obesity." *N Engl J Med.* 2003 May 22;348(21):2082–90.

22. J.H. O'Keefe Jr. and L. Cordain, "Cardiovascular disease resulting from a diet and lifestyle at odds with our Paleolithic genome: how to become a 21st-century hunter-gatherer." *Mayo Clin Proc.* 2004 Jan;79(1):101–8.

23. S. Lindberg, et al., "A Palaeolithic diet improves glucose tolerance more than a Mediterranean-like diet in individuals with ischaemic heart disease." *Diabetologia.* 2007 Sep;50(9):1795–807.

24. T. Jonsson, et al., "Beneficial effects of a Paleolithic diet on cardiovascular risk factors in type 2 diabetes: a randomized cross-over pilot study." *Cardiovasc Diabetol.* 2009 Jul 16;8:35.

25. S. Jew, "Evolution of the human diet: linking our ancestral diet to modern functional foods as a means of chronic disease prevention." *J Med Food.* 2009 Oct;12(5):925–34.

26. K.M. Smith and N.R. Sahyoun, "Fish consumption: recommendations versus advisories, can they be reconciled?" *Nutr Rev.* 2005 Feb;63(2):39–46.

27. K.L. Stanhope, et al., "Consumption of fructose and high fructose corn syrup increase postprandial triglycerides, LDL-cholesterol, and apolipoprotein-B in young men and women." *J Clin Endocrinol Metab.* 2011 Oct;96(10):E1596–605.

The HOPE Solution—H=High Fiber

1. A.L. Miller, "The pathogenesis, clinical implications, and treatment of intestinal hyperpermeability." *Alt Med Rev.* 1997;2(5):330–7.

2. www.webmd.com/diet/fiber-health-benefits-11/fiber-heart

3. M.A. Pereira, et al., "Dietary fiber and risk of coronary heart disease: a pooled analysis of cohort studies." *Arch Intern Med.* 2004 Feb 23;164(4):370–6.

4. K.J. Joshipura, et al., "The effect of fruit and vegetable intake on risk for coronary heart disease." *Ann Intern Med.* 2001 Jun 19;134(12):1106–14.

5. M.W. Gillman, et al., "Protective effect of fruits and vegetables on development of stroke in men." *JAMA.* 1995 Apr 12;273(14):1113–7.

6. L.A. Bazzano, et al., "Dietary fiber intake and reduced risk of coronary heart disease in US men and women: the National Health and Nutrition Examination Survey I Epidemiologic Follow-up Study." *Arch Intern Med.* 2003 Sep 8;163(16):1897–904.

7. S. Liu, et al., "Fruit and vegetable intake and risk of cardiovascular disease: the Women's Health Study." *Am J Clin Nutr.* 2000 Oct;72(4):922–8.

8. F.J. He, et al., "Increased consumption of fruit and vegetables is related to a reduced risk of coronary heart disease: meta-analysis of cohort studies." *J Hum Hypertens.* 2007 Sep;21(9):717–28.

9.   D.S. Ludwig, et al., "Dietary fiber, weight gain, and cardiovascular disease risk factors in young adults." *JAMA*. 1999 Oct 27;282(16):1539–46.

10.   American Heart Association. 2001 Heart and Stroke Statistical Update. Dallas, Tex: American Heart Association, 2000.

The HOPE Solution—O=Omega-3s

1.   W.S. Harris, et al., "Omega-3 fatty acids and coronary heart disease risk: clinical and mechanistic perspectives." *Atherosclerosis*. 2008 Mar;197(1):12–24.

2.   N. Hussein, et al., "Long-chain conversion of [13C]linoleic acid and alpha-linolenic acid in response to marked changes in their dietary intake in men." *J Lipid Res*. 2005 Feb;46(2):269–80.

3.   P.M. Kris-Etherton, et al., "Polyunsaturated fatty acids in the food chain in the United States." *Am J Clin Nutr*. 2000 Jan;71(1 Suppl):179S–88S.

4.   A.P. Simopoulos, "Omega-3 fatty acids in health and disease and in growth and development." Am J Clin Nutr. 1991 Sep;54(3):438–63.

5.   A.P. Simopoulos, "The importance of the ratio of omega-6/omega-3 essential fatty acids." *Biomed Pharmacother*. 2002 Oct;56(8):365–79.

6.   R. De Caterina, "n-3 fatty acids in cardiovascular disease." *N Engl J Med*. 2011 Jun 23;364(25):2439–50.

7.   J. Dyerberg, et al., "Eicosapentaenoic acid and prevention of thrombosis and atherosclerosis?" *Lancet*. 1978 Jul 15;2(8081):117–9.

8.   W.S. Harris, "Tissue n-3 and n-6 fatty acids and risk for coronary heart disease events." *Atherosclerosis*. 2007 Jul;193(1):1–10.

9.   F.B. Hu, et al., "Fish and omega-3 fatty acid intake and risk of coronary heart disease in women." *JAMA*. 2002 Apr 10;287(14):1815–21.

10.   M.L. Burr, et al., "Effects of changes in fat, fish, and fibre intakes on death and myocardial reinfarction: diet and reinfarction trial (DART)." *Lancet*. 1989 Sep 30;2(8666):757–61.

11.   Gruppo Italiano per lo Studio della Sopravvivenza nell'Infarto miocardico. "Dietary supplementation with n-3 polyunsaturated fatty acids and vitamin E after myocardial infarction: results of the GISSI-Prevenzione trial." *Lancet*. 1999 Aug 7;354(9177):447–55.

12.   L. Tavazzi, et al., "Effect of n-3 polyunsaturated fatty acids in patients with chronic heart failure (the GISSI-HF trial): a randomised, double-blind, placebo-controlled trial." *Lancet*. 2008 Oct 4;372(9645):1223–30.

13.   M. Yokoyama, et al., "Effects of eicosapentaenoic acid on major coronary events in hypercholesterolaemic patients (JELIS): a randomised open-label, blinded endpoint analysis." *Lancet*. 2007 Mar 31;369(9567):1090–8.

14.   Simopoulos, "The importance of the ratio of omega-6/omega-3 essential fatty acids."

15.   F. Thies, et al., "Association of n-3 polyunsaturated fatty acids with stability of atherosclerotic plaques: a randomised controlled trial." *Lancet*. 2003 Feb 8;361(9356):477–85.

16.   J. Goodfellow, et al., "Dietary supplementation with marine omega-3 fatty acids improve systemic large artery endothelial function in subjects with hypercholesterolemia." *J Am Coll Cardiol*. 2000 Feb;35(2):265–70.

17.   J.N. Din, et al., "Omega 3 fatty acids and cardiovascular disease—-fishing for a natural treatment." *BMJ*. 2004 Jan 3;328(7430):30–5

18.   T. Huang, et al., "High consumption of Ω-3 polyunsaturated fatty acids decrease plasma homocysteine: a meta-analysis of randomized, placebo-controlled trials." *Nutrition*. 2011 Sep;27(9):863–7.

19.   P.M. Kris-Etherton, et al., "Omega-3 fatty acids and cardiovascular disease: new recommendations from the American Heart Association." *Arterioscler Thromb Vasc Biol*. 2003 Feb 1;23(2):151–2.

20.   N. Kromann and A. Green: "Epidemiological studies in the Upernavik district, Greenland. Incidence of some chronic diseases 1950–1974." *Acta Med Scand*. 1980;208(5):401–6.

21.   L. Ferrucci, et al., "Relationship of plasma polyunsaturated fatty acids to circulating inflammatory markers." *J Clin Endocrinol Metab*. 2006 Feb;91(2):439–46.

22.   A.P. Simopoulos, "Omega-s fatty acids in inflammation and autoimmune diseases." *J Am Coll Nutr*. 2002 Dec;21(6):495–505.

23.   Din, et al., "Omega 3 fatty acids and cardiovascular disease."

24.   R. Wall, et al., "Fatty acids from fish: the anti-inflammatory potential of long-chain omega-3 fatty acids." *Nutr Rev*. 2010 May;68(5):280–9.

25.   J.M. Schwab and C.N. Serhan, "Lipoxins and new lipid mediators in the resolution of inflammation." *Curr Opin Pharmacol*. 2006 Aug;6(4):414–20.

26.   Kris-Etherton, et al., "Omega-3 fatty acids and cardiovascular disease."

27.   E. Guallar, et al., "Mercury, fish oils, and the risk of myocardial infarction." *N Engl J Med*. 2002 Nov 28;347(22):1747–54.

28.   www.epa.gov/mercury/advisories.htm

29.   www.fda.gov/OHRMS/DOCKETS/ac/02/briefing/3872_Advisory%201.pdf

30.   R.B. Singh, et al., "Randomized, double-blind, placebo-controlled trial of fish oil and mustard oil in patients with suspected acute myocardial infarction: the Indian experiment of infarct survival—4." *Cardiovasc Drugs Ther*. 1997 Jul;11(3):485–91.

31.   M. de Lorgeril, et al., "Mediterranean diet, traditional risk factors, and the rate of cardiovascular complications after myocardial infarction: final report of the Lyon Diet Heart Study." *Circulation*. 1999 Feb 16;99(6):779–85.

32.   W.J. Bemelmans, et al., "Effect of an increased intake of alpha-linolenic acid and group nutritional education on cardiovascular risk factors: the Mediterranean Alpha-linolenic Enriched Groningen Dietary Intervention (MARGARIN) study." *Am J Clin Nutr*. 2002 Feb;75(2):221–7.

33.   H. Natvig, et al., "A controlled trial of the effect of linolenic acid on incidence of coronary heart disease: The Norwegian vegetable oil experiment of 1965–66." *Scand J Clin Lab Invest Suppl*. 1968;105:1–20.

34.   Simopoulos, "Omega-3 fatty acids in inflammation and autoimmune diseases."

35.   De Caterina, "n-3 fatty acids in cardiovascular disease."

36.   www.dhaomega3.org/FAQ/Is-DHA-better-for-cardiovascular-care-than-EPA-What-should-I-focus-on

37.   Kris-Etherton, et al., "Omega-3 fatty acids and cardiovascular disease."

38. A.P. Simopoulos, et al., "Workshop on the Essentiality of and Recommended Dietary Intakes for Omega-6 and Omega-3 Fatty Acids." *J Am Coll Nutr.* 1999 Oct;18(5):487–9.

39. W.S. Harris and C. Von Schacky, "The Omega-3 Index: a new risk factor for death from coronary heart disease?" *Prev Med.* 2004 Jul;39(1):212–20.

40. C. Von Schacky, et al., "The effect of dietary omega-3 fatty acids on coronary atherosclerosis. A randomized, double-blind, placebo-controlled trial." *Ann Intern Med.* 1999 Apr 6;130(7):554–62.

41. J.E. Teitelbaum and W. Allan Walker, "Review: the role of omega 3 fatty acids in intestinal inflammation." *J Nutr Biochem.* 2001 Jan;12(1):21–32.

42. D.S. Barbosa, et al., "Decreased oxidative stress in patients with ulcerative colitis supplemented with fish oil omega-3 fatty acids." *Nutrition.* 2003 Oct;19(10):837–42.

43. B.G. Feagan, et al., "Omega-3 free fatty acids for the maintenance of remission in Crohn's disease: the EPIC Randomized Controlled Trials." *JAMA.* 2008 Apr 9;299(14):1690–7.

44. Q. Li, et al., "n-3 polyunsaturated fatty acids prevent disruption of epithelial barrier function induced by proinflammatory cytokines." *Mol Immunol.* 2008 Mar;45(5):1356–65.

45. J.E. Teitelbaum, et al., "Review: the role of omega 3 fatty acids in intestinal inflammation." *J Nutr Biochem.* 2001 Jan;12(1):21–32.

46. L.E. Willemsen, et al., "Polyunsaturated fatty acids support epithelial barrier integrity and reduce IL-4 mediated permeability in vitro." *Eur J Nutr.* 2008 Jun;47(4):183–91.

The HOPE Solution—P=Probiotics

1. S.R. Gill, et al., "Metagenomic analysis of the human distal gut microbiome." *Science.* 2006 Jun 2;312(5778):1355–9.

2. M.L. Phillips, et al., "Gut reaction: environmental effects on the human microbiota." *Environ Health Perspect.* 2009 May;117(5):A198–205.

3. J. Penders, et al., "Factors influencing the composition of the intestinal microbiota in early infancy." *Pediatrics.* 2006 Aug;118(2): T511–21.

4. Ibid.

5. D. Mariat, et al., "The Firmicutes/Bacteroidetes ratio of the human microbiota changes with age." BMC Microbiol. 2009 Jun 9;9:123.

6. T. Mitsuoka, "Intestinal flora and human health." *Asia Pac J Clin Nutr.* 1996;5(1):2–9.

7. W. Valtonen, "Infection as a risk factor for infarction and atherosclerosis." *Ann Med.* 1991;23(5):539–43.

8. C.J. Weidermann, et al., "Association of endotoxemia with carotid atherosclerosis and cardiovascular disease: prospective results from the Bruneck Study." J Am Coll Cardiol. 1999 Dec;34(7):1975–81.

9. A. Krack, et al., "The importance of the gastrointestinal system in the pathogenesis of heart failure." *Eur Heart J.* 2005 Nov;26(22):2368–74.

10. M.H. Floch and A.S. Kim, Eds., Probiotics: A Clinical Guide. Thoroughfare, NJ: SLACK Inc., 2010, p. 141.

The HOPE Solution—Supplements

1. L-Glutamine Monograph. *Alt Med Rev.* 2001;6(4):406–10.

2. A.L. Miller, "The pathogenesis, clinical implications, and treatment of intetstinal hyperpermeability." *Alt Med Rev.* 1997;2(5):330–7.

3. B.J. Lee, et al., "Coenzyme Q10 supplementation reduces oxidative stress and increase antioxidant enzyme activity in patients with coronary artery disease." *Nutrition.* 2011 Oct 11.

4. J.M. Hodgson, et al., "Coenzyme Q10 improves blood pressure and glycaemic control: a controlled trial in subjects with type 2 diabetes." *Eur J Clin Nutr.* 2002 Nov;56(11):1137–42.

5. M.F. Holick, et al., "High prevalence of vitamin D inadequacy and implications for health." *Mayo Clin Proc.* 2006 Mar;81(3):353–73.

6. T.J. Wang, et al., "Vitamin D deficiency and risk of cardiovascular disease." *Circulation.* 2008 Jan 29;117(4):503–11.

7. J.R. Guyton, "Niacin in cardiovascular prevention: mechanisms, efficacy, and safety." *Curr Opin Lipidol.* 2007 Aug;18(4):415–20.

8. www.umm.edu/altmed/articles/vitamin-c-000339.htm

9. R. di Giuseppe, et al., "Regular consumption of dark chocolate is associated with low serum concentrations of C-reactive protein in a healthy Italian population." *J Nutr.* 2008 Oct;138(10):1939–45.

10. D. Taubert, et al., "Effects of low habitual cocoa intake on blood pressure and bioactive nitric oxide: a randomized controlled trial." *JAMA.* 2007 Jul 4;298(1):49–60.

The HOPE Solution—Functional Testing

1. D.I. Phillips et al., "Understanding oral glucose tolerance: comparison of glucose or insulin measurements during the oral glucose tolerance test with specific measurements of insulin resistance and insulin secretion." *Diabet Med.* 1994 Apr;11(3):286–92.

2. www.vitamindcouncil.org/about-vitamin-d/vitamin-d-deficiency

3. W. Davis, "Effect of a combined therapeutic approach of intensive lipid management, omega-3 fatty acid supplementation, and increased serum 25 (OH) vitamin D on coronary calcium scores in asymptomatic adults." *Am J Ther.* 2009 Jul–Aug;16(4):326–32.

4. L. Papatheodorou and N. Weiss, "Vascular oxidant stress and inflammation in hyperhomocysteinemia." *Antioxid Redox Signal.* 2007 Nov;9(11):1941–58.

5. L.D. Botto and Q. Yang, "5,10-Methylenetetrahydrofolate reductase gene variants and congenital anomalies: a HuGE review." *Am J Epidemiol.* 2000 May 1;151(9):862–77.

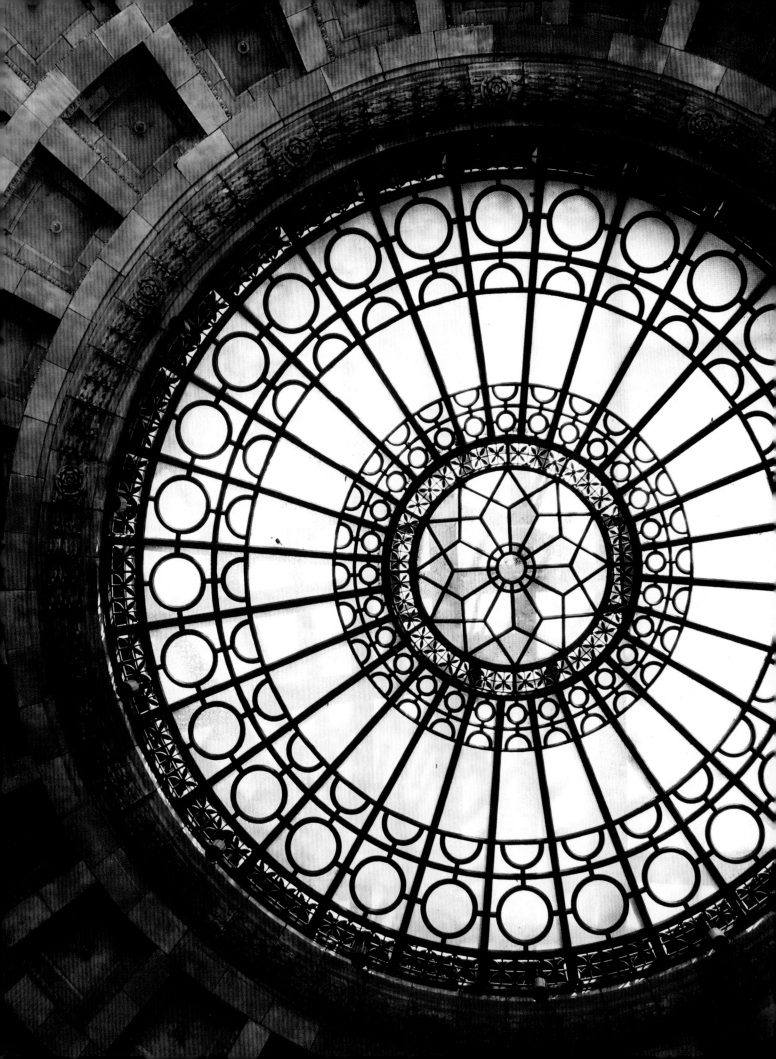

index

E

Echocardiograms (ECHO), 155
Edema, 82
EDTA (ethylenediaminetetraacetic acid), 211, 213
EDTA chelation therapy, 211, 213
Eggplant Roulades (recipe), 292–295, 390
Ellis, Dave, 158
Endothelial dysfunction, 18, 51, 150, 175–187
    and atherosclerosis, 175–179, 181
    and homocysteine, 182
    oxidative stress, 175, 180
    testing for, 182
    tips for reducing, 183
    triggers of, 180
Endotoxemia
    defined, 67
    diet-induced, 141
    and low-grade inflammation, 33
    metabolic, 67–68, 149
    and obesity, 99
Endotoxins, 67
    and atherosclerosis, 273–274
    lipopolysaccharide, 67, 68
Enteric nervous system, 167
EnteroLab, 142, 239, 280
Enzymes, 275
EPA, 154, 267
Epigenome, 145
Epinephrine, 201–202
Epithelial lining, 129
Essential fatty acids, 154
Estrogen metabolites, 189–190, 192–193
Estrogen(s), 191
Ethylenediaminetetraacetic acid (EDTA), 211, 213
Eustress, 159
Exercise, stress and, 171
Exorphins, 83, 84

F

Fasting blood sugar test, 278
Fasting insulin test, 60, 279
Fasting plasma glucose test, 60
Fat. See Body fat; Dietary fats

Fatigue, diet and, 253
Fatty acids, 154, 262. See also Dietary fats; specific fatty acids
Fecal bacteriotherapy, 152–153
Fiber
    and blood sugar levels, 72–74
    from carbohydrates, 238–239
    and cholesterol levels, 34, 36
    and gut-heart connection, 69
    and heart health, 150, 258, 260
    and inflammation, 114
    in Love Your Heart Eating Plan, 260
    in low-carb diets, 242
    in SAD vs. Paleolithic diets, 227
    soluble and insoluble, 257–259
    supplements, 260
Fibrates drugs, 37, 120
Fibromyalgia, 201, 202
Fight-or-flight response, 159–160
Firmicutes, 98
Fish contaminants, 266–267
Fish oils, 25, 26, 154
Fish oil supplements, 25, 26, 267, 269–270
Flow-mediated dilation (FMD), 182
Fluid retention, 46
Foam cells, 18, 150
Folic acid, 182
Food addiction, 199–200
Food processing, 230
Food Pyramid, 125
Food sensitivities, 116, 134, 280
Food Sensitivity Test, 142–143
Foxx, Redd, 174
Framingham Heart Study, 230
Free radicals, 151
Fruits
    and blood pressure, 48
    fiber from, 239
    importance of, 154, 155
    in Paleo diet, 243
    teaspoons of sugar in, 385
    tracking sugar from, 248
Functional testing, 277–280

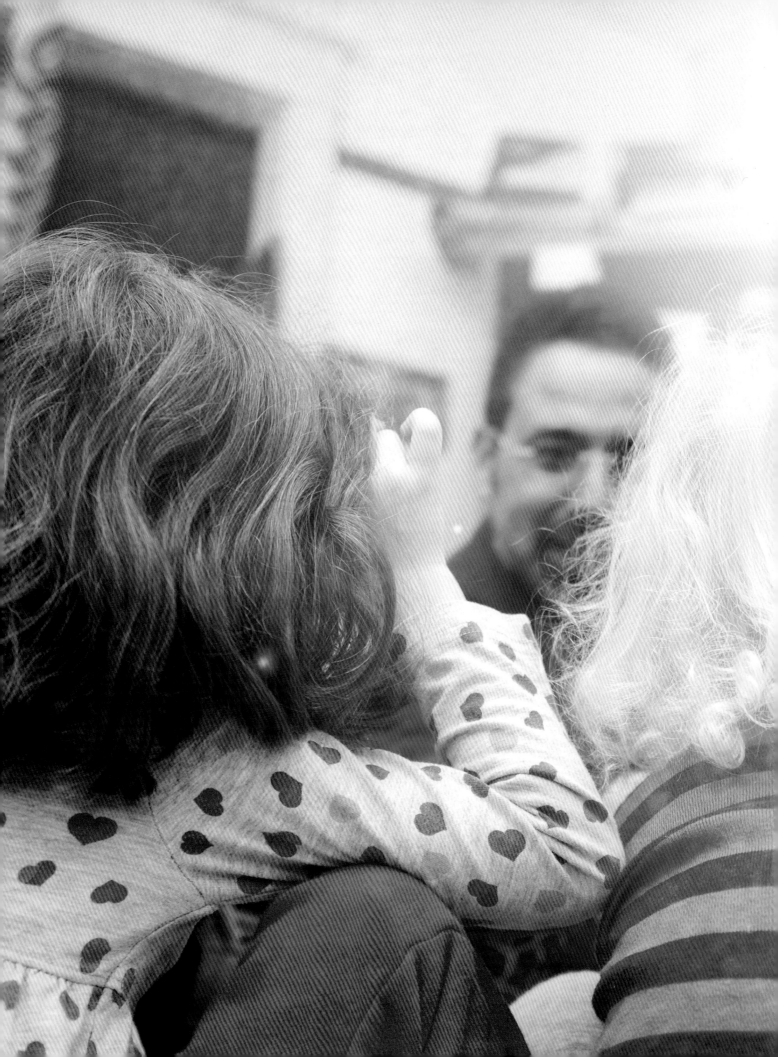

credits

Credits – Illustrations

Page 12, Centers for Disease Control, National Vital Statistics Systems and the US Census Bureau

Page 12, Centers for Disease Control, Behavioral Risk Factor Surveillance System

Page 16, Adam Questell A KYU Design

Page 19, Adam Questell A KYU Design

Page 22, Adam Questell A KYU Design

Page 27, Adam Questell A KYU Design

Page 28–29, Adam Questell A KYU Design

Page 30–31, Adam Questell A KYU Design

Page 35, Adam Questell A KYU Design

Page 44–45, Adam Questell A KYU Design

Page 62, Adam Questell A KYU Design

Page 66–67, Adam Questell A KYU Design

Page 136, Adam Questell A KYU Design

Page 161, Adam Questell A KYU Design

Page 179, Adam Questell A KYU Design

Page 181, Adam Questell A KYU Design

Page 229, Adam Questell A KYU Design, adapted from J Med Food. 2009 Oct;12(5):925–34.

Page 259, Adam Questell A KYU Design

Page 268–269, Adam Questell A KYU Design

Credits – Photography

Book front liner, michael black | BLACK SUN ® & John Stuart Photography

Page 3, John Stuart Photography

Page 10, michael black | BLACK SUN ®

Page 20, michael black | BLACK SUN ®

Page 39, michael black | BLACK SUN ®

Page 42, michael black | BLACK SUN ®

Page 55, michael black | BLACK SUN ®

Page 58, michael black | BLACK SUN ®

Page 71, provided by author

Page 90, michael black | BLACK SUN ®

Page 104, michael black | BLACK SUN ®

Page 108, michael black | BLACK SUN ®

Page 123, provided by author

Page 128, michael black | BLACK SUN ®

Page 158, michael black | BLACK SUN ®

Page 174, michael black | BLACK SUN ®

Page 188, michael black | BLACK SUN ®

Page 206, michael black | BLACK SUN ®

Page 226, michael black | BLACK SUN ®

Page 236, michael black | BLACK SUN ®

Page 244, michael black | BLACK SUN ®

Page 256, michael black | BLACK SUN ®

Page 288–289, michael black | BLACK SUN ®

Page 290, michael black | BLACK SUN ®

Page 291, michael black | BLACK SUN ®

Page 292–293, michael black | BLACK SUN ®

Page 294 x4, michael black | BLACK SUN ®

Page 295, michael black | BLACK SUN ®

Page 296–297, michael black | BLACK SUN ®

Page 298, michael black | BLACK SUN ®

Page 299, michael black | BLACK SUN ®

Page 300–301, michael black | BLACK SUN ®

Page 302 x2, michael black | BLACK SUN ®

Page 303, michael black | BLACK SUN ®

Page 304–305, michael black | BLACK SUN ®

Page 306 x3, michael black | BLACK SUN ®

Page 307, michael black | BLACK SUN ®

Page 308–309vmichael black | BLACK SUN ®

Page 310, michael black | BLACK SUN ®

Page 311, michael black | BLACK SUN ®

Page 312–313, michael black | BLACK SUN ®

Page 314 x4, michael black | BLACK SUN ®

Page 315, michael black | BLACK SUN ®

Page 316–317, michael black | BLACK SUN ®

Page 318, michael black | BLACK SUN ®

Page 319 x3, michael black | BLACK SUN ®

Page 320–321, michael black | BLACK SUN ®

Page 322 x3, michael black | BLACK SUN ®

Page 323, michael black | BLACK SUN ®

Page 324–325, michael black | BLACK SUN ®

Page 326, michael black | BLACK SUN ®

Page 327 x3, michael black | BLACK SUN ®

Page 328–329, michael black | BLACK SUN ®

Page 330 x3, michael black | BLACK SUN ®

Page 331, michael black | BLACK SUN ®

Page 332–333, michael black | BLACK SUN ®

Page 334, michael black | BLACK SUN ®

Page 335 x3, michael black | BLACK SUN ®

Page 336–337, michael black | BLACK SUN ®

Page 338 x3, michael black | BLACK SUN ®

Page 339, michael black | BLACK SUN ®

Page 340–341, michael black | BLACK SUN ®

Page 342, michael black | BLACK SUN ®

Page 343 x3, michael black | BLACK SUN ®

Page 344–345, michael black | BLACK SUN ®

Page 346 x3, michael black | BLACK SUN ®

Page 347, michael black | BLACK SUN ®

Page 348–349, michael black | BLACK SUN ®

Page 350, michael black | BLACK SUN ®

Page 351 x2, michael black | BLACK SUN ®

Page 352–353, michael black | BLACK SUN ®

Page 354 x3, michael black | BLACK SUN ®

Page 355, michael black | BLACK SUN ®

Page 356–357, michael black | BLACK SUN ®

Page 358, michael black | BLACK SUN ®

Page 359 x4, michael black | BLACK SUN ®

Page 360–361, michael black | BLACK SUN ®

Page 362 x2, michael black | BLACK SUN ®

Page 363, michael black | BLACK SUN ®

Page 374, michael black | BLACK SUN ®

Page 376–377, provided by doctors

Page 378, michael black | BLACK SUN ®

Page 384, michael black | BLACK SUN ®

Page 388, michael black | BLACK SUN ®

Page 398, michael black | BLACK SUN ®

Page 414, michael black | BLACK SUN ®

Page 430, Daniel Wilkenson for BLACK SUN ®

Book back liner, michael black | BLACK SUN ®

Credits – Quotes

Page 10, Dalai Lama XIV

Page 20, Franklin P. Adams

Page 42, Augusten Burroughs

Page 58, Siddhartha Gautama

Page 90, Winston S. Churchill

Page 108, Vincent van Gogh

Page 128, Virgil

Page 158, Dave Ellis

Page 174, Redd Foxx

Page 188, Siddhartha Gautama

Page 206, William Shakespeare

Page 226, Plato

Page 236, Maimonides

Page 244, Morgan Spurlock

Page 256, Deepok Chopra

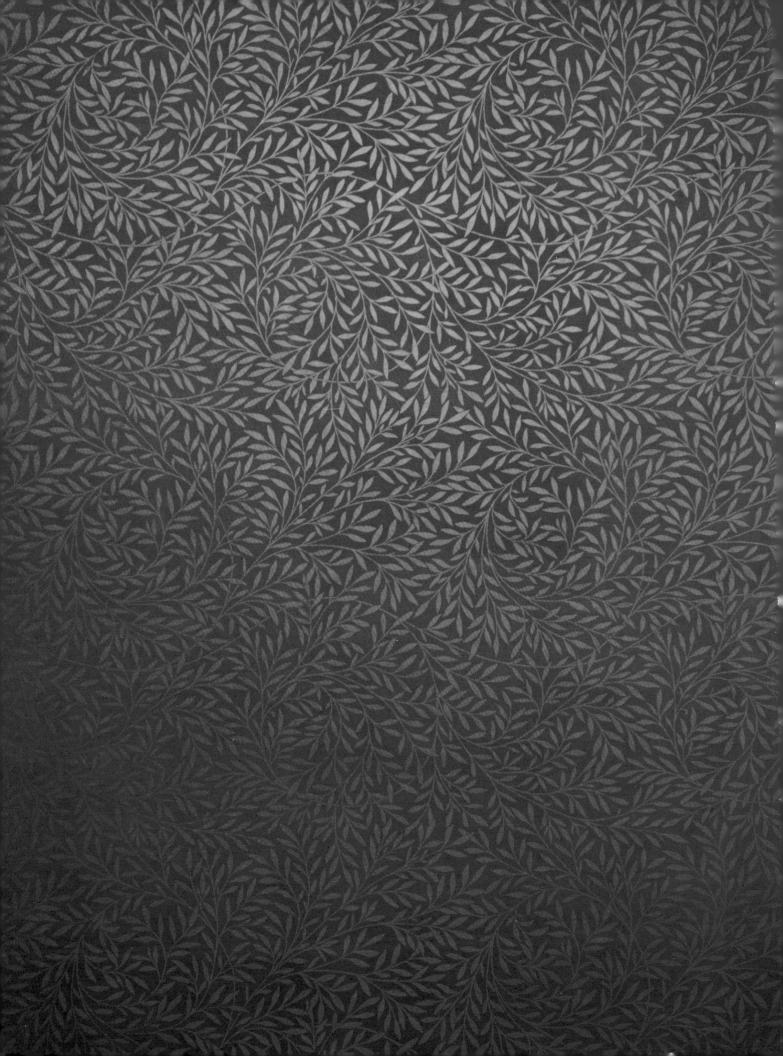